Evidence-Based
Rehabilitation
A Guide to Practice

Evidence-Based
Rehabilitation
A Guide to Practice

Edited by

Mary Law, PhD, OT(C)
McMaster University
Hamilton, Ontario
Canada

Jackie Bosch, MSc, OT(C)
Winnie Dunn, PhD, OTR, FAOTA
Angela Everett, BHSc(OT)
Jill Foreman, BHSc(OT)
Lori Letts, MA, OT(C)
Jennie Q. Lou, MD, MSc, OTR
Angela Mandich, PhD
Linda Miller, PhD
Donna Nicholson, PTReg(C), OTReg(C)

Ian Philp, BASc
Nancy Pollock, MSc, OT(C)
Julie Richardson, MSc
Sarah Rochon, MSc(T), OT(C)
Debra Stewart, MSc, OT(C)
Linda Tickle-Degnen, PhD, OTR/L
Diane Watson, PhD, MBA, BScOT
Muriel Westmorland, MHSc

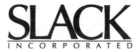

An innovative information, education and management company
6900 Grove Road • Thorofare, NJ 08086

Printed in the United States of America.

Library of Congress Cataloging-in-Publication Data

Evidence-based rehabilitation : a guide to practice / edited by Mary
Law.
    p. cm.
Includes bibliographic references and index.
  ISBN 1-55642-453-1
  1. Medical rehabilitation. 2. Evidence-based medicine. 3.
Occupational therapy. I. Law, Mary C.
  RM930.E934 2002
  617'.03--dc21

                    2002002608

Published by: SLACK Incorporated
                 6900 Grove Road
                 Thorofare, NJ 08086 USA
                 Telephone: 856-848-1000
                 Fax: 856-853-5991
                 www.slackbooks.com

Contact SLACK Incorporated for more information about other books in this field or about the availability of our books from distributors outside the United States.

Last digit is print number: 10   9   8   7   6   5   4   3   2

DEDICATION

To my parents, who fostered my curiosity.

CONTENTS

Dedication v
Acknowledgments. ix
About the Editor xi
Contributing Authors xiii
Preface xv

Section I   Introduction to Evidence-Based Practice

Chapter 1   Introduction to Evidence-Based Practice 3
             Mary Law, PhD, OT(C)

Chapter 2   Development of Evidence-Based Knowledge 13
             Winnie Dunn, PhD, OTR, FAOTA and Jill Foreman, BHSc(OT)

Chapter 3   Becoming an Evidence-Based Practitioner 31
             Nancy Pollock, MSc, OT(C) and Sarah Rochon, MSc(T), OT(C)

Section II   Finding the Evidence

Chapter 4   Outcomes in Evidence-Based Practice 49
             Angela Mandich, PhD; Linda Miller, PhD; and Mary Law, PhD, OT(C)

Chapter 5   Searching for the Evidence 71
             Jennie Q. Lou, MD, MSc, OTR

Section III Assessing the Evidence

Chapter 6   Evaluating the Evidence. 97
             Mary Law, PhD, OT(C) and Ian Philp, BASc

Chapter 7   Systematically Reviewing the Evidence 109
             Mary Law, PhD, OT(C) and Ian Philp, BASc

Chapter 8   The Effectiveness of Cognitive-Behavioral Interventions with
             People with Chronic Pain: An Example of a Critical Review
             of the Literature 127
             *Debra Stewart, MSc, OT(C); Mary Law, PhD, OT(C); Nancy Pollock,
             MSc, OT(C); Lori Letts, MA, OT(C); Jackie Bosch, MSc, OT(C); Muriel
             Westmorland, MHSc; and Angela Everett, BHSc(OT)*

Chapter 9   Evaluating the Evidence: Economic Analysis 171
             Diane Watson, PhD, MBA, BScOT

Section IV   Using the Evidence

Chapter 10   Building Evidence in Practice 185
             Mary Law, PhD, OT(C)

Chapter 11   Practice Guidelines, Algorithms, and Clinical Pathways 195
             Donna Nicholson, PTReg(C), OTReg(C)

Chapter 12   Communicating Evidence to Clients, Managers, and Funders. . . . 221
              Linda Tickle-Degnen, PhD, OTR/L

Chapter 13   Research Dissemination and Transfer of Knowledge 255
              Mary Law, PhD, OT(C) and Ian Philp, BASc

Chapter 14   Health Care Delivery of Rehabilitation Services for
              Postacute Stroke: Home Care Versus Institutional Care—
              What is the Evidence? 269
              Julie Richardson, MSc

Appendix A   *Outcome Measures Rating Form* *287*

Appendix B   *Outcome Measures Rating Form Guidelines*. *299*

Appendix C   *Critical Review Form for Quantitative Studies* *305*

Appendix D   *Guidelines for Critical Review Form: Quantitative Studies*. *309*

Appendix E   *Critical Review Form for Qualitative Studies* *323*

Appendix F   *Guidelines for Critical Review Form: Qualitative Studies*. *329*

Appendix G   *Instructions for the Use of the Functional Independence Measure*
              Decision Trees *339*

Appendix H   *Clinical Pathway Example* *341*

Appendix I   *Variance Record Example* *345*

Appendix J   *Client Outcomes Example* *347*

Appendix K   *Key Indicator Record Example*. *349*

Appendix L   *Template for the Development of Clinical Pathways:*
              Key Indicators *351*

Appendix M   *Template for the Development of Clinical Pathways: Timeline* . . . *353*

Appendix N   *Developing Outcomes* *355*

Index. *357*

Instructors: *Evidence-Based Rehabilitation: A Guide to Practice Instructor's Manual*
is also available from SLACK Incorporated. Don't miss this important companion to
Evidence-Based Rehabilitation: A Guide to Practice. To obtain the Instructor's Manual,
please visit *http://www.efacultylounge.com*.

Acknowledgments

I have been very fortunate to have an excellent group of authors who have willingly shared their expertise in writing chapters of this book. Their contributions are thoughtful, challenging, and structured to promote learning. I thank each one of them. My work in this area has been stimulated and supported by colleagues and students at McMaster University, Hamilton, Ontario, Canada. I particularly wish to acknowledge the Occupational Therapy Evidence-Based Practice Research Group in the School of Rehabilitation Science at McMaster University. Together, we have explored many issues in evidence-based practice, and I am grateful for this partnership. Special thanks to my mother-in-law, Doris M. Law, for the art on the cover of the book.

About the Editor

Mary Law, PhD, OT(C), is a professor, associate dean (health sciences), and director of the School of Rehabilitation Science at McMaster University in Hamilton, Ontario, Canada. Mary is currently codirector of CanChild Centre for Childhood Disability Research, an internationally acclaimed, multidisciplinary research centre. Her clinical and research interests include the development, validation, and transfer into practice of outcome measures; evaluation of interventions for children with disabilities; development of evidence-based practice; and the study of environmental factors that affect the participation of children with disabilities.

CONTRIBUTING AUTHORS

Jackie Bosch, MSc, OT(C) is a research fellow in the Canadian Cardiovascular Collaboration and an assistant clinical professor at the School of Rehabilitation Science at McMaster University, Hamilton, Ontario, Canada.

Winnie Dunn, PhD, OTR, FAOTA is professor and chair of the Occupational Therapy Education Program, School of Allied Health, University of Kansas Medical Center, Kansas City.

Angela Everett, BHSc(OT) is an occupational therapist at Hamilton Health Sciences, Hamilton, Ontario, Canada.

Jill Foreman, BHSc(OT) is an occupational therapist in private practice in Hamilton, Ontario, Canada.

Lori Letts, MA, OT(C) is an assistant professor at the School of Rehabilitation Science, McMaster University, Hamilton, Ontario, Canada.

Jennie Q. Lou, MD, MSc, OTR is an associate professor in the Occupational Therapy Department, Nova Southeastern University, Fort Lauderdale, FL.

Angela Mandich, PhD is an assistant professor at the School of Occupational Therapy, University of Western Ontario, London, Canada.

Linda Miller, PhD is an associate professor at the School of Occupational Therapy, University of Western Ontario, London, Canada.

Donna Nicholson, PTReg(C), OTReg(C) is the manager of Professional Practice & Research, Ottawa-Carleton Community Care Access Centre (OC-CCAC) and has worked with CCACs across Ontario to facilitate the development of clinical pathways.

Ian Philp, BASc, at the time of writing this book, was a student in the Arts and Science Program at McMaster University, Hamilton, Ontario, Canada. He has since graduated and is currently working overseas.

Nancy Pollock, MSc, OT(C) is an associate professor at the School of Rehabilitation Science, McMaster University, Hamilton, Ontario, Canada and an investigator at CanChild Centre for Childhood Disability Research, McMaster University.

Julie Richardson, MSc is an assistant professor at the School of Rehabilitation Science, McMaster University, Hamilton, Ontario, Canada.

Sarah Rochon, MSc(T), OT(C) is an assistant clinical professor at the School of Rehabilitation Science, McMaster University, Hamilton, Ontario, Canada.

Debra Stewart, MSc, OT(C) is a clinical lecturer and professional associate at the School of Rehabilitation Science, McMaster University, Hamilton, Ontario, Canada and an associate member of the CanChild Centre for Childhood Disability Research, McMaster University.

Linda Tickle-Degnen, PhD, OTR/L is an associate professor at Sargent College of Health and Rehabilitation Sciences, Boston University, MA.

Diane Watson, PhD, MBA, BScOT is the assistant director for the Institute for Health Services and Policy Research at the Canadian Institutes for Health Research, Ottawa, Canada.

Muriel Westmorland, MHSc is an associate professor at the School of Rehabilitation Science, McMaster University, Hamilton, Ontario, Canada.

PREFACE

*"Science is not formal logic—it needs the free play of the mind in as great a
degree as any other creative art. It is true that this is a gift which can hardly be
taught, but its growth can be encouraged in those who already possess it."*

—Max Born (1882-1970)

Evidence-based practice has been one of the most debated topics in health care over the
past decade. Initially developed in the area of medicine, evidence-based practice is now part
of every health care discipline and professional education program. While everyone agrees
that it is important to use evidence in practice, the challenges of finding, evaluating, and using
evidence are substantial. My goal in editing this text is to provide information to students and
practitioners in rehabilitation that aids in the development of evidence-based practice.

The book is designed to outline the concepts, methods, and strategies underpinning evidence-based rehabilitation. There are four sections within the text: *Section I, Introduction to
Evidence-Based Practice*, describes the basic concepts of evidence-based rehabilitation and
discusses how knowledge is developed within a discipline. The role of most reflective practice in supporting evidence-based practice is outlined; *Section II, Finding the Evidence*, centers on outcomes in evidence-based rehabilitation and methods to search for evidence. The
evaluation, critical appraisal, and systematic review of evidence is highlighted in *Section III,
Assessing the Evidence*. An example of a completed systematic review of evidence in the area
of rehabilitation practice illustrates these methods. *Section IV, Using the Evidence*, discusses
strategies that build evidence in practice and communicate evidence to clients, managers,
funders, and practitioners. The relationship between practice guidelines and evidence-based
practice is described in Chapter 11. An example of a descriptive critical review of an area of
rehabilitation services is provided to stimulate discussion and learning regarding the transfer
of knowledge into practice and policy.

A companion instructor's manual has been developed for this book. The manual provides
information about the key objectives of each chapter and ideas for teaching content and
exploring the learning activities in the book.

I hope that rehabilitation students, practitioners, and educators will explore the issues and
methods raised in this book and find it useful in building professional knowledge. We wel-
come your thoughts and comments about the book's content.

Mary Law, PhD, OT(C)

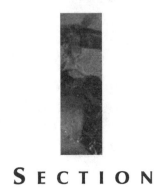

S E C T I O N

Introduction to
Evidence-Based Practice

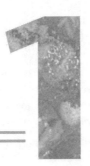

Introduction to Evidence-Based Practice

Mary Law, PhD, OT(C)

LEARNING OBJECTIVES

After reading this chapter, the student/practitioner will be able to:

- Distinguish between the various definitions of evidence-based practice and recognize the key elements of each.
- Critique some of the misconceptions surrounding evidence-based practice.
- Recognize the nature of evidence-based practice in rehabilitation.
- Understand and explain the key aspects of evidence-based rehabilitation, including awareness, consultation, judgment, and creativity.

"I have used this intervention for many years, and now researchers have shown that it is not effective. How do I know whether I should believe them and stop using this treatment?"

"The program in which I work is starting a new service designed to improve the work tolerance and function of injured clients. We will need to demonstrate that the outcomes of this new program are excellent. How do I identify assessment tools to evaluate client outcomes after receiving the program?"

"Several studies have shown that a short, intensive therapy intervention may be more effective than therapy for a longer period of time. What are the cost implications of this type of service delivery?"

DEFINING EVIDENCE-BASED PRACTICE

Any rehabilitation practitioner could ask these questions. The implication of such questions is the need for high quality information on which to base clinical and managerial decisions. These issues point to the need for practice based on available evidence. Evidence-based practice in rehabilitation has emerged as one of the most influential concepts in the past decade.

The very mention of evidence-based practice brings out different reactions from rehabilitation practitioners. The whole concept of this practice often seems daunting to the beginner—finding applicable evidence, evaluating it, and putting its recommendations into practice is no small feat! However, if done right, evidence-based practice is not a burden but a very powerful tool that helps practitioners provide a higher level of care to their clients and families. Evidence-based practice is often perceived as an "all-or-nothing" approach but, in reality, it can be put into practice in stages through setting priorities for action. The fears that surround evidence-based practice are largely unfounded and are based largely on a misunderstanding of the concept. Indeed, evidence-based practice is probably one of the most misunderstood concepts in health care today because of its newness and the degree to which it breaks from traditional practice. This chapter aims to provide a number of working definitions of evidence-based practice and to debunk the myths surrounding it.

Initial Definitions

Numerous attempts have been made to conclusively define evidence-based practice by the health care community, some of which are cited here. Evidence-based medicine and evidence-based practice are often used interchangeably to mean the same thing. Technically, evidence-based medicine refers only to the "medical" field, whereas evidence-based practice encompasses more aspects of health care, including rehabilitation.

Of all of the attempts to define evidence-based practice in the literature, the most influential and most widely quoted is probably Sackett, Rosenberg, Gray, Haynes, and Richardson's article, "Evidence-Based Medicine: What It Is and What It Isn't," which was published in the *British Medical Journal* in 1996. The collected expertise of these five authors is formidable. The most well-known author is Dr. David Sackett, coauthor of *Evidence-Based Medicine: How to Practice and Teach Evidence-Based Medicine*, one of the definitive first texts on the subject. Another author, R. Brian Haynes, works at McMaster University in Canada where the concept of evidence-based medicine was first developed and where much subsequent work has been done.

In their article, Sackett et al. (1996) offer this definition of evidence-based practice:

Evidence-based medicine is the conscientious, explicit, and judicious use of current best evidence in making decisions about the care of individual patients. The practice of evidence-based medicine means integrating individual clinical expertise with the best available external clinical evidence from systematic research.

This definition has been carefully worded to strike a fine balance between "clinical expertise" and "external clinical evidence." One of the greatest obstacles to the spread of evidence-based practice is that some established practitioners are opposed to it on ideological grounds. They object to evidence-based practice on the grounds that it pays no heed to the experience and expertise that professionals have been developing throughout entire careers. This is one of the main misconceptions about evidence-based practice. It does not ignore clinical skill; in fact, it welcomes it. Evidence-based practice tries to root out assessment procedures and interventions that have worked their way into accepted practice but which may not be the most beneficial for the client. The argument for evidence-based practice is simple: If there is a better way to practice, therapists should find it. This means critically evaluating what is already done to see if it could be improved, making evidence-based practice a heavily client-centred approach to providing care. However, evidence-based practice in no way advocates throwing the clinical experience of established practitioners out the window. If anything, that experience is more important, for knowledgeable practitioners are the ones who will know how best to implement evidence-based practice's findings. Evidence-based practice's central message here is one of flexibility and of being able to blend the old ways with the fruits of research and new knowledge. As Sackett et al. (1996) go on to say, "By individual clinical expertise we mean the proficiency and judgment that individual clinicians acquire through clinical experience and clinical practice."

In essence, evidence-based practice is based on a self-directed learning model, whereby practitioners must not only continue learning but also continue evaluating their techniques and practice in light of this learning to see what can be improved. This is, in the truest sense of the form, the ability to critically examine, evaluate, and apply knowledge and then assess one's own findings. Strange as it may sound, practitioners must maintain a humble attitude about their own practice patterns to excel at evidence-based practice. The ability to admit one's own errors and oversights and to critically assess one's own prior work is crucial because knowing one's own limitations (and when to look for help) is the basis of evidence-based practice. If you maintain this attitude, evidence-based practice's use of the "best external evidence" allows you to tap into the work of thousands of professionals around the world in order to find the best possible interventions for your clients. As Sackett et al. (1996) say, "By best available external clinical evidence we mean clinically relevant research, often from the basic sciences of medicine, but especially from patient-centered clinical research..."

Thus the definition offered by Sackett et al. (1996) is an acknowledgment that health care is an imperfect science that requires both overarching clinical guidelines and individual judgment in equal parts. Evidence-based practice works with the interplay of these two factors, making it a powerful tool that practitioners can use to guide their clinical decisions.

Another useful definition of evidence-based practice comes from another expert in the field, Dr. Trisha Greenhalgh. Dr. Greenhalgh is a senior lecturer in Primary Health Care at University College London, England and the director of that institution's Unit for Evidence-Based Practice and Policy. She has contributed a great deal to popularizing evidence-based practice in accessible language and wrote a series in the *British Medical Journal* entitled, "How to Read a Paper," a wonderfully helpful guide for those new to evidence-based practice. Greenhalgh's article series was turned into a book entitled *How to Read a Paper: The Basics of Evidence-Based Medicine*, which is an excellent companion for those struggling with the more technical aspects of evaluating journal articles. She offers a simple definition of evidence-based practice: "Evidence-based medicine requires you to read the right papers at the right time and then to alter your behaviour (and, what is often more difficult, the behaviour of other people) in light of what you have found" (Greenhalgh, 1997, p. 2).

A more detailed definition comes from Rosenberg and Donald (1995) in their paper, "Evidence-Based Medicine: An Approach to Clinical Problem Solving." They write that evidence-based medicine/practice is, "the process of systematically finding, appraising, and using contemporaneous research findings as the basis for clinical decisions. Evidence-based medicine asks questions, finds and appraises the relevant data, and harnesses that information for everyday clinical practice" (p. 1122).

The definition offered by Rosenberg and Donald (1995) not only outlines evidence-based practice, it also provides a step-by-step method of going about it. The four steps are questioning, searching, evaluating, and implementing and should be a constant cycle for the dedicated practitioner of evidence-based practice. At any moment, practitioners will likely be faced with a number of problems to which they must apply evidence-based practice, and they will be at various stages of the process at different times.

MYTHS SURROUNDING EVIDENCE-BASED PRACTICE

Despite attempts to publicise the realities surrounding evidence-based practice, there continue to be some "myths" surrounding it (Table 1-1), which Sackett et al. (1996) touch upon and debunk in their article. The misconception that evidence-based practice is either "already in place" or "impossible to practice" is their first target. Addressing the first point, Sackett et al. point out that while completely keeping up with the health research literature is impossible for any person, many practitioners take little or no time in their weekly routine to examine journals and publications, preferring instead to rely completely on their initial training to guide their practice.

Evidence-based practice doesn't mean that every clinical situation will send a practitioner slavishly running to the library, but it does mean that when a new situation presents itself, a clinician should employ research skills to find an answer and pass this information on to colleagues. Unfortunately, this isn't always the case; many clinicians rely solely on the expertise of others, which, while it can be helpful, is inherently based on the quirks of individual experience. As previously stated, a balance between the two sources of information can hardly hurt practitioners in making more accurate and more insightful diagnoses. This argument also meshes with Sackett et al.'s (1996) further point that evidence-based practice is not impossible to put into place. In fact, they specifically state that "studies show that busy clinicians who devote their scarce reading time to selective, efficient, client-driven searching, appraisal and incorporation of the best available evidence can practice evidence-based medicine." Practicing evidence-based practice isn't a matter of inundating one's self with evidence—it's a matter of deftly locating and snatching the evidence from the ever-growing pile of research and rehabilitation knowledge.

Another point often raised against evidence-based practice is that it is "cookie-cutter" medicine or devoid of the need for individual clinical judgment. This criticism returns to the earlier fears of evidence-based practice making clinicians' expertise irrelevant, and Sackett et al. (1996) again attempt to clarify the goals of evidence-based practice. As they state, "exter-

Table 1-1
MYTHS OF EVIDENCE-BASED PRACTICE

Myth	*Reality*
• Evidence-based practice already exists	• Many practitioners take little or no time to review current medical findings
• Evidence-based practice is impossible to put into place	• Even extremely busy practitioners can initiate evidence-based practice through little work
• Evidence-based practice is cookie-cutter medicine	• Evidence-based practice requires extensive clinical expertise
• Evidence-based practice is a cost-cutting mechanism	• Evidence-based practice emphasizes the best available clinical evidence for each client's situation

nal clinical evidence can inform, but can never replace, individual clinical expertise; this expertise will assist the practitioner in deciding whether the external evidence applies to the individual client at all and, if so, how it should be integrated into a clinical decision." As previously mentioned, no supporter of evidence-based practice has argued for the removal of regular training for practitioners; they have merely suggested that the training include information on how evidence-based practice fits into the clinical equation.

Lastly, Sackett et al. (1996) debunk the concept that evidence-based practice is merely a malicious tool of health-policy makers—either introduced to cut costs or insisting that each clinical intervention be backed by a randomized controlled trial (RCT). Both issues miss the point of evidence-based practice—to bring the best available clinical evidence to each client's situation. Using the best available evidence does not reduce the need for costly interventions; it simply attempts to ensure that each client gets the treatment appropriate for his or her condition. Furthermore, evidence-based practice insists that each case is treated with the best available evidence and is not so haughty that it rejects anything that isn't a RCT outright. Because of this strength of evidence-based practice, it can be applied now in all forms of health care. This fact is discussed by Pamela Duncan in her article on evidence-based physical therapy (1997).

One final definition of evidence-based practice must be considered, and it comes from Cook and Levy's 1998 article, "Evidence-Based Medicine: A Tool for Enhancing Critical Care Practice." They touch on an aspect of evidence-based practice that others often overlook, namely that "EBM is a style of practice and teaching which may also help plan future research" (Cook & Levy, 1998). This is likely one of the greatest forgotten strengths of evidence-based practice. Not only does evidence-based practice enable the use of the current best evidence in treatment, it can also be used to direct research advances. This conception of evidence-based practice closely links applied practice with the research aspects of health care. Evidence-based practice is a force for integration, bringing these two often separate domains together and aiming to further streamline the process of generating new clinical knowledge.

Table 1-2
IMPORTANT CONCEPTS IN EVIDENCE-BASED REHABILITATION

- Awareness
- Consultation
- Judgment
- Creativity

In concluding this examination of fundamental ideas of evidence-based practice, it must be said that none of these definitions captures exactly what evidence-based practice is all about, but all definitions can contribute in some way to our understanding of the concept. Until evidence-based practice has established a safe place within accepted clinical practice, it will continue to be challenged by those who doubt its relevance, strength, and credibility. However, if evidence-based practice can be integrated into the common practitioner's repertoire of tools, we will see a shift toward more analytical, certain, and ultimately effective clinical practice in health care.

EVIDENCE-BASED REHABILITATION

One of the goals of this book is to assist students in becoming better practitioners and caregivers through using evidence-based techniques. The previous discussion of evidence-based practice provides a theoretical understanding of the concept. The remainder of the chapter focuses on a discussion of evidence-based rehabilitation (EBR), which students may find more applicable and more relevant to their future work.

EBR is a subset of evidence-based clinical practice, which has been discussed at length. Let's look at some ideas that will help us to ascertain the key aspects of good EBR (Table 1-2).

Awareness

The first definition is from the Health Informatics Research Unit (HIRU) at McMaster University, which states, "Evidence-based clinical practice (EBCP) is an approach to health care practice in which the clinician is aware of the evidence that bears on her clinical practice, and the strength of that evidence" (Health Information Research Unit, 2002).

The HIRU makes an important point—the clinician *must be aware* of the evidence related to his or her practice. This does not mean that he or she must read every new journal that comes out cover-to-cover, but he or she should find ways of staying up-to-date with what new research is happening in his or her field. There are many ways to do this, from journals that specifically summarize research advances to web sites that bring information together to online discussion groups and chat forums in which practitioners can interact. Instead of awareness of everything without comprehension, the goal is *focused awareness*, or a knowledge of where to look. Each practitioner must find his or her own natural way to stay up-to-date. This is important because striving for excellence means giving the best to each client and his or her family.

Consultation

A second definition comes from J. A. Muir Gray's (1997) book on evidence-based health care, in which he points out, "Evidence-based clinical practice is an approach to decision making in which the clinician uses the best evidence available, in consultation with the patient, to decide upon the option which suits that patient best." Muir Gray's definition is a reminder of one of the most important aspects of health care—transparency. Practitioners have a specialized set of skills and knowledge, and an essential part of their job has always been to be good communicators. Their role is to work together with the client to ascertain the problem(s) and how it can be resolved in the easiest possible terms. With the advent of evidence-based rehabilitation, that job remains the same, albeit somewhat more complex. Evidence-based practice is a method for distilling information from the findings of others and, equally, a vehicle for educating the client. Practitioners who are able to adeptly explain the practice of evidence-based rehabilitation to their clients, how they have found the clinical data they are using, and what they are doing with it will be the most successful. This opens the process up to the client, so they can see what the practitioner is doing. Evidence-based practice turns the focus toward the community, with the practitioner working as an educator as well as a service provider.

Judgment

Although evidence-based practice and evidence-based rehabilitation represent a major advance in the field of rehabilitation, they should not be embraced blindly. At the 60th Annual Assembly of the American Academy of Physical Medicine and Rehabilitation, keynote speaker Dr. Joel DeLisa (1999) made these remarks about evidence-based practice and rehabilitation, "However, there are problems in the 'evidence' of evidence-based medicine... the laudable goal of making clinical decisions based on evidence can be impaired by the restricted quality and scope of what is collected as 'best available evidence'" (p. 7).

The problems or limits to the evidence in evidence-based practice cannot and should not be ignored. As DeLisa (1999) points out:

> *Derived almost exclusively from randomized trials and meta-analysis... the results [of EBP work in rehabilitation] show comparative efficacy of treatment for an "average" randomized patient and are not for pertinent subgroups formed by cogent clinical features such as severity of symptoms, illness, comorbidity, and other clinical nuances. (p. 7)*

Practitioners must possess good clinical judgment to differentiate how to apply the recommendations of evidence-based practice and how they must be tailored to the specifics of each client's situation.

Creativity

A final definition of evidence-based health care, which lends itself to evidence-based rehabilitation, comes from an article in the *Journal of the American Medical Association*, which summarizes a discussion on the practice of evidence-based medicine. The definition that comes from this round table is that evidence-based health care is "a conscientious, explicit, and judicious use of the current best evidence to make a decision about the care of patients" (Marwick, 1997). Using the best effort in a "conscientious, explicit, and judicious" way will not always be straightforward, and practitioners will have to use their creative skills to meet the challenges of real life. Learning evidence-based practice is both a science and an art and, as such, must be melded to the already existing body of skills that a practitioner has in his or her repertoire. Evidence-based rehabilitation may sound like "cookie-cutter" practice but, in actuality, it requires a great deal of creativity and insight to work correctly. Ultimately, evidence-based practice allows practitioners to "write their own textbook," so to speak, and teach themselves what they need to do. This makes creativity essential.

CONCLUSION

Evidence-based rehabilitation is an important part of current practice. Practicing confident, resourceful, and creative rehabilitation is an art and must be developed over time. It is hoped that this book will serve to speed that process for many practitioners as they formulate their own definition of evidence-based rehabilitation.

Take-Home Messages

Evidence-Based Practice (EBP)
- There are misunderstandings of EBP because of the way in which it breaks with traditional practice; it can be seen as a powerful tool, not a burden.
- EBP maintains a fine balance between clinical expertise and external clinical evidence.
- EBP is based on a self-directed learning model.
- EBP can support a strongly client-centred approach to rehabilitation.
- Clinical experience remains crucial because knowledgeable practitioners will best implement their findings based on evidence.
- EBP makes use of the current best methods of treatment.

Evidence-Based Rehabilitation (EBR)
- EBR is a subset of the clinical practice of EBP.
- Awareness: The clinician must be aware of the evidence that has to do with practice and maintain *focused awareness*.
- Consultation: Specialized set of skills and knowledge to be a good communicator; the practitioner works as an educator/service provider.
- Judgment: The practitioner differentiates between cases about how to apply recommendations of EBP; tailored to specifics of each client's situation.
- Creativity: EBR requires creativity and insight as the practice and application of the best available evidence is not always straightforward.

WEB LINKS

Definitions of Evidence-Based Practice
www.shef.ac.uk/~scharr/ir/def.html
This site has an extensive selection of definitions for EBP, including many found in this chapter. It also has links to other resources for learning more about the essential aspects of EBP.

Evidence-Based Medicine Learning Resources
www.herts.ac.uk/lis/subjects/health/ebm.htm
This site features a large section of definitions of EBP and a list of links to centres and institutes that work with EBP, giving an overview of the work being done in the field.

PT Manager
www.ptmanager.com
PT Manager describes itself as "The Rehabilitation Leadership and Management Electronic Community" and has a number of resources related to rehabilitation on the web. Although they do not have a page dedicated to EBP, PT Manager is committed to the idea, having hosted several conferences on the subject.

Evidence-Based Health Informatics
http://hiru.mcmaster.ca/overview.htm#Evidence_based_Health_Informatics
This page from the HIRU site at McMaster University provides information on the idea of evidence-based rehabilitation, as well as the preferences and outcomes it has delivered for Rehabilitation.
Another similar initiative can be found at The Centres for Health Evidence at the following address: www.cche.net/about.

LEARNING AND EXPLORATION ACTIVITIES

The purpose of this segment is to introduce the concept of EBP through the exploration of key definitions found in the literature. The following exercises guide the student through a process of thinking critically about the definition of EBP and applying this knowledge to possible clinical scenarios. The work done in these exercises should be saved by the students as a good reference during their study of EBP.

1. Defining Evidence-Based Practice
   a. What is your concept of EBP? What was your conception before you read this chapter? Make a chart and list both side by side, then attempt to locate where the gaps were in your knowledge. Then address the follow-up questions by thinking on a wider scale: How could misinformation about EBP be misleading to other practitioners? What should be done?
   b. Build upon the ideas uncovered in the previous step by writing your own definition of EBP. You can incorporate parts of the definitions given above if you'd like, but make sure that the definition is meaningful and makes sense to you. Keep this definition written down somewhere and look at it again once you have finished working through this book. Has your definition changed? Why?
   c. In small groups, write a definition of EBP, listing the most crucial aspects. Prepare a short (5 minute) presentation about your definition, and present it to the rest of the class. This can include creative elements (dramatic, artistic, etc.). Your goal is to get the message across and make it stick in the minds of your audience.

2. Evidence-Based Rehabilitation
   a. The four principles of EBR outlined in the chapter—awareness, consultation, judgment, and creativity—serve as good guideposts for practitioners using EBR, but they are not perfect. Can you think of any other guideposts for yourself? If not, can you further define what is meant from each of the original guideposts?

b. Briefly list the differences and similarities between evidence-based medicine and EBR. What are the key dissimilarities? How are EBM and EBR the most different? How are they the most similar? Why? What will need to happen before EBR gains the prestige already held by EBM?

REFERENCES

Cook, D. J., & Levy, M. M. (1998). Evidence-based medicine: A tool for enhancing critical care practice. *Crit Care Clin, 14*(3), 353-358.

DeLisa, J. A. (1999). Issues and challenges for psychiatry in the coming decade. *Arch Phys Med Rehabil, 80*, 1-12.

Duncan, P. W. (1997). Evidence-based medicine. *Physiother Res Int, 2,* 271-272.

Greenhalgh, T. (1997). *How to read a paper: The basics of evidence-based medicine.* London: BMJ Press.

Health Information Research Unit. (2002). How to teach evidence-based clinical practice 2002. Retrieved February 14, 2002, from McMaster University, Health Information Research Unit web site, from http://hiru.mcmaster.ca.

Marwick, C. (1997). Proponents gather to discuss practicing evidence-based medicine. *JAMA, 278*(7), 531-532.

Muir Gray, J. A. (1997). *Evidence-based health care: How to make health policy and management decisions.* London: Churchill Livingstone.

Rosenberg, W., & Donald, A. (1995). Evidence-based medicine: An approach to clinical problem solving. *British Medical Journal, 310*(6987), 1122-1126.

Sackett, D. L., Rosenberg, W. M., Gray, J. A., Haynes, R. B., & Richardson, W. S. (1996). Evidence-based medicine: What it is and what it isn't. *British Medical Journal, 312*(7023), 71-72.

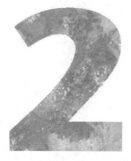

Development of Evidence-Based Knowledge

Winnie Dunn, PhD, OTR, FAOTA and Jill Foreman, BHSc(OT)

LEARNING OBJECTIVES

After reading this chapter, the student/practitioner will be able to:
- Recognize and understand the multiple levels at which knowledge develops within a discipline.
- Define the different periods of development for the practitioner and explain the corresponding relationship with the development of knowledge.
- Understand the subsequent responsibilities and challenges of the practitioner as an individual, a member of a discipline, and a representative of a discipline.

INTRODUCTION

It is easy to believe that the knowledge of a particular discipline has been there for all time, was established quickly by experts who were defining the discipline, and was carried forth by all subsequent generations as stable and clear factors that characterize the discipline's perspectives and work. With this belief, persons would only have to acquire the knowledge, skills, and viewpoints of the discipline so they can use the information and then pass it along.

In fact, knowledge develops at many levels within one's own discipline and in concert with other disciplines that are interested in similar ideas. Additionally, as each new insight emerges, people have the opportunity to understand in a new way and simultaneously to consider what new dilemmas this insight reveals. There are many issues that people cannot even conceive are present until certain other knowledge becomes clear to them.

Knowledge is a collection of ideas and facts about a topic. People tend to say they have knowledge when information and ideas have stood the test of time and experience. Evidence is information that makes a conclusion apparent, and it is the accumulation of these conclusions that leads to new insights. The accumulation of evidence typically advances knowledge in a particular area, and knowledge, in turn, introduces other possibilities for gathering evidence. Although people generally refer to formal research as evidence for professional practice, in actuality, each professional act provides evidence that accumulates into that professional's knowledge base.

An Example

It was standard practice in the United States during the early 1900s to institutionalize persons with disabilities (i.e., people with disabilities were housed in large government-funded facilities and provided basic care for their survival). This practice was based on the belief that persons who were mentally or physically deficient could not contribute to and could not care for themselves; therefore, we needed to get them isolated from society and care for them.

People then began to demonstrate that individuals with disabilities could learn. This insight led people to question their beliefs about individuals with disabilities: Could they take care of themselves and contribute to society? People began to consider what the possibilities were for persons who could learn; they had to reconsider the standard practice of institutionalization, which by its very nature kept people with disabilities from participating in certain activities, including contributing to society and learning to care for themselves. Some members of the society began to press for persons with disabilities to be moved out of institutions so they could become members of communities and realize their potential (i.e., the deinstitutionalization movement).

Deinstitutionalization operationalized the knowledge about persons with disabilities having the potential to learn and, therefore, the possibility to contribute to society. When communities began to move people out of institutions, everyone realized that the communities did not have the infrastructure in place to support these new community members. Communities needed housing for all these persons; this issue had been irrelevant when people with disabilities were housed in large institutions. The community members who had worked in the institutions were now displaced from their work, creating an economic shift in the community. Communities were certainly able to tackle these challenges, but prior to deinstitutionalization there was no opportunity to see these issues; therefore, there was no opportunity to develop knowledge. As each insight occurred, other opportunities for insight presented themselves.

A century later, it can be seen that those who had the courage to challenge institutional-ization beliefs and practices began a process of changing services for persons with disabili-ties forever. Those who provided institutional care could not have conceived of some of our current practices (e.g., buildings that are accessible to everyone) because these innovations were too divergent from their beliefs and practices.

Evidence-based knowledge serves a generative function in the evolution of information for practice. It invites us to simultaneously gain insight to solve a current problem and see the dilemmas that are only visible from the next vantage point.

Purpose

The purpose of this chapter is to introduce the ways that evidence-based knowledge develops within a discipline. Primarily, there are three vantage points for knowledge devel-opment. First, the individual professional travels through a developmental process beginning with preservice educational preparation and continuing through the "expert" phase of the professional career path. Second, professionals develop and share information with each other within their own disciplines. Finally, professionals develop and share information across disciplines to inform a wider circle of thinkers. We will discuss each of these in turn and consider what our responsibilities are in the development of evidence-based knowledge.

The Individual Professional

Responsibilities

Individual professionals are responsible for facilitating knowledge development as insights emerge in daily practice. In order to accomplish this, professionals must first devel-op awareness of their own beliefs. It is essential to recognize that knowledge is not a prereq-uisite for a belief (Quine & Ullian, 1978). Beliefs emerge from experiences, viewpoints of those we trust, and sociocultural influences. Awareness of individual beliefs is important because beliefs form a filter through which professionals view and, therefore, interpret events and information. When beliefs are undefined, professionals are unaware of the reasons for their choices in practice (i.e., they act on interpretations that are guided surreptitiously by their beliefs), masking alternative interpretations.

For example, therapists may believe in the benefits of a therapeutic modality based on practice experience and a mentor's fervor for the method, while scientific knowledge of how the modality works may be scarce. Conductive education techniques are an example of this. Conductive education has been used with children who have cerebral palsy, although there is little evidence to support its efficacy (Bairstow, Cochrane, & Rusk, 1991; Bochner, Center, Chapparo, & Donelly, 1999; Lonton & Russell, 1989; Reddihough, King, Coleman, & Catanese, 1998). Therapists have a belief in the power of movement and therapeutic interac-tion and have experienced changes in children's movements subsequent to using these meth-ods. Therefore, they have a predisposition toward believing that conductive education will be an effective method, although reports are sparse and varied. Reddihough et al. (1998) stud-ied 34 children with cerebral palsy and found that those receiving conductive education made similar progress to children in alternative intervention groups. Bochner et al. (1999) report-ed that results of conductive education were quite variable with children who have motor disabilities, with some children showing no changes and others learning specific motor skills; however, they also cited lack of generalization of skills as a problem.

The example of conductive education illustrates what Quine and Ullian (1978) describe: "the intensity of a belief cannot be counted on to reflect its supporting evidence" (p. 7). When developing evidence-based practice, professionals must remain aware of the power of personal beliefs, be open to identifying the source and nature of the beliefs, and be willing to search for evidence-based knowledge to inform their practice techniques separate from their beliefs. Many professional practices begin with an experienced professional acting out a hunch; this willingness to discover new possibilities is appropriate as long as we take the next steps to evaluate effectiveness.

Evaluating effectiveness is the second responsibility for professionals (Feyerbend, 1993). The ability to continually question current information and seek new answers is often described as lifelong learning for the individual; this process forms the basis of evidence-based practice for the profession. The third responsibility is a willingness to use information to abandon ineffective methods and/or erroneous ideas and beliefs in favor of more effective options. This responsibility is challenging to fulfill because it requires professionals to entertain the possibility that their particular framework for thinking and problem solving needs adjustment. Beliefs and conceptual frameworks are interwoven; if one's framework doesn't change, the beliefs within that framework will be difficult to alter (Kuhn, 1996).

For example, rehabilitation professionals educated within a medically-based framework may have difficulty abandoning the belief that "doing something to or for the patient is best" as part of the "professional as expert" conceptual framework. A client-centered framework suggests that professionals collaborate with the client and family, and it has been shown to be an effective approach (Dunst, Deal, & Trivette, 1996; Rosenbaum, King, Law, King, & Evans, 1998). However, it requires professionals to reconstruct their beliefs to acknowledge the client and family as active participants in planning.

To meet the responsibility of knowledge development for evidence-based practice, professionals must also share their emerging insights and broader beliefs with others. Open dialogue and the ability to request feedback in practice encourages the development of efficacious practices. It enables professionals to remain flexible in their approach to practice challenges and facilitates ongoing improvements in practices (Feyerbend, 1993). Finally, professionals must participate in activities that are effective in their practices. In order to implement effective practices, professionals must conduct critical reviews of the literature, participate in quality reviews, and/or participate in formal data collection activities. Vigilance in collecting data enables patterns to emerge, hypotheses to be tested, and decisions to be made based on information actually available within the practice. There is potential to gather evidence-based data for a variety of audiences (e.g., for the professional's own practice, for the discipline, for the consumer, for the payer). With each audience, the evidence is gathered as a means of convincing the professionals that interventions are effective, providing support for the viability of the discipline, demonstrating changes to consumers, and/or to convincing payers that they are using their resources to purchase valuable services.

Phases of Professional Development

Professionals do not leave their educational preparation and enter work fully equipped to meet all of the responsibilities of serving as evidence-based professionals. The course of one's career affords different possibilities (Table 2-1).

Table 2-1

PROFESSIONAL KNOWLEDGE DEVELOPMENT

Preservice Experience
- Becomes aware of own beliefs and learns initial strategies for questioning beliefs

Novice Professional Period
- Begins to generalize ideas, determines effective and ineffective methods for practice, and tests knowledge and beliefs

Experienced Professional Period
- Establishes methods for evaluating effectiveness, hypothesizes successful therapeutic techniques, and shares with colleagues

Expert Professional Period
- Participates in formal methods of collecting data and evaluating interventions, shares knowledge more globally, and critiques work of others

---

Preservice Experiences

Through preservice experiences, students learn the knowledge base of the discipline and are exposed to the available evidence for current interventions. In this initial stage, the professional learns how to use the available evidence to construct preliminary clinical reasoning strategies and decision-making guides. The knowledge development for preservice students occurs within the current thought paradigms of the discipline, thereby focusing their learning to include current knowledge and evidence (Kuhn, 1996; Schell, 1998). Preservice professionals meet the first and second responsibilities of becoming evidence-based professionals (i.e., they become aware of their beliefs and learn initial strategies for questioning those beliefs in the interest of effectiveness).

Novice Professional Period

In the novice period, professionals learn how others apply knowledge and evaluate evidence. Novice professionals try ideas and evaluate their effectiveness in individual situations. It is during this period of development that professionals begin to generalize ideas across peoples and settings, determining effective and ineffective methods for practice, thus building a resource of professional experiences that guides future decisions. The novice professional period provides opportunities to test the knowledge and beliefs that professionals have acquired through educational preparation, increasing clarity and generalizability of knowledge for practice. This period forms the foundation for clinical reasoning as knowledge and personal beliefs, now grounded in experience, begin to merge.

Experienced Professional Period

With further experience, professionals begin to create a personal "database" from all their professional experiences and learning. The experienced professional period enables the individual to establish methods for evaluating the effectiveness of selected interventions based on their personal database (Feyerbend, 1993). Professionals working within particular settings will be able to evaluate the effectiveness of therapeutic interventions on functional outcomes achieved by clients in that setting. The experienced professional is better able to hypothesize those therapeutic techniques that will be most successful for clients admitted with particular functional concerns due to the breadth and depth of the professional practice to inform these decisions. As professionals generate evidence in practice, they also begin to share their personal "evidence" with other professionals; sharing facilitates development of collective knowledge about effective practices. This collective knowledge can be shared in team meetings, focus groups, and professional conference presentations for specific areas of practice.

Expert Professional Period

In the expert professional period, professionals participate in more formal methods of collecting data and evaluating effectiveness of interventions. Professionals may solicit funding to conduct research within their service setting or population. For example, professionals may participate in a randomized controlled trial to try to determine which of two intervention methods is most effective, or they may publish a case study to illustrate a client's experience with a particular disability. The knowledge gained through this research allows professionals to make findings more globally available to other professionals. When expert professionals share in more public forums, they can impact evidence-based practice knowledge development by inviting less advanced colleagues to benefit from the expert's insights. This period also includes critiquing the work and insights of others to advance knowledge for the discipline (Feyerbend, 1993; Quine & Ullian, 1978).

PROFESSIONALS WITHIN A DISCIPLINE

Just as for individual development, professionals within a discipline have collective responsibilities to contribute to evidence-based knowledge. These include challenging current beliefs, sharing information with colleagues, introducing new ideas, and formally testing hypotheses for their new ideas.

The growth of knowledge in a discipline is possible only when the members and interested others challenge current beliefs and theories. By challenging current theory, a discipline ensures thoroughness and refinement and fosters further development of knowledge. Knowledge development within a professional community requires its members to constantly push the limits imposed by current working paradigms. By encouraging professionals to participate in dialogues about knowledge development and understanding, both the discipline and the individual professionals evolve (Feyerbend, 1993), creating a generative cycle.

Individuals within a discipline relate their practice knowledge base to theories of the profession. Theories within the profession guide practice decisions and practice experiences, in turn informing the theory. It is valuable to recognize the challenge that members have in introducing new ideas to a professional group with established theories that form the basis for current research and communication within the profession. One may expect new ideas to be encouraged because new ideas serve to further develop professional knowledge. However, new ideas also challenge the foundation of current activities, which can be threatening to the stability of professional beliefs (Feyerbend, 1993).

Professionals within a discipline are responsible for designing and implementing formal methods for testing hypotheses that grow out of the cycle of practice-construct dialogue. Professionals need to have current beliefs to begin, but these ideas need to be challenged in some way in order to advance current forms of professional practice and, ultimately, refine the constructs and beliefs. Thus, tension between research and practice is inevitable and a necessary struggle for the advancement of knowledge (Quine & Ullian, 1978). For researchers to understand how to propose change, they must understand that issues arise in practice that seem contradictory to currently held beliefs. New data can be generated to inform more advanced thinking, thus advancing the discipline's body of knowledge. How a professional community adopts or rejects innovative or controversial information determines its evolution and viability (Chinn & Brewer, 1993).

PROFESSIONALS ACROSS DISCIPLINES

Evidence-based knowledge development must also occur in collaboration with other disciplines that are interested in similar ideas. There are many professional practice problems that simply cannot be solved with a single discipline's perspective. When the knowledge of a variety of disciplines is shared, there emerges many more possibilities for knowledge development. To enable the sharing of knowledge across disciplines, members of professional communities have several responsibilities.

First, professionals must remain open to other points of view. Collaboration among professionals requires teamwork with a desire to share and receive new ideas. Second, it is important to remain aware of how decisions made by a variety of disciplines may impact families and individuals being served. The paradigm of family-centered care provides a good example of this need for collaboration. Professionals employing this paradigm encourage and support family involvement regardless of the expertise of any particular discipline. For family-centered care to be effective, professionals then need to identify the unique and complementary knowledge that will enable a family to act on their goals without creating undue burden on the family (e.g., an undue burden would be each discipline designing their own intervention plans, expecting the family to carry them out).

The third responsibility professionals have is to recognize and facilitate awareness about the similarities and differences in approaches to problem solving and knowledge development for each discipline. Clear communication between professionals about investigation approaches and methods is necessary to ensure effective collaboration across disciplines. The fourth responsibility in advancing collective evidence-based knowledge among disciplines is to collaboratively conduct research. Professionals can work together to design and implement formal methods for testing hypotheses that grow out of the interdisciplinary dialogue. Research can focus on problems that are best tested from an interdisciplinary perspective.

For example, several disciplines contribute to knowledge about barrier-free design (sometimes called *universal design* or *universal access*). Individuals with backgrounds in occupational therapy, physiotherapy, architecture, interior design, environmental psychology, human ecology, and urban and regional planning all have knowledge and skills related to barrier-free design. The collective knowledge of these professionals expands the possible solutions for designing a barrier-free environment (Cooper, Cohen, & Hasselkus, 1991; Steinfeld & Shea, 1993).

Finally, professionals from across disciplines must recognize uncomfortable places as opportunities for knowledge development. It is naturally difficult for individuals with different theoretical paradigms to collaborate with each other; however, each discipline evolves from the reflection of colleagues from other disciplines. The product of interdisciplinary collaboration can advance knowledge for each discipline and for collective knowledge in an area of interest.

An Example Illustrating the Contribution of Research and Evidence to Developing Evidence-Based Knowledge for Practice and Knowledge Development

All of the ideas presented in this chapter and throughout this book are platitudes if there is no evidence that knowledge development and evolution actually occur in these ways. Those of us who are further along on our professional journeys have a sense of knowledge development from our own lived experiences, but it is inefficient for a discipline to rely on "living it" to see the power of the knowledge development. As disciplines mature, we must be willing to conduct formal analyses of knowledge development; this not only includes the facts and data from studies, but also the evolution of insights at each new point in the knowledge development process. Without scholars willing to wonder, muse, and hypothesize about the meaning of information, all the data in the world would not advance knowledge. Additionally, we need practitioners who are open to new ideas and who question current practice so that hypotheses can be tested and refined.

A powerful example from the occupational therapy (and related disciplines) literature comes from the development of knowledge about sensory integration. This area of knowledge development illustrates all levels of evolution: individual scholars moving from novice to expert, the discipline increasingly incorporating advancing knowledge into the collective thinking, and the impact of occupational therapy's work on other disciplines' knowledge development.

Early Developments and Insights

Occupational therapy has a long history of relying on the neuroscience literature to guide our thinking about assessment and intervention. Many early theorists have discussed the importance of nervous system operations for the production of adaptive human behaviors (Ayres, 1955; Blashy & Fuchs, 1959; Bobath & Bobath, 1955; Cruickshank, Bice, & Wallen, 1957; Fay, 1948; Rood, 1952). These scholars were peers in the 1950s so much of their work was interdependent. For this discussion, we shall focus specifically on the evolution of sensory integration knowledge, which we primarily attribute to Dr. A. Jean Ayres.

Dr. Ayres' early thinking arose from her study of neuroscience during doctoral and postdoctoral work (Sieg, 1988). At that time, she also had experience working with children and adults with various central nervous system conditions (Cruickshank, 1974). Therefore, from an individual perspective, we would say Dr. Ayres was in her experienced professional period (see Table 2-1). As you recall from earlier in the chapter, this means she would have created a personal database for decision making and would be sharing her perspectives with others. She was also seeking formal doctoral and postdoctoral education at this time, foreshadowing her intent to enter the expert professional period, which we will discuss later.

Dr. Ayres was fascinated by what she observed in children with cerebral palsy and learning disabilities. From her studies and her professional experiences she began to hypothesize about the nature of these children's performance difficulties. She emphasized visual motor functions and perceptual and proprioceptive facilitation to improve upper extremity function (Henderson, Llorens, Gilfoyle, Myers, & Prevel, 1974). She wrote several articles to share her ideas with others (Ayres, 1954, 1958, 1960, 1963), as do most people in the experienced professional period.

At the discipline level, Dr. Ayres was generating an impact in two ways. First, she was beginning to change the course of occupational therapy thinking. Secondly, those in related disciplines who also had an interest in children's perceptual motor skills considered Dr. Ayres a visionary scholar. Dr. William Cruickshank, a noted scholar of education and psychology and one of Dr. Ayres' peers, stated in reviewing Dr. Ayres early work, "…the writings of Jean Ayres… have been instrumental in setting new directions for a total discipline, or at least have directed the profession of occupational therapy in two areas that are historically and functionally different… prior to 1955" (1974, p. viii).

Testing Hypotheses to Gain New Perspectives

After publishing her ideas and insights on children's perceptual motor skills and completing her postdoctoral education, Dr. Ayres began to test her theoretical ideas with larger samples and sound measurement methods.

These actions represent the expert professional period of her individual career path. She was quite prolific in writing during this period, reporting on her findings, interpreting the results in light of her own and the work of other scholars, and making more refined hypotheses for subsequent research.

In order to test some of the theoretical constructs, Dr. Ayres identified available methods and constructed some of her own methods of measuring children's sensory, perceptual, motor, and praxis abilities. In her 1965 article, "Patterns of Perceptual Motor Dysfunction in Children," she reported on her first of several factor analytic studies, a creative and insightful work for the time. Using data from 100 children with perceptual deficits and 50 typically developing children, Dr. Ayres hypothesized that there were five syndromes representing dysfunction, including apraxia, tactile and visual perception, tactile defensiveness, bilateral integration, and poor figure ground perception.

With this study and subsequent work to refine these patterns, Dr. Ayres began to validate theoretical constructs that would provide a specific focus for occupational therapy research for the next four decades and beyond. Simultaneously, this work has influenced work in related disciplines by informing them of occupational therapy's significant and unique contributions and advancing knowledge to their work as well.

In a series of factor analytic studies (Ayres, 1965, 1966a, 1966b, 1969a, 1969b, 1971, 1972a, 1972b), Dr. Ayres continued to elucidate perceptual motor and sensory integrative constructs. She and colleagues standardized the Southern California Sensory Integrative Tests, which enabled professionals to identify specific types of sensory integrative performance problems.

By 1972, Dr. Ayres had identified five types of sensory integrative dysfunction:

→ Visual/tactile/kinesthetic form and space perception

→ Motor planning and tactile perception

→ Tactile perception, hyperactivity, distractibility, and tactile defensiveness

→ Postural and ocular muscle control

→ Auditory language functions

In her studies, she increasingly refined her measures so that she could illustrate these categories of performance problems with more clarity. Because she had demonstrated the presence of several of these factors across study populations, she spoke with more confidence about their integrity and applicability to assessment and intervention planning in practice situations. Dr. Ayres also conducted other studies to examine the effectiveness of interventions based on her hypotheses (Ayres, 1972a, 1976). These intervention studies informed therapists how they might apply her ideas in their practice.

The Second Generation Develops Insights

As Dr. Ayres traversed through her expert professional period, she was influencing many younger therapists with her ideas. The knowledge that Dr. Ayres developed and validated through her research moved into occupational therapy curricula as core knowledge, and sensory integration theory and practice began to be inherent in service planning for children. As these "second generation" colleagues moved from their novice period into their experienced professional period, they began making and testing hypotheses of their own.

Armed with the tools that Dr. Ayres provided (i.e., the data, the tests, new knowledge, expert insights), occupational therapists serving children began to emphasize sensory integration factors when evaluating and designing intervention programs. Occupational therapy graduate students and scholars who were studying Dr. Ayres' work began to design and implement intervention studies to evaluate the effectiveness of a sensory integrative approach in therapy. (Note: Since our purpose here is to examine the knowledge development process and not provide a comprehensive review of this literature, please review Fisher, Murray, & Bundy [1991] for an in-depth reporting of the work during this period.)

This was a prolific period for testing hypotheses and generating insights about the role of sensory integration in persons' performance. Dr. Ayres had provided such a rich foundation of ideas that what began as a few musings and insights had now become a whole body of ideas to consider. Because Dr. Ayres was so vigilant at disseminating her ideas in writing and in presentations, the possibility of advancing knowledge multiplied geometrically with this new cohort of novices emerging to experienced professionals. For example, Ottenbacher (1982) found 49 articles reporting on research about sensory integrative interventions. His meta-analysis revealed a positive effect for sensory integrative interventions, but only eight of the articles met his criteria for inclusion in the review process. Other studies reported more equivocal results (Feagans, 1983; Ferry, 1981; Ottenbacher & Short-DeGraff, 1985), suggesting that further work still needed to be done to demonstrate the appropriate application of sensory integrative constructs for evidence-based practice.

Another important event in knowledge development at the discipline level occurred during this time. Because there was more information available about the constructs and application (both effective and ineffective) of sensory integration, scholars from other disciplines began to consume this knowledge, with mixed results. For example, Arendt, MacLean, and Baumeister (1988) published a critique of sensory integration therapy as it might be applied to persons with mental retardation and reported that it would be inappropriate to apply these methods based on the available evidence. The editor recognized the provocative nature of this topic and invited five scholars in occupational therapy to respond to this article. The entire series of articles is published in one volume, providing an excellent example of scholarly discourse. From a knowledge-development perspective, critiques such as this are not possible until knowledge has developed to the point that others can study it and consider their perspectives on the ideas.

It was also during this period that scholars conducted clinical trials of sensory integration interventions (Humphries, Snider, & McDougall, 1993; Humphries, Wright, McDougall, & Vertes, 1990; Humphries, Wright, Snider, & McDougall, 1992; Kaplan, Polatajko, Wilson, & Faris, 1993; Polatajko, Kaplan, & Wilson, 1992; Polatajko, Law, Miller, Schaffer, & Macnab, 1991; Wilson & Kaplan, 1994; Wilson, Kaplan, Fellowes, Gruchy, & Faris, 1992). These research teams reported similar results (i.e., that sensory integration therapy was equally effective as other interventions [e.g., perceptual motor, tutoring, traditional interventions], not more effective at affecting sensorimotor outcomes and that results on the impact of sensory integration on academic performance were equivocal).

These studies reflect the maturation of therapists' thinking about sensory integration and its increasing visibility in the larger professional arenas. There was more interest and pressure to demonstrate the usefulness of these "new" ideas. Those outside the "web of belief" were appropriately asking questions about the claims of effectiveness. It was time for researchers to study the nature and scope of sensory integration practices and for those in practice to understand when sensory integration interventions would be the appropriate or inappropriate choice to make. This process of refinement had an important impact on knowledge generation in that it illuminated the possible limitations of this knowledge for particular intervention practices. It is critical that both effective and ineffective methods become clear in the research; this establishes the parameters for proper use of knowledge and invites scholars to reconceptualize the nature and meaning of their constructs for use in practice and in subsequent research.

The "Renaissance Period"

So here we are more than a decade later from all this activity. We have another cohort of occupational therapy professionals who are in their experienced professional period, only this time they have been able to study not only the knowledge that Dr. Ayres provided but also all the knowledge that the first cohort provided (who are now in their expert professional periods). This breadth of information *and* distance from the original seeds of knowledge provide a new vantage point for considering the ideas. Additionally, the culture of scholarly endeavors has matured as well, affording new tools and strategies for testing the fidelity of knowledge and the effectiveness of its application in practice.

Great things are happening, as they do when knowledge has the time to settle in, and scholars can take a fresh look with new tools. Occupational therapy scholars have been studying neuroscience and sensory integration knowledge and are adding clarity to some of Dr. Ayres' original ideas, as well as proposing new ideas for consideration. As an indicator of the available accumulating knowledge, Miller and Lane (2000) produced a three-part series of articles that provided a taxonomy of definitions related to sensory integration and sensory processing, inviting scholars to use consistent terms for this burgeoning body of knowledge.

As one example of knowledge being reformulated, Dr. Ayres discussed tactile defensiveness and gravitational insecurity as conditions in which the person was unable to tolerate touch and movement input, respectively (Ayres, 1972b). Researchers of today are revisiting one's inability to process sensory input as part of modulating the amount and type of information a person might need for creating adaptive responses. They are using the knowledge developed thus far and applying contemporary methods of research to characterize sensory modulation as a range of responses to sensory events (Baranek, Foster, & Berkson, 1997; Dunn, 2000), thus broadening original ideas and observations.

We have also broadened ideas about the domain of study. In the early years, sensory integration concepts and treatment methods were the focus of the research but, in more recent years, scholars have identified constructs that are more properly classified in the larger context of sensory processing. While sensory integration is a component of sensory processing (i.e., the nervous system's capacity to process sensory input [Miller & Lane, 2000, p. 2]), the term *sensory processing* encompasses the application of broader neuroscience constructs to the human experience (i.e., the way the nervous system receives, modulates, integrates, and organizes incoming sensory information [Miller & Lane, 2000]). Studies of children with poor coping skills (Williamson & Szczepanski, 1999), poor regulatory abilities (DeGangi, 2000), autism (Baranek et al., 1997; Kientz & Dunn, 1997), and fragile X syndrome (Belser & Sudhalter, 1995) provided evidence that a broader consideration was appropriate.

Additionally, studies of intervention in natural settings (Case-Smith & Bryan, 1999; Kemmis & Dunn, 1996) have suggested that some of the findings of ineffectiveness of sensory integration interventions may be related to a too narrow perspective.

With a broader perspective, it becomes imperative for scholars to conduct studies with scholars from other disciplines. Furthermore, scholars from other disciplines are finding sensory processing knowledge from the literature themselves and using knowledge from occupational therapy to inform their research programs.

For example, DeGangi, Sickel, Wiener, and Kaplan (1996) studied fussy babies by combining occupational therapy methods and psychophysiological methods and found that there are distinct patterns of performance indicating hyper-responsivity to stimuli. Baranek et al. (1997) conducted a factor analysis of behaviors of children and adults with developmental disabilities and found two factors that both supported the idea of sensitivities to sensory input. Miller and colleagues (MacIntosh, Miller, Shyu, & Hagerman, 1999; Miller et al., 1998) have reported behavioral and psychophysiological data indicating poor sensory modulation in children with fragile X syndrome and identified a distinct pattern of performance they call *sensory modulation disorder*. Dunn and colleagues (Dunn, 1994; Dunn & Brown, 1997; Dunn & Westman, 1997; Ermer & Dunn, 1998; Kientz & Dunn, 1997) have reported on distinct patterns of children's responses to sensory events in daily life based on disabilities such as autism and attention deficit hyperactivity disorder (ADHD). Belser and Sudhalter (1995) found distinct arousal difficulties in children with fragile X syndrome when compared to children with autism and ADHD, and they hypothesized about their ability to modulate input for responding.

Personal Reflection—Winnie Dunn

My professional development has occurred during the periods I have briefly described. As a novice in 1972, I had the advantage of Dr. Ayres' work from the onset of my studies to be an occupational therapist. Looking back, I certainly had no idea that I, as a novice, was part of this *new direction* (as Dr. Cruickshank called it). I just thought of sensory integration as part of occupational therapy knowledge. At that time, the role of researcher was a distant and disconnected one from practice. I certainly began to realize the power of this knowledge evolution as I attended workshops and studied. If someone had told me then that I would be contributing to this body of knowledge, I would have laughed and dismissed the comment. That is the way of novices—we don't have insight about the impact we have on others and ourselves, nevertheless the impact occurs.

For me, it was the plague of a practice dilemma for which I could not find an answer in my books and references. I was completely focused on solving my dilemma without any awareness that THIS WAS the beginning of my research career. It was many years later that I was able to identify with my "researcher self."

In the last few years, as I have studied sensory processing and developed the sensory profile tools for research and practice, I came upon some of my work pages from my novice period. I found a diagram I had been trying to formulate that contained the same constructs that I reported in an article in 1997 (Dunn, 1997). What strikes me is that it took me more than 20 years to achieve clarity about these ideas; yet, it also strikes me that I had these ideas more than 20 years ago!

I relay this experience because many novices feel discouraged, feeling that they will never learn and know what their mentors do. I invite you to be aware of the raw material ideas you produce during your novice period; perhaps we need to plant those seeds early so that we can release them to the public at a later date. Pay attention to your own development and how it affects you, the persons you serve, and your profession. Yes, YOU affect knowledge development with every action you take. Experts are sometimes encumbered by their own history, making it difficult to see knowledge a new way—in the role of the novice entering the world of knowledge development.

SUMMARY

In this chapter we considered how knowledge develops. There are simultaneous activities occurring that enable knowledge to emerge and evolve. Individual professionals develop along their respective career paths, profiting from the work that has come before them and gathering their own information and insights along the way. As individuals in a profession gather and discuss their ideas, collective insights form as hypotheses that can be formulated and tested. As data become available, professionals reformulate their hypotheses and gain new insights. Interdisciplinary discourse also advances knowledge by adding perspectives to evolving ideas. These are the processes that occur to produce evidence for practice.

There is still a lot to discover about the nature of sensory integration constructs and their appropriate application in practice. With the wealth of colleagues attending to this body of knowledge, I have no doubt that this journey will continue and be a fruitful source of knowledge development. It is through the persistent processes of professionals moving from novice to expert and disciplines evolving that this will occur.

Take-Home Messages

- Knowledge develops at many different levels—simultaneously within a discipline and in collaboration with other disciplines.
- The tension between practice and knowledge is inevitable and acts in a positive way as the source for the advancement of knowledge.
- The role of the individual professional within a discipline area passes through four distinct stages: preservice experience, novice professional period, experienced professional period, and expert professional period.
- An understanding of how knowledge develops must include a recognition of the three different vantage points for knowledge (individual professional; professional within a discipline; professionals across disciplines).
- Novices can enact a positive influence on knowledge development by becoming aware of their research self and encouraging new ideas.
- There are different responsibilities for the practitioner in each of the three different vantage points for the development of knowledge:

    Individual Professional
    - Remaining aware of influence of own personal beliefs
    - Evaluating effectiveness through questioning current information and seeking answers
    - Willing to use this information to abandon ineffective practices

Professional Within a Discipline
- Challenging current beliefs and sharing information with colleagues
- Introducing new ideas and formally testing hypotheses

Professionals Across Disciplines
- Conducting research collaboratively and being open to other points of view
- Remaining aware of how decisions are being made by a variety of disciplines may impact families
- Facilitating awareness of various approaches to problem solving between disciplines

LEARNING AND EXPLORATION ACTIVITIES

The purpose of this chapter is to introduce the different vantage points at which knowledge develops and to demonstrate how these levels interact in practice.

1. Select one of the following topics of rehabilitation practice that interests you: (1) treatment of acute low back pain; (2) outcomes of medical versus stroke units for person experiencing a stroke; or (3) home-based treatment for persons with arthritis. Complete the following activities for the topic you have selected:

    a. Using your current knowledge and a literature search, construct a preliminary clinical reasoning strategy to guide treatment and practice for this topic area. Focus on what you know as a student and the elements of practice that should be put into place based on the evidence that you find.

    b. Interview a practitioner in the same topic area. Ask him or her to tell you about his or her clinical reasoning strategy to guide practice.

    c. Compare the results of what you found and what you discussed with the practitioner. Are the two approaches congruent? If not, what are the differences? Why might these differences occur, and how do they relate to the development of knowledge in rehabilitation practice?

REFERENCES

Arendt, R., MacLean, W., & Baumeister, A. (1988). Critique of sensory integration therapy and its application in mental retardation. *Am J Ment Retard, 92*, 401-411.

Ayres, A. J. (1954). Ontogenetic principles in the development of arm and hand functions. *Am J Occup Ther, 8*(3), 95-99, 121.

Ayres, A. J. (1955). Proprioceptive facilitation elicited through the upper extremities: Part 3: Special applications to occupational therapy. *Am J Occup Ther, 9*(3), 121-126.

Ayres, A. J. (1958). The visual motor function. *Am J Occup Ther, 12*(3), 130-138.

Ayres, A. J. (1960). Occupational therapy for motor disorders resulting from impairment of the central nervous system. *Rehabilitation Literature, 21*, 302-310.

Ayres, A. J. (1963). The development of perceptual motor abilities: A theoretical basis for treatment of dysfunction. *Am J Occup Ther, 17*(6), 221-225.

Ayres, A. J. (1965). Patterns of perceptual motor dysfunction in children. *Percept Mot Skills, 20*, 335-368.

Ayres, A. J. (1966a). Interrelations among perceptual motor abilities in a group of normal children. *Am J Occup Ther, 20*(6), 288-292.

Ayres, A. J. (1966b). Interrelationships among perceptual motor functions in children. *Am J Occup Ther, 20*(2), 68-71.

Ayres, A. J. (1969a). Relation between Gesell development quotients and later perceptual motor performance. *Am J Occup Ther, 23*(1), 11-17.

Ayres, A. J. (1969b). Deficits in sensory integration in educationally handicapped children. *J Learn Disabil, 2*, 160-168.

Ayres, A. J. (1971). Characteristics of types of sensory integrative dysfunction. *Am J Occup Ther, 25*(7), 329-334.

Ayres, A. J. (1972a). Improving academic scores through sensory integration. *J Learn Disabil, 5*, 338-343.

Ayres, A. J. (1972b). Types of sensory integrative dysfunction among disabled learners. *Am J Occup Ther, 26*(1), 13-18.

Ayres, A. J. (1976). *The effect of sensory integrative therapy on learning disabled children: The final report of a research project.* Los Angeles, CA: University of Southern California.

Bairstow, P., Cochrane, R., & Rusk, I. (1991). Selection of children with cerebral palsy for conductive education and the characteristics of children judged suitable and unsuitable. *Dev Med Child Neurol, 33*(11), 941-942.

Baranek, G., Foster, L., & Berkson, G. (1997). Sensory defensiveness in persons with developmental disabilities. *Occupational Therapy Journal of Research, 17*(3), 173-185.

Belser, R., & Sudhalter, V. (1995). Arousal difficulties in males with fragile X syndrome: A preliminary report. *Developmental Brain Dysfunction, 8*, 270-279.

Blashy, M., & Fuchs, R. (1959). Orthokinetics: A new receptor facilitation method. *Am J Occup Ther, 13*(5), 226-234.

Bobath, K., & Bobath, B. (1955). Tonic reflexes and righting reflexes in the diagnosis and assessment of cerebral palsy. *Cerebral Palsy Review, 16*(5), 4-10.

Bochner, S., Center, Y., Chapparo, C., & Donelly, M. (1999). How effective are programs based on conductive education? A report of two studies. *Journal of Intellectual and Developmental Disability, 24*(3), 227-242.

Case-Smith, J., & Bryan, T. (1999). The effects of occupational therapy with sensory integration emphasis on preschool-age children with autism. *Am J Occup Ther, 53*(5), 489-497.

Chinn, C., & Brewer, W. (1993). The role of anomalous data in knowledge acquisition: A theoretical framework and implications for science instruction. *Review of Educational Research, 63*(1), 1-49.

Cooper, B. A., Cohen, U., & Hasselkus, B. R. (1991). Barrier-free design: A review and critique of the occupational therapy perspective. *Am J Occup Ther, 45*(4), 344-350.

Cruickshank, W. (1974). Foreword. In A. Henderson, L. Llorens, E. Gilfoyle, C. Myers, & S. Prevel (Eds.), *The development of sensory integrative theory and practice: A collection of the works of A. Jean Ayres.* Dubuque, IA: Kendall/Hunt Publishing.

Cruickshank, W., Bice, H., & Wallen, N. (1957). *Perception and cerebral palsy.* Syracuse, NY: Syracuse University Press.

DeGangi, G. (2000). *Pediatric disorders of regulation in affect and behavior: A therapist's guide to assessment and treatment.* San Diego, CA: Academic Press.

DeGangi, G., Sickel, R., Wiener, A., & Kaplan, E. (1996). Fussy babies: To treat or not to treat? *British Journal of Occupational Therapy, 59*(10), 457-464.

Dunn, W. (1994). Performance of typical children on the sensory profile: An item analysis. *Am J Occup Ther, 48*(11), 967-974.

Dunn, W. (1997). A conceptual model for considering the impact of sensory processing abilities on the daily lives of young children and their families. *Infants and Young Children, 9*(4), 23-35.

Dunn, W. (2000). The sensations of everyday life: Empirical, theoretical, and pragmatic considerations. *Am J Occup Ther, 55*(6), 608-620.

Dunn, W., & Brown, C. (1997). Factor analysis on the sensory profile from a national sample of children without disabilities. *Am J Occup Ther, 51*, 490-495.

Dunn, W., & Westman, K. (1997). The Sensory Profile: The performance of a national sample of children without disabilities. *Am J Occup Ther, 51*, 25-34.

Dunst, C. J., Deal, A. G., & Trivette, C. M. (1996). *Supporting & strengthening families: Methods, strategies and practices, Volume 1.* Cambridge, MA: Brookline Books, Inc.

Ermer, J., & Dunn, W. (1998). The Sensory Profile: A discriminant analysis of children with and without disabilities. *Am J Occup Ther, 52*(4), 283-290.

Fay, T. (1948). The neurophysical aspects of therapy in cerebral palsy. *Arch Phys Med, 29*(6), 327-334.

Feagans, L. (1983). A current view of learning disabilities. *J Pediatr, 102*(4), 487-493.

Feyerbend, P. (1993). *Against method* (3rd ed.). London, England: Verso.

Ferry, P. C. (1981). On growing new neurons: Are early intervention programs effective? *Pediatrics, 67*(1), 38-41.

Fisher, A. G., Murray, E. A., & Bundy, A. C. (1991). *Sensory integration theory and practice.* Philadelphia, PA: F. A. Davis Company.

Henderson, A., Llorens, L., Gilfoyle, E., Myers, C., & Prevel, S. (1974). *The development of sensory integrative theory and practice: A collection of the works of A. Jean Ayres.* Dubuque, IA: Kendall/Hunt Publishing.

Humphries, T., Snider, L., & McDougall, B. (1993). Clinical evaluation of the effectiveness of sensory integrative and perceptual motor therapy in improving sensory integrative function in children with learning disabilities. *Occupational Therapy Journal of Research, 13*(3), 163-182.

Humphries, T., Wright, M., McDougall, B., & Vertes, J. (1990). The efficacy of sensory integration therapy for children with learning disability. *Physical and Occupational Therapy in Pediatrics, 10*(3), 1-17.

Humphries, T., Wright, M., Snider, L., & McDougall, B. (1992). A comparison of the effectiveness of sensory integrative therapy and perceptual-motor training in treating children with learning disabilities. *J Dev Behav Pediatr, 13*(1), 31-40.

Kaplan, B. J., Polatajko, H. J., Wilson, B. N., & Faris, P. D. (1993). Reexamination of sensory integration treatment: A combination of two efficacy studies. *J Learn Disabil, 26*(5), 342-347.

Kemmis, B., & Dunn, W. (1996). Collaborative consultation: The efficacy of remedial and compensatory interventions in school contexts. *Am J Occup Ther, 50*(9), 709-717.

Kientz, M., & Dunn, W. (1997). A comparison of the performance of children with and without autism on the Sensory Profile. *Am J Occup Ther, 51*(7), 530-537.

Kuhn, T. (1996). *The structure of scientific revolutions* (3rd ed.). Chicago, IL: University of Chicago Press.

Lonton, A. P., & Russell, A. (1989). Conductive education—magic or myth? *Z-Kinderchir, 44*(Suppl 1), 21-23.

MacIntosh, D., Miller, L., Shyu, V., & Hagerman, R. (1999). Sensory modulation disruption, electrodermal responses, and functional behaviors. *Dev Med Child Neurol, 41*, 608-615.

Miller, L., & Lane, S. (2000). Toward a consensus in terminology in sensory integration theory and practice, part 1: Taxonomy of neurophysiological processes. *Sensory Integration Special Interest Section Quarterly, 23*(1), 1-4.

Miller, L., McIntosh, D., McGrath, J., Shyu, V., Lampe, M., Taylor, A., et al. (1998). Electrodermal responses to sensory stimuli in individuals with fragile X syndrome: A preliminary report. *Am J Med Genet, 83*, 268-279.

Ottenbacher, K. (1982). Sensory integration therapy: Affect or effect? *Am J Occup Ther, 36*, 571-578.

Ottenbacher, K., & Short-DeGraff, M. (1985). *Vestibular processing dysfunction in children.* Binghamton, NY: Haworth Press, Inc.

Polatajko, H., Kaplan, B., & Wilson, B. (1992). Sensory integration treatment for children with learning disabilities: Its status 20 years later. *Occupational Therapy Journal of Research, 12*(6), 323-341.

Polatajko, H., Law, M., Miller, J., Schaffer, R., & Macnab, J. (1991). The effect of a sensory integration program on academic achievement, motor performance, and self-esteem in children identified as learning disabled: Results of a clinical trial. *Occupational Therapy Journal of Research, 11*(3), 155-174.

Quine, W., & Ullian, J. (1978). *The web of belief* (2nd ed., pp. 9-34). New York, NY: McGraw-Hill.

Reddihough, D. S., King, J., Coleman, G., & Catanese, T. (1998). Efficacy of programmes based on conductive education for young children with cerebral palsy. *Dev Med Child Neurol, 40*(11), 763-770.

Rood, M. (1952). Neurophysiological mechanisms utilized in the treatment of neuromuscular dysfunction. *Am J Occup Ther, 10*(4), 220-225.

Rosenbaum, P., King, S., Law, M., King, G., & Evans, J. (1998). Family-centred service: A conceptual framework and research review. *Physical and Occupational Therapy in Pediatrics, 18*(1), 1-20.

Schell, B. (1998). Clinical reasoning: The basis of practice. In M. Neistadt & E. Crepeau (Eds.), *Willard and Spackman's occupational therapy* (9th ed.). Philadelphia, PA: Lippincott, Williams & Wilkins.

Sieg, K. (1988). A. Jean Ayres. In B. Miller, K. Sieg, F. Ludwig, S. Shortridge, & J. Van Deusen (Eds.), *Six perspectives on theory for practice of occupational therapy* (pp. 95-142). Rockville, MD: Aspen Publishers.

Steinfeld, E., & Shea, S. (1993). Enabling home environments. Identifying barriers to independence. *Technology and Disability, 2*(4), 69-79.

Williamson, G., & Szczepanski, M. (1999). Coping frame of reference. In P. Kramer & J. Hinojosa (Eds.), *Frames of reference for pediatric occupational therapy* (pp. 431-468). Philadelphia, PA: Lippincott, Williams & Wilkins.

Wilson, B. N., & Kaplan, B. J. (1994). Follow-up assessment of children receiving sensory integration treatment. *Occupational Therapy Journal of Research, 14*(4), 244-266.

Wilson, B. N., Kaplan, B. J., Fellowes, S., Gruchy, C., & Faris, P. (1992). The efficacy of sensory integration treatment compared to tutoring. *Physical and Occupational Therapy in Pediatrics, 12*(1), 1-36.

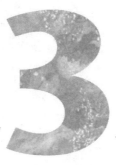

Becoming an Evidence-Based Practitioner

Nancy Pollock, MSc, OT(C) and Sarah Rochon, MSc(T), OT(C)

LEARNING OBJECTIVES

After reading this chapter, the student/practitioner will be able to:

- Understand the relationship that reflexivity plays in evidence-based practice.
- Recognize the role of reflection in helping novice practitioners to evaluate, understand, and apply their experience.
- Define the various components of the E model and how it acts as an organizing framework for decision-making.
- Recognize the role that technology plays in improving opportunities for evidence-based practice.

Three-year-old Michael is playing with his toy cars, absorbed in a private game during free play time at his preschool. Heather, his occupational therapist, crashes her toy car into his and shouts, "Watch out mister. I'm driving here!" Michael glances briefly at Heather and then angrily pushes her car away and turns his back. Kristen, a student occupational therapist, is puzzled by the therapist's actions. Why did she do that? Why did Heather intentionally provoke Michael and act so aggressively? En route to their next visit, Kristen asks Heather why.

As occupational therapists and physical therapists, we repeatedly encounter this type of situation. Clients, families, students, and team members ask us why we do what we do. The reflective practitioner welcomes this question and enjoys the process of uncovering the reasoning underlying his or her actions. For many therapists, this reflection is what makes their work stimulating, challenging, and satisfying. For others, however, particularly student therapists, this uncertainty can be frustrating and unsettling. The clinical reasoning process that underlies the decisions we make as therapists has been well described in recent literature (Mattingly & Fleming, 1994; Shepard, Hack, Gwyer, & Jensen, 1999). However, it remains for the most part an interior process, one that is hard to access and, therefore, hard to teach to others. Expert therapists have a difficult time describing the factors that influence the actions and decisions they routinely take with clients. The knowledge and experience they bring to the particular situation is called *tacit knowledge* (i.e., knowledge that is embedded in their thinking) (Schön, 1983). They don't have to consciously think about it; it is automatic. The recent work in our fields on clinical reasoning has given language to that thinking process and helps to make it accessible to novice practitioners and learners (Mattingly, 1991a, 1991b; Rochon, 1994). Why did Heather crash into Michael's car? What factors did she consider before taking that action? On what evidence did she base this decision?

In this chapter, we will explore the premise that a prerequisite to becoming an evidence-based practitioner is being a reflective practitioner and embracing the process of trying to become mindful of, understand, and articulate why we do what we do. Our practice, however, is not based solely on research evidence. Evidence is an important ingredient that should be considered in our clinical reasoning, but it is only one factor. There are many other factors that influence what we do. We will discuss the relationship between clinical reasoning and evidence-based practice and present a model to assist in the reasoning process. Finally, we will provide some clinical examples to illustrate the ideas and some exercises to apply the concepts described here.

THE REFLECTIVE PRACTITIONER

As health care professionals, it is incumbent upon us to develop and use more than just our technical skills. We must make decisions and base our actions on many factors, which interact in complex ways. Theoretical grounding, previous experience, client wishes, environmental conditions, research evidence, and resource constraints are but a few of the factors that influence our decision-making. There are very rarely right decisions or actions in our practices; more likely there are best decisions or actions. In our efforts to use best practice, the process of reflection can be a powerful learning tool. Reflection is a metacognitive process (i.e., we are thinking about our thinking) (Argyris & Schön, 1974). As therapists, our thinking is likely focused on our clinical reasoning. Why did we make the decisions we did, on what did we base them, what can we hypothesize about why they were effective, and what do we anticipate will happen next time? As busy clinicians, however, we often don't have the time to pause and think about the reasons underlying our actions. We are too busy doing to think about why we do what we do. It is when we are questioned or challenged, for example, by a student during fieldwork or by a client who responds in a surprising way to an intervention that we are triggered to pause and reflect.

A reflective practitioner, as first described by Schön (1983), is one who uses reflection-in-action. Many clinical situations are dealt with by the experienced practitioner in a routine way, basing actions on prior experience, assumptions, and understanding. It is when the practitioner is surprised by an unexpected outcome or challenged by a new situation that he or she must move into a phase of reflection to re-examine the problem, the assumptions, and how he or she has been thinking about the situation. In our earlier example, Kristen asking why is the stimulus for Heather's reflection. Schön (1987) argues that reflection represents the "art" of practice and knowledge and evidence the "science." Professionals practicing today require both the art and the science. Rogers (1983), in describing the art of practice, stated, "Artistry involves the orchestration of broad strategies for grappling effectively with the uncertainties inherent in clinical practice" (p. 614). It is this orchestration, which is applied automatically by the expert therapist, that may be uncovered through a reflective process.

As novice practitioners, we need rules to help us organize our thoughts, observations, and actions (Benner, 1984; Dreyfus & Dreyfus, 1986). At this stage of development as a clinician, we can only attend to a few elements of the therapeutic interaction at one time, and there is a tendency to focus on objective findings. The complexities of the relationships among the client, the environment, the therapist, and the expectations are typically beyond the capacity of the novice. In contrast, the expert therapist maintains these rules but shifts them to the background and simultaneously integrates and understands a multiplicity of factors also influencing the interaction (Slater & Cohn, 1991). What can be done to help move the novice along the continuum?

Experience, of course, is a strong mediator of the reasoning process, but it can only be acquired over time. Recognizing that novices need rules, we can find some guidance around what rules to apply (Benner, 1984; Hirschhorn, 1991). We can devise an organizing framework for decision-making that can support best practice decisions. We call our decision-making framework the *E model*. The novice practitioner can use the E model to anticipate situations and decisions and frame intervention plans and recommendations. For the more experienced practitioner, the E model can serve as a tool for reflection, a more systematic way of uncovering the tacit knowledge and "givens" that unwittingly shape practice.

> *As a recent physical therapy graduate, Carolyn began her practice on a developmental assessment team in a children's hospital. Children were seen over a 3-day period by a multidisciplinary team for assessment, then recommendations were shared with the family. She was fortunate to work with some experienced clinicians who helped her get started. After assessing a few children together with her supervisor, she was on her own. She was feeling reasonably confident that she was able to engage the children in the assessment process, manage their behaviour, complete some standardized assessments correctly, and make some good observations along the way. Prior to attending the feedback meeting with the team and family, she reviewed her findings with her supervisor. It all seemed to make sense and then the supervisor asked, "So, what will you recommend? Does he need therapy?" Carolyn didn't know how to answer or even how to start thinking about the question. What rules could she apply? What evidence could she use to help her make that decision? What considerations should she take into account? What did all these assessment findings really mean anyway?*

THE E MODEL

There are many factors that Carolyn needed to consider in deciding whether to recommend therapy. We have organized these factors into five categories: **E**xpectations, **E**nvironment, **E**xperience, **E**thics, and **E**vidence, hence the name: **E** model. Within each category, we will describe the factors in more detail and suggest some tools that can help the novice or expert therapist to explore the ideas within the category.

Expectations

The first set of expectations to take into consideration are those of the client. Our fields have moved increasingly to more client-centred models of practice in which the client is a true partner in the therapy process (Law, 1998). One of the central tenets of client-centred practice is that the client articulates the goals or expectations of the therapy process. The client defines the outcomes of therapy that are most important to his or her functioning. What is it that the client would like to be able to do as a result of intervention? The client brings the expertise about his or her life situation, values and beliefs, roles and expectations; therefore, he or she must be the one to articulate the goals. The therapist brings the expertise about how to work together to achieve those goals, but the destination is defined by the client.

In recent years, specific tools and measures have been developed to help us understand the clients' expectations and to assist them in articulating their goals. The Canadian Occupational Performance Measure (Law et al., 1998) uses a semistructured interview process to understand client priorities and the client's perception of current performance and satisfaction with performance and to set goals. This instrument enables the therapist to get a clear sense of the outcomes the client is expecting from therapeutic intervention.

The McMaster-Toronto Arthritis (MACTAR) Patient Preference Disability Questionnaire (Tugwell et al., 1987), which is another example of a client-centred measure, helps clients with arthritis articulate what is important to them and how their lives have been impacted by their illness or disability. These types of individualized assessments help therapists to understand what the client is experiencing and his or her expectations. With this information, therapists can move forward into a more meaningful partnership with the client. An understanding of the client's expectations is a key factor in one's decision-making process and should be one of the first things that is considered.

Another source of expectations is our knowledge of theory. As complex as theories can appear, they guide a clinician's thinking (Beckstand, 1986; Cooper & Saarinen-Rahikka, 1986; Rochon, 1994). They serve to explain one's observations, to enhance understanding of relationships, and to predict future events. Our models of practice evolve from theories that are translated into practical guidelines for action. There has been an increased focus in our disciplines on theory over the past three decades. We are either writing more about theory, developing new theories, or applying theories from other disciplines in new ways. Practice in the 1970s and 1980s was predominated by models derived from sensory integration theory, neurodevelopmental theory, and psychoanalytical theory (McColl, Law, & Stewart, 1993). Today, motor learning theory, dynamic systems, and metacognitive theories have come to the forefront (Larin, 1995; Law, Missiuna, Pollock, & Stewart, 2001). Models of practice, which guide our actions, continue to be developed from these more contemporary theoretical bases. Theories help to explain behaviour and predict outcomes, allowing us to formulate a set of assumptions or expectations that can guide our actions (Cooper & Saarinen-Rahikka, 1986; Hunt, 1977, 1980, 1988; Rochon, 1994; Rochon & Worth, 1995; Tammivaara & Shepard, 1990). Assumptions are the building blocks of theories. They are if-then statements.

Practitioners use theory in practice by applying these assumptions in guiding action. If a person is stumbling, then they are drunk, have ataxia, have improper shoes, have sensory deficits, or are tripping over obstacles in the environment. All of these assumptions are testable and lead the practitioner to the specific and proper assessment process to test each hypothesis. What you assess will be guided by the theory you use, and the interpretation of the results leading to intervention will be directly shaped by the guiding theory.

Environment

Decisions are never made in a vacuum. The environment exerts a powerful influence on our beliefs, thoughts, and actions. In a therapeutic relationship, environmental factors may exist at a macro level (e.g., the influences of health reform and health care funding on resource allocation, payment schemes, and access and eligibility for services). Cultural and social norms and values will influence plans and recommendations. Certain actions may be very acceptable within one culture and inconceivable within another. The physical location of the service delivery will influence the decision-making process, the role of the therapist, and the reality of the recommendations. Will the client be seen in a clinic; in his or her home, school, or workplace; or in a hospital or long-term care facility? Who is present in the client's immediate environment? Can you see the client directly, or will it be best to use a consultation or mediator model of service? Will you also be working with a spouse, a teacher, a health care team, or an extended family? What resources does the client have access to in his or her environment? Does he or she live in a remote community or a major urban centre? Are there extra costs, materials, or equipment associated with different treatment approaches? Are there language or communication barriers? It is essential that we think through all of the physical, cultural, social, political, and institutional aspects of the environment when making decisions and recommendations. Recommendations will only be effective if they are appropriate to current environmental contexts.

Experience

The experience one gathers over the years is a powerful force influencing decision making. Experience may encompass our education, both our professional preparation at an undergraduate or graduate level and our continuing education. These formal experiences set the stage for development of new ideas, reflection on current knowledge, and incorporation of this new knowledge into one's repertoire of skills (Benner, 1984). Less structured experiences occur constantly as we work. We begin to see similarities across groups of clients. We recognize patterns and, based on experience, can add meaning to these patterns. We encounter surprises or unexpected outcomes that challenge our assumptions and stimulate us to find new knowledge or perspectives that we can then bring to our next encounter (Schön, 1983). We network with colleagues, attend rounds, discuss a case, or work in a small learning group or tutorial. Thinking about these experiences is a prime mover in progressing along the novice-to-expert continuum. It is not enough to simply have experience by virtue of number of years worked, but it is the use of the experience as a learning tool that will make it of value. Reflection is a significant tool to enable the richness of learning from experience, but it is limited by one's own subjective reality.

A more objective means of using our growing experience in a systematic fashion is to use outcome measurement and precise documentation of our practice. Outcome measures allow us to examine the impact of what we do with individual clients, but they additionally allow us to examine trends, to look for recurring patterns, and to support the decisions we make. In this way we can truly use the experience we gain over time to benefit future clients. We can turn experiential anecdotes into powerful evidence on which to base decisions. The quest for appropriate outcome measures to use in our practice has always been challenging, but recent developments have significantly reduced this difficulty. Exponential growth in the number of well-developed tools in the rehabilitation field is extremely encouraging. Many of the newer measures have concordance with more current theoretical perspectives as well, thus allowing examination of outcomes at the level of activity and participation (e.g., the School Function Assessment) (Coster, Deeney, Haltwanger, & Haley, 1998). Texts (Cole, Finch, Gowland, Mayo, & Basmajian, 1994; Van Deusen & Brunt, 1997) and web-based sources (www. ericae.net) provide reviews of current measures. A CD-ROM program called *All About Outcomes: An Education Program to Help You Understand, Evaluate, and Choose Adult Outcome Measures* (Law et al., 2000) walks the user through a decision-making process to determine the appropriate focus for measurement and then provides critical reviews of possible measures. With these recent and powerful developments, it is now possible to discover and routinely use the best available outcome measures with clients no matter your location or situation.

Cumulative evidence from the systematic use of outcome measurement is an extremely powerful tool in responsible and credible practice. The current thrust in rehabilitation practice on outcome data demands our attention. Emphasis on how to interpret and use the results of outcome measurement in our practice is now emerging. For example, Stratford, Binkley, and Riddle (1996) have provided assistance in determining clinically important differences and interpretation of measurement results.

There have been many recent developments in our field that can support us in broadening, documenting, and deriving meaning from our experience. Internet technology allows us to chat with colleagues around the world and to participate in courses from the comfort of home. Email allows for discussion groups, on-line tutorials, and learning strategies such as interactive journalizing to be used at a distance (Tryssenaar, 1995). Although an individual's experience can only be gained over time, the amassing of critical information and provocation for critical thinking is greatly enhanced by these 21st century technologies that support dialogue about experiences and their relevance to future action.

Ethics

The role of ethics in decision making, particularly in health care, has assumed a more central role, both in the professional literature and in the popular literature (Somerville, 2000). As science has advanced, the available options and the complexities of the decisions health care providers must make has increased tremendously. In rehabilitation, decisions are not usually life or death decisions but, more typically, involve issues of access, confidentiality, determination of the primary client, and potential conflicts of interest. Resource limitations lead to decisions about who qualifies for service and, at times, the nature of service that is possible. Therapists often find themselves in the position of advocating on behalf of individual clients with program managers and third party payers. Weighing the needs of the individual against the collective needs of a population is very difficult and requires careful consideration. Deciding whether to recommend therapy when working in a private, user-pay system requires the therapist to be very confident that the recommendation stems from the best possible evidence that this therapy will be of benefit to the client and is not merely a revenue generation method.

Fortunately, as our professions have evolved and matured, more resources have been developed to help guide therapists in making difficult decisions (Brockett, Geddes, Salvatori,

& Westmorland, 1997; Geddes, Finch, & Larin, 1999). Provincial, state, and national regulatory bodies and professional associations have codes of ethics that elucidate principles for ethical decision making. These codes compel us to act with an ethic of truth and rightness, putting the needs of our clients first and respecting the boundaries of our knowledge and scope of practice (Canadian Association of Occupational Therapists, 2001).

Another aspect of ethics that a reflective practitioner considers is one's personal philosophy of practice and understanding of one's role as a therapist. These core values will influence every interaction with clients and every decision taken. Do you work from a biomedical model of practice? Do you believe that your role as a therapist is to fix the problem for the client? Do you involve the family in therapy? Do you work in partnership with clients? Do you feel your role is to create an environment in which the client can make the changes he or she wants to or is able to make? These are examples of the types of questions that are important to ask one's self in order to be clear and objective about one's thinking. Clinical reasoning is not situationally specific; it draws on the values, beliefs, philosophies, and culture of the reasoner. We will suggest some exercises later in the chapter that can help to uncover these personal values and beliefs.

Evidence

The use of evidence in clinical decision making is probably the factor in the E model that has experienced the greatest change over the past decade. The idea of a more explicit use of evidence in decision making began with the emergence of evidence-based medicine (EBM) (Sackett & Haynes, 2000). Historically, clinical decision making had been strongly influenced by the practitioner's education and by the opinions of experts in the field. This new idea of EBM demanded that physicians take responsibility for being up-to-date on the latest research evidence and use this information in making their decisions. EBM spread to other health disciplines and is now accepted as a key part of practice. Evidence-based practice is possible now because of several advances in our fields. First, of course, is the advancing volume of available evidence. While there are many areas of rehabilitation for which we do not have any solid evidence, there has been a substantial increase in both the quality and the quantity of research available to guide our decision making. Opportunities for access have also developed. The advent of the Internet has allowed practitioners access to on-line literature searching and some full text journal articles from anywhere in the world.

A second, more difficult barrier to the use of evidence—that of the need for critical appraisal of the evidence—is also being overcome through the many sources for critical and systematic reviews of the current research evidence. Journals with a singular focus on evidence-based practice are being published. International efforts such as the Cochrane Collaboration provide high quality systematic reviews of existing evidence about health care interventions. Professional associations are making critical reviews available to their members. Web sites devoted to the dissemination of systematic reviews are available in physical therapy (http://ptwww.cchs.usyd.edu.au/pedro) and occupational therapy (www.fhs.mcmaster.ca/rehab). Research units with a focus on a particular area of practice (www.fhs.mcmaster.ca/canchild) are producing critical reviews for dissemination to practitioners and consumers. Our professional education programs are including a strong focus on evidence-based practice so that the practitioners of tomorrow will be well equipped to access, appraise, and use the evidence in their decision making.

With all the information to consider, how does one put the E model into practice? Let's return to the example of Carolyn, the newly graduated physical therapist working on the developmental clinic. Although she believed that she didn't have any framework for deciding whether to recommend therapy to the family or not, the E model could provide her with the guidance she needs. The consideration of Expectations, Environment, Experience, Ethics, and Evidence can lead to Excellence in her clinical decision making.

USING THE E MODEL

To illustrate the use of the E Model in practice, we will return to Kristen, Michael, and Heather. Kristen, the student occupational therapist, is wondering why Heather, the occupational therapist, acted so aggressively with Michael, crashing her car into his and yelling in a play session at the preschool. Three-year-old Michael was diagnosed with autism 4 months ago. He began attending a community preschool, and a referral was made through the child development centre for occupational therapy and speech language pathology.

Expectations

Heather conducted a Canadian Occupational Performance Measure (COPM) (Law et al., 1998) with Michael's parents and with the preschool teacher. They identified the development of more social play interactions as a primary goal for Michael. Heather is familiar with the work of Greenspan and Wieder (1998), which is based on psychoanalytical theories of social and emotional development and their application to children with autism. Within this model of practice, known as *Floor Time*, it is essential that the adult assumes the role of player, plays alongside the child as he or she interacts with favourite toys or activities, and, if required, interrupts the child's play space in whatever way necessary to cause some kind of a reaction. This is the first step toward the development of communication. Michael has typically ignored Heather in her attempts to play alongside him, so she decided that she needed to provoke a reaction through the crashing of cars and shouting. She did receive a reaction from Michael, if only a sense of annoyance. It is a beginning and matches the expectations she had based on her understanding of theory and fits with the stated expectations of his parents and teacher.

Environment

Michael's parents had identified other areas of concern on the COPM, including the development of some self-help skills and improvement in Michael's ability to sleep through the night. These are issues that can be tackled best at home with the parents. The play issue, however, is perfectly suited to the preschool environment. The majority of time spent at the preschool is oriented toward play. There are a myriad of materials, toys, opportunities for play, and—the most important ingredient—other children with whom to play. Heather used the Test of Playfulness (Bundy, 1997) with Michael to determine the environmental barriers and supports to his play in the preschool environment. In this way, she can approach this goal within a naturalistic environment and educate those that work with Michael about ways in which they can influence his play development.

Experience

Heather has worked with children with developmental challenges for several years and has continued her education, taking courses in the areas of autism and pervasive developmental disorders. She is familiar with sensory integration therapy as applied to this population and has some knowledge of applied behavioural analysis methods (Linderman & Stewart, 1999; Lovaas & Smith, 1988). This has allowed her to make an informed choice about her approach to the development of Michael's play. She is also using a systematic approach to measuring the outcomes of therapy. The COPM will provide a measure of progress from the parents' and teacher's perspectives; however, the changes expected in Michael are subtle, so Heather has chosen to use goal attainment scaling as well to be able to note smaller steps across time (King, McDougall, Palisano, Gritzan, & Tucker, 1999). While the changes she has seen in other children who are similar to Michael are dramatic for that particular child, they are relatively small and most norm-referenced measures are not sensitive enough to capture the changes.

Ethics

Michael is fortunate to qualify for a publicly funded service; therefore, decisions about access are not relevant in this case. Heather is employed by the child development centre, and the mandate includes both in-centre and outreach services. There is also clarity in this situation about who is the primary client, as the philosophy of the child development centre is family centred.

Evidence

Heather has been keeping up-to-date on the latest evidence about the effectiveness of different therapies for children with autism. While large randomized trials do not exist for many of the approaches, there is new evidence coming forward. Research results for the use of applied behavioural analysis (ABA) methods have shown some positive changes in the participants, but it tends to be in acquisition of specific skills and doesn't seem to be generalizing to areas such as play (Smith, Groen, & Wynn, 2000). Also, the ABA studies have evaluated a very intensive model of intervention (30 to 40 hours per week), and this is not realistic for Michael in his current situation. The sensory integration literature is mixed (Vargas & Camilli, 1999). Large randomized trials have not shown differential positive outcomes when compared to other types of therapy in children with learning disabilities; however, there have been some promising results from single subject trials of sensory modulation approaches applied to children with autism (Case-Smith & Bryan, 1999; Linderman & Stewart, 1999). Heather is applying some of these ideas as she consults with the parents and preschool staff about changes they can make in Michael's environment to facilitate his participation. The evidence for the Floor Time approach is also preliminary in nature (Greenspan & Wieder, 1997); however, Heather is using this approach and monitoring its effects with Michael through her goal attainment scaling.

Heather is an excellent role model for Kristen, the student occupational therapist. Although Heather has a great deal of tacit knowledge that went into her decision to crash her car into Michael's, she is able to explain the basis of her decision and demonstrate for Kristen in a systematic way the many layers that lie beneath an apparently simple, if puzzling, action. It is Heather's ability to reflect on and explain her actions that lends credibility to her practice and provides a novice therapist with some tools for thinking.

SUMMARY

As we enter the era of evidence-based practice, there is a concern that the pendulum will swing too far. While we must continue to produce high quality research, access and interpret the evidence, and apply the findings to our particular clinical questions, it will be important to remember that evidence is just one piece of the puzzle. Evidence must be considered and contribute to our decision making along with a consideration of other factors, including expectations from clients and theoretical models, the environmental context, prior experiences, and ethical practice. A competent practitioner is conscious of all these factors and weighs them carefully in making recommendations.

Take-Home Messages

- A prerequisite to becoming an evidence-based practitioner is to become a reflective practitioner.
- Evidence is only one factor of the clinical reasoning process, and the best decisions are made with a conscious and appropriate consideration of other factors.
- The clinical reasoning process is difficult to access because it is an interior process; the tacit knowledge used in decision making is characterized as embedded knowledge.
- The E model (expectations, environment, experience, ethics, evidence) is a decision-making framework used to guide decision making and to reflect on decisions.

Expectations are shaped by:
- A client who articulates the goals and expectations of the therapy process.
- Knowledge of theory, which allows for the formulation of a set of assumptions and subsequent models of practice.

Environment will strongly influence decisions and recommendations:
- Including physical, social, cultural, political, and institutional aspects of the environment.
- Recommendations will only be effective if they are appropriate to current environmental context.

Experience (formal and informal):
- Reflection is a significant tool to learn from one's experiences, but it may be limited by personal subjectivity.
- Objectivity can be gained through using outcome measures and precise documentation; growth of new measures and web-based sources can assist this process.
- The use of cumulative evidence from the systematic use of outcome measurement represents an important tool in rehabilitation practice.

Ethics are assuming a more central role:
- Often related to issues of limited resources and the therapist as advocate.
- Ethical decisions are guided by the increasing development of regulatory bodies and a recognition of personal philosophy.

Evidence is experiencing the greatest change with emergence of evidence-based practice:
- The development of evidence-based practice is made possible by increasing access to evidence and the development of more systematic reviews offering critical appraisals of research.

- Professional education programs are continuing to develop an emphasis on evidence-based practice, thereby giving important tools to future practitioners

LEARNING AND EXPLORATION ACTIVITIES

Exercises to Facilitate Reflection

The ability to reflect on one's practice is not easy. While acknowledged as important, it is sometimes hard to know how to get started. The following are some exercises that can help both students and practising therapists to reflect systematically about their thinking and the basis it holds for the decisions they make everyday in practice. The first exercise is best done alone, the second with a trusted learning partner, and the third with a group of colleagues.

1. Values Clarification

This exercise is based on the contention that human behaviour is shaped by the beliefs and values held by the individual. Thus, behaviours taken as therapists are shaped by their own beliefs and values. We are, however, often unaware of these values and, therefore, unable to analyze their influence on our practice. Many fields of endeavour—from business practices to personal relationships—recommend exercises to allow for clarification of one's personal values (Levoy, 1997; Pfeiffer & Jones, 1973; Rochon & Worth, 1995; Senge, Roberts, Ross, Smith, & Kleiner, 1994). This exercise, adapted from several of these works, should be done as an individual and can help you to uncover your own values and analyse their impact on your work with clients.

From the following list of values (both work and personal), select the 15 that are most important to you. Feel free to add important values that are missing from the list in the spaces at the end.

Step 1: Make a List of Your Most Strongly Held Values—Choose 15

___advancement	___fame	___working alone
___power	___excellence in prac-	___competition
___challenges	tice	___pleasure
___collaborating with	___the affections of	___helping myself
others	others	___wisdom
___peace of mind	___professional growth	___decisiveness
___community recogni-	___supervising others	___self-respect
tion	___stability and pre-	___excitement
___meaningful work	dictability	___freedom
___new learning	___physical activity	___integrity
___being sure of myself	___family connections	___the gratitude of
___achievement	and time	others
___friendship	___economic security	___personal growth
___leadership	___efficiency	___cooperation
___helping others	___thought-provoking	___responsibility
___loyalty	work	___privacy
___financial gain	___improving society	___creativity
___ethical practice	___honesty	___cooperation
___security	___independence	___sophistication
___change and variety	___knowledge acquisi-	
	tion	

Step 2: Reduce the List

Now that you have identified 15 values, imagine that you can only have five. Which 10 would you give up? What is left? Now try to reduce your list to only three.

Step 3: Analysis

Take a look at the three values remaining on your list. Consider the three following questions and write a paragraph relating to each to capture your reaction. What do you think these values say about you as a person? What do they say about you as a therapist? What picture develops regarding the kind of work you value most?

2. Letter to a Learning Partner

This exercise is best applied by students during their fieldwork experiences or by novice therapists. You will need a partner to work with on this exercise. It will be important to choose someone with whom you feel comfortable and trust so that you can have open dialogue and share your ideas without fear or criticism. This dialogue will span an expanded period of time, so choose your learning partner accordingly.

Over the course of a few weeks, you are going to write several letters to your partner. Ideally, your partner will do the same, thus using you to help him or her reflect on practice. The letters are written about your reactions to significant experiences during your clinical encounters. They will be snapshots of your reactions at one point in time. At each interval, you will describe what occurred, how you felt about the experience, and what conclusions you drew at that moment. At the end of the overall time period, you will be guided through your own analysis of the letters as a group.

Before starting, you and your partner must decide whether both of you are participating and how long you are contracting to work together. It may be for 1 week, the course of the clinical practice, or for all practice at preset intervals. You may also set some rules for feedback that will be followed, perhaps regarding the need for a balance for frankness and respectfulness of communication style.

Definition of significant experience: a significant experience is one that has emotional impact. You may recognize that it has occurred because it makes you stop and think, makes your heart skip a beat, rocks your sense of rightness or confidence, makes you blush, or makes your stomach lurch. Whatever your reaction, it makes you take notice. Such experiences are often called *aha moments*.

Step 1: Writing the Letters

Right after a significant experience occurs, jot it down. If possible, immediately take 10 minutes to write your letter. If you can't do it right away, use your jotting to jog your memory at some later time. Do not take any longer than that, as the exercise is intended to capture your immediate reaction. Try to choose different types of experiences to write about over the course of the contracted time.

Format for each Letter:
Dear _____,
Write a few sentences to describe briefly what happened using action language.
To get started, complete the following sentences:
"I felt..."
"I have felt this way before when..."
"From this experience, I think the following is true..."

Complete your letter quickly, put it away, and repeat the exercise at least five or six times over the course of a few weeks or longer, depending on the terms of your contract with your partner. Once you have collected at least five letters, the analysis can occur.

Step 2: Analysis

This step is done in conjunction with your learning partner. Each partner does this step separately, then compares each other's reaction to the same set of letters. Read over one person's collection of letters. Is there anything that jumps out at you? Are there insights there that surprise you? What do you think these tell you about the person? What values seem to emerge? In the experiences described, were any values shaken or reinforced? What does it seem that he or she believes about effective practice? Were there any particular situations in which the person seemed to feel most comfortable? Are there types of clients where he or she seemed to feel most skilled? Do you see any patterns? How do your conclusions hold up with the passage of time?

As the writer, consider these questions: How do you react to the feedback from your partner? Do you agree/disagree with his or her conclusions? Were there things that you felt were true at the time that you now question? What has happened in the interim to change your thinking? Have your perspectives broadened or narrowed? When do you feel most vulnerable? When do you feel most capable? What does this tell you about factors that shape your practice as a therapist (Hunt, 1988; Rochon, 1994; Wilkins, Pollock, Rochon & Law, 2001)?

3. Video Case Analysis

This is an exercise that can work very well with a group of learners or therapists and uses videotaping and analysis of the tape.

Step 1: Planning

One therapist will be the subject of the video. That therapist chooses a client and seeks his or her consent to participate in a videotaped case analysis. Prior to taping the client, the therapist answers some questions on the videotape, either alone or through an interview conducted by a colleague.

On the tape, briefly describe the client who will be taped, then answer these questions:
- What are the client's current goals for therapy?
- What are the immediate goals for this session?
- What assumptions have you made about the client?
- What theoretical approach or practice model are you using?
- What hypotheses do you have about the client?
- What do you expect to happen in the therapy session and why?

Step 2: Videotape the therapy session with the client

Step 3: Analysis

Show the tape to your colleagues and discuss what happened, how it relates to your prior assumptions, and how it differed from your expectations and why. Draw some conclusions and summarize your insights. How will this impact your next encounter with this client? What general insights can you take to all of your client encounters (Salvatori, Baptiste & Ward, 2000; Slater & Cohn, 1991)?

REFERENCES

Argyris, C., & Schön, D. (1974). *Theory in practice: Increasing professional effectiveness*. San Francisco, CA: Jossey-Bass.

Beckstand, J. (1986). The notion of a practice theory and the relationship of scientific and ethical knowledge to practice. In L. H. Nicoll (Ed.), *Perspectives on nursing theory* (pp. 481-488). Boston, MA: Little Brown.

Benner, P. (1984). *From novice to expert: Excellence and power in clinical nursing practice*. Menlo Park, CA: Addison-Wesley Publishing.

Brockett, M., Geddes, L., Salvatori, P., & Westmorland, M. (1997). Moral development or moral decline? A discussion education for the health care professions. *Medical Teacher, 19*, 301-309.

Bundy, A. (1997). The test of playfulness. In L. D. Parham & L. S. Fazio (Eds.), *Play and occupational therapy for children* (pp. 58-60). St. Louis, MO: Mosby.

Canadian Association of Occupational Therapists. (2001). *CAOT code of ethics*. Ottawa, Ontario: Author.

Case-Smith, J., & Bryan, T. (1999). The effects of occupational therapy with sensory integration emphasis on preschool age children with autism. *Am J Occup Ther, 53*, 489-497.

Cole, B., Finch, E., Gowland, C., Mayo, N., & Basmajian, J. (1994). *Physical rehabilitation outcome measures*. Toronto, Ontario: CPA.

Cooper, B., & Saarinen-Rahikka, H. (1986). Interrelationships of theory, clinical models, and research. *Physiotherapy Canada, 38*, 97-100.

Coster, W., Deeney, T., Haltwanger, J., & Haley, S. (1998). *School function assessment*. San Antonio, TX: The Psychological Corporation.

Dreyfus, H. L., & Dreyfus, S. E. (1986). *Mind over machine: The power of human intuition and expertise in the era of the computer*. New York, NY: Free Press.

Geddes, L., Finch, E., & Larin, H. (1999). *Ethical issues relevant to physical therapy*. Hamilton, Ontario: McMaster University.

Greenspan, S., & Wieder, S. (1997). Developmental patterns and outcomes in infants and children with disorders in relating and communicating: A chart review of 200 cases of children with autism spectrum disorders. *J Learn Disabil, 26*, 342-347.

Greenspan, S., & Wieder, S. (1998). *The child with special needs*. Reading, MA: Perseus Books.

Hirschhorn, L. (1991). Organizing feelings towards authority: A case study of reflection-in-action. In D. Schön (Ed.), *The reflective turn: Case studies in and on educational practice* (pp. 111-125). New York, NY: Teachers College Press.

Hunt, D. E. (1977). Theory to practice as persons in relation. *Ontario Psychologist, 9*, 52-62.

Hunt, D. E. (1980). How to be your own best theorist. *Theory Into Practice, 19*, 287-293.

Hunt, D. E. (1988). *Beginning with ourselves: In practice, theory, and human affairs*. Cambridge, MA: Brookline Books.

King, G., McDougall, J., Palisano, R., Gritzan, J., & Tucker, M. (1999). Goal attainment scaling: Its use in evaluating pediatric therapy programs. *Physical and Occupational Therapy in Pediatrics, 19*, 31-52.

Larin, H. (1995). Motor learning: Theories and strategies for the practitioner. In S. K. Campbell (Ed.), *Physical therapy for children* (pp. 167-182). Philadelphia, PA: Saunders.

Law, M. (1998). *Client-centered occupational therapy*. Thorofare, NJ: SLACK Incorporated.

Law, M., Baptiste, S., Carswell, A., McColl, M., Polatajko, H., & Pollock, N. (1998). *Canadian Occupational Performance Measure* (3rd ed.). Ottawa, Ontario: CAOT Publications.

Law, M., King, G., Russell, D., Stewart, D., Hurley, P., & Bosch, E. (2000). *All about outcomes: An educational program to help you understand, evaluate, and choose adult outcome measures* [CD ROM]. Thorofare, NJ: SLACK Incorporated.

Law, M., Missiuna, C., Pollock, N., & Stewart, D. (2001). Foundations for occupational therapy practice with children. In J. Case-Smith (Ed.), *Occupational therapy for children* (4th ed., pp. 39-70). St. Louis, MO: Mosby.

Levoy, G. (1997). *Callings: Finding and following an authentic life.* New York, NY: Three Rivers Press.

Linderman, T., & Stewart, D. (1999). Sensory-integrative-based occupational therapy and functional outcomes in young children with pervasive developmental disorders: A single subject study. *Am J Occup Ther, 53,* 145-152.

Lovaas, O. I., & Smith, T. (1988). Intensive behavioural treatment with young autistic children. In B. B. Lahey & A. E. Kazdin (Eds.), *Advances in child psychology* (pp. 285-324). New York, NY: Plenum Press.

Mattingly, C. (1991a). What is clinical reasoning? *Am J Occup Ther, 45,* 975-986.

Mattingly, C. (1991b). The narrative nature of clinical reasoning. *Am J Occup Ther, 45,* 998-1005.

Mattingly, C., & Fleming, M. H. (1994). *Clinical reasoning: Forms of inquiry in therapeutic practice.* Philadelphia, PA: F. A. Davis Company.

McColl, M. A., Law, M., & Stewart, D. (1993). *Theoretical basis of occupational therapy: An annotated bibliography of applied theory in the professional literature.* Thorofare, NJ: SLACK Incorporated.

Pfeiffer, J. W., & Jones, J. (1973). *A handbook of structured experiences for human relations training.* La Jolla, CA: University Associates.

Rochon, S. (1994). *Theory from practice: A reflective curriculum for occupational therapists.* Unpublished master's thesis, McMaster University, Hamilton, Ontario, Canada.

Rochon, S., & Worth, B. (1995). *Working together to meet the challenges of change: A transition workshop for middle managers.* Hamilton, Ontario: Chedoke-McMaster Hospitals.

Rogers, J. (1983). Clinical reasoning: The ethics, science, and art. *Am J Occup Ther, 37,* 601-616.

Sackett, D., & Haynes, B. (2000). *Evidence-based medicine: How to practice and teach EBM* (2nd ed.). New York, NY: Churchill-Livingstone.

Salvatori, P., Baptiste, S., & Ward, M. (2000). Development of a tool to measure clinical competence in occupational therapy: A pilot study. *Can J Occup Ther, 67,* 51-60.

Schön, D. A. (1983). *The reflective practitioner: How professionals think in action.* New York, NY: Basic Books.

Schön, D. A. (1987). *Educating the reflective practitioner.* New York, NY: Basic Books.

Senge, P. M., Roberts, C., Ross, R., Smith, B., & Kleiner, A. (1994). *The fifth discipline fieldbook.* New York, NY: Doubleday.

Slater, D. Y., & Cohn, E. S. (1991). Staff development through analysis of practice. *Am J Occup Ther, 45,* 1038-1044.

Shepard, K. F., Hack, L. M., Gwyer, J., & Jensen, G. M. (1999). Describing expert practice in physical therapy. *Qualitative Health Research, 9,* 746-758.

Smith, T., Groen, A., & Wynn, J. (2000). Randomized trial of intensive early intervention for children with pervasive developmental disorder. *Am J Ment Retard, 105,* 269-285.

Somerville, M. (2000). *The ethical canary: Science, society, and the human spirit.* New York, NY: Viking Press.

Stratford, P., Binkley, J., & Riddle, D. (1996). Health status measures: strategies and analytic methods for assessing change scores. *Phys Ther, 76,* 1109-1123.

Tammivaara, J., & Shepard, K. (1990). Theory: The guide to clinical practice and research. *Phys Ther, 70,* 578-582.

Tryssenaar, J. (1995). Interactive journals: An educational strategy to promote reflection. *Am J Occup Ther, 49,* 695-702.

Tugwell, P., Bombardier, C., Buchanan, W., Goldsmith, C., Grace, E., & Hanna, B. (1987). The MAC-TAR Patient Preference Disability Questionnaire: An individualized functional priority approach for assessing improvements in physical disability clinical trials in rheumatoid arthritis. *J Rheumatol, 14*, 446-451.

Van Deusen, J., & Brunt, D. (1997). *Assessment in occupational therapy and physical therapy.* Philadelphia, PA: Saunders.

Vargas, S., & Camilli, G. (1999). A meta-analysis of research on sensory integration treatment. *Am J Occup Ther, 53*, 189-198.

Wilkins, S., Pollock, N., Rochon, S., & Law, M. (2001). Implementing client-centred practice: Why is it so difficult to do? *Can J Occup Ther, 68*(2), 70-79.

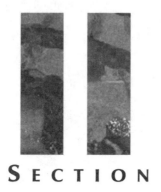

SECTION

Finding the Evidence

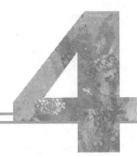

Outcomes in Evidence-Based Practice

Angela Mandich, PhD; Linda Miller, PhD; and Mary Law, PhD, OT(C)

LEARNING OBJECTIVES

After reading this chapter, the student/practitioner will be able to:
- Identify and understand the conceptual models of disablement and how outcome measurement relates to these models.
- Distinguish between descriptive and inferential statistics and understand how these apply to outcome measurements.
- Define and understand evidence-based terminology.

Therapists wonder:

What constitutes evidence?

What outcomes are really necessary to demonstrate the effectiveness of my intervention?

I know it works, but how do I demonstrate that to the health care stakeholders?

How do I develop my knowledge and become more evidence-based?

What is a p value anyway?

Consumers ask:

How do I know the intervention is going to work?

How is this therapy going to help me put on my shirt?

Administrators ask:

Where is the evidence?

Is the intervention cost effective?

Why should we pay for this service?

INTRODUCTION

Challenging questions such as these are being posed by health care stakeholders and reflect the current trend toward evidence-based practice. Indeed, evidence-based practice is gaining momentum, and practitioners are required to demonstrate the effectiveness of their interventions in a climate in which health care funding is decreasing and consumer demands for best practice are increasing (Evidence-Based Medicine Working Group, 1992). Leaders in the area of evidence-based practice acknowledge this trend, stating, "Clients expect interventions that are effective, provided by competent therapists, and appropriate to their needs and preferences" (Law & Baum, 1998, p. 132).

Building a practice that is evidence-based will not only demonstrate the value of the service to health care stakeholders, but it will also serve to strengthen the scientific foundation of the discipline (Kitson, 1999). The purpose of this chapter is to provide the practitioner with the skills to understand and work toward evidence-based outcomes. Establishing evidence based on observable outcomes requires practitioners to become familiar with the current models of rehabilitation and the common forms of clinical evidence that stem from these models to understand the concepts and terminology of measurement, and to understand how data are displayed and analyzed.

MEASURING HEALTH OUTCOMES:
BEYOND THE ABSENCE OF DISEASE

Practitioners are committed to providing interventions that are based on scientific evidence and best practice (Altman, 1994; Estabrooks, 1999; Sackett, Straus, Richardson, Rosenberg, & Haynes, 2000; Taylor, 2000). In order to do this, it is imperative that practitioners keep abreast of current research, incorporate this research into practice, and measure outcomes that are valid and well-documented (Wood, 1998). As such, clinical research must be based on outcomes that are specific, measurable, attainable, and time-limited. Such a process enlists the use of quantitative and qualitative methods, depending on the desired outcomes (Bax, 1997). Each method contributes to our knowledge and understanding of clinical practice. Various methods offer a unique perspective, and the specific methods applied are often dictated by the clinical questions being asked (Berg, 1998). Outcomes of health care form the basis for decision making and service provision and are pivotal to evidence-based practice (Taylor, 2000).

Historically, the biomedical model has significantly influenced outcome measurement. The biomedical model defines health as the absence of disease. Subsequently, outcome measurement has been focused at the impairment or physical level of the individual. Current models of rehabilitation reflect a paradigm shift and define health in broader terms, acknowledging that social, psychological, and environmental factors contribute to health and quality of life (World Health Organization, 1980, 2001). The World Health Organization (WHO) (2001) and the National Center for Medical Rehabilitation Research (NCMRR) (1993) have developed models based on this broader definition of health. Such models can be used to conceptualize outcomes and assist practitioners in defining outcome measures of importance.

Conceptualizing the Outcomes: Models of Rehabilitation

Medical models have emphasized outcomes that focus on treating and curing the disease or disorder. Subsequently, little emphasis has been placed on how the disease affects the individual at a functional or societal level. Such models have been based on traditional concepts of motor control, emphasize neuromaturational and reflex-hierarchical factors, and target intervention at the level of the physical impairments. However, contemporary models of motor learning and control acknowledge the contributions of physical, social, and psychological well-being and emphasize the importance of the interaction between the individual and the environment (Shumway-Cook & Woollacott, 2000). Contemporary practice models have emphasized other variables beyond the physical components of the individual and acknowledge that the interaction of the person and environment is integral to performance (Law et al., 1996). Contemporary models acknowledge that significant sources of evidence include measures of client satisfaction, functional capacity, and measures of quality of life. Such models are congruent with contemporary theoretical notions that acknowledge that behavior arises from a dynamic interaction of the multiple subsystems and that environmental factors play a key role (Kamm, Thelen, & Jensen, 1990; Thelen, 1979).

Current models are comprehensive and facilitate clear descriptions of outcome measures at various levels and enable clarification of roles between professionals. Models proposed by WHO and NCMRR reflect contemporary views of health and provide frameworks for conceptualizing outcome measures. These models assist practitioners in defining clear intervention outcomes.

International Classification of Functioning Model

Recently, WHO (2001) has introduced a new classification system for understanding functioning and disability: the International Classification of Functioning (ICF) Model. This new model provides a framework for structuring outcome measures and elucidating the relationships among impairments, activities, and participation, nested in the environmental context.

Emphasis is placed on the influence of the environmental factors and their impact, both positive and negative, on the three dimensions of body functions and structures, activities, and participation. Practitioners can target outcomes at the level of the various dimensions and establish relevant goals and observable outcome measures on which these are based. Outcomes may be targeted at the body function (impairment) level (e.g., improving range of motion, reducing tone), but the practitioner may also want to establish outcome measures that demonstrate to the client or the insurer payer how targeting at that level will directly or indirectly influence performance at the activity or at the participation level (i.e., increasing range of motion may provide the foundational skills for the individual to put on his or her sweater). Table 4-1 provides definitions of and illustrates some examples of desired outcomes at each level. The following clinical case example illustrates the use of this model to define outcomes.

Case Example 1

Steven, an 8-year-old boy, was referred to therapy with a diagnosis of developmental coordination disorder. Steven was having difficulties with handwriting, tying his shoes, playing ball, and riding his bike. The therapist completed an initial assessment and determined that Steven's coordination difficulties were due to poor balance, problems with bilateral coordination, manual dexterity, and the persistence of abnormal reflex patterns.

Goal of Therapy
1. Improved righting reactions
2. Improved strength and range of motion
3. Improved balance and coordination
4. Improved manual dexterity

Theoretical Approach
A neurodevelopmental approach emphasizes the development of normal patterns of movement. Development of these foundational skills will improve functional performance.

Examples of Intervention Strategies
Handling and facilitation techniques, use of a therapy ball.

Targeted Outcome
Impairment level:
- Increased range of motion
- Reduced abnormal tone
- Increased patterns of normal movement

Activity level:
- Improved writing skills
- Ability to ride his bike

Participation level:
- Inclusion in playground games activities with peers

This case example illustrates how the theoretical orientation of the practitioner can influence the type of intervention provided and, thus, the outcomes that are measured. Although in this case the intervention was targeted at the level of body function, it is important that the therapist explain the relationship between these underlying abilities and task performance. Did the improvement in body function lead to observable, improved performance at the activity or participation level? Can Steven ride a bike and print neatly?

To establish clear outcomes, practitioners can use the ICF model. By clarifying and describing clear and observable outcomes, practitioners will be able to evaluate interventions, influence practice, and provide clinical evidence for the effectiveness of the intervention.

Table 4-1

ICIDH-2: DEFINITIONS OF THE DIMENSIONS CONSIDERED IN THE CONTEXT OF A HEALTH CONDITION

Dimensions	Definitions	Limitations	Examples of Target Outcomes
Body functions and structure	Body functions are the physiological functions of the body systems.; body structures are the anatomical parts of the body, such as organs, limbs, and their components	Impairments are problems in body function or structure such as a significant deviation or loss	• Range of motion • Balance • Memory • Sensory abilities • Problem solving • Visual tracking • Praxis • Midline crossing • Bilateral integration
Activity	The performance of a task or action by an individual	Activity limitations are difficulties an individual may have in the performance of activities	• Walking • Self-care activities • Play skills • Leisure activities • Work-related tasks • Vocational training
Participation	An individual's involvement in life situations in relation to health conditions; body functions; and structures, activities, and contextual factors	Participation restrictions are problems an individual may have in the manner or extent of involvement in life situations	• Attitudes • Beliefs • Accessible issues • Advocacy • Lived experiences • Fulfillment of social roles

Contextual factors: An integral component of the classification, consisting of environmental factors and personal factors

The National Center for Medical Rehabilitation Research Model

NCMRR (1993) also provides a framework for considering outcome measures. They developed a model that is an amalgam of the work of Nagi (1965) and the ICF model previously described. The NCMRR provides a five-component classification system that is a useful framework for intervention and outcome measurement. Table 4-2 provides a definition of the classification system and examples of outcomes at each level.

Similar to the ICIDH-2 model, the NCMRR model highlights the interactions of the individual and the environmental context. The individual is placed at the centre of the rehabilitation process. This model emphasizes outcome measures at the physical, functional, and societal level. This system can also be used as a framework for defining outcomes, as illustrated in the following case example.

Case Example 2

Susan, a 48-year-old woman with rheumatoid arthritis, was referred to therapy for intervention. Susan's symptoms included swollen, painful joints; decreased range of motion; and decreased functional ability in tasks of daily living.

Goal of Therapy
Reduce or prevent dysfunction.

Theoretical Approach
Biomechanical approach.

Examples of Intervention Strategies
- Range of motion exercises
- Adapting/grading of activities
- Therapeutic activities (e.g., stacking cones)
- Heat modalities

Targeted Outcome
  Impairment level:
  - Decrease joint swelling and pain
  - Increase range of motion
  Functional limitations:
  - Improve hand grasps
  Disability:
  - Improve self-care
  Societal:
  - Inclusion in social roles (e.g., Monday night bridge club)

Summary

Increasingly, the health care system is demanding that practitioners be accountable and provide empirical evidence for their interventions. This challenges practitioners to choose outcome measures that are specific, observable, measurable, and congruent with the needs

	Table 4-2		
THE NATIONAL CENTER FOR MEDICAL REHABILITATION MODEL CLASSIFICATION SYSTEM			
Domain	*Definitions*	*Level of Impact*	*Examples of Target Outcomes*
Pathophysiology	Interruption of normal physiological and developmental processes or structures	Cell and tissue level	Central nervous system sites
Impairment	Loss and/or abnormality of cognitive, emotional, physiological, or anatomical structures or function; includes secondary impairments not attributable to the initial pathophysiology	Organ and organ systems	• Range of motion • Balance • Strength • Tone • Memory • Sensory abilities • Problem solving • Visual tracking • Praxis • Midline crossing • Bilateral integration
Functional limitations	Restriction or lack of ability to perform an action in the manner or range consistent with the purpose of an organ or organ system	Function of organ and organ systems	• Sitting • Reaching • Organizational skills • Attention to task • Shifting pegs
Disability	Inability or limitation in performing tasks and roles to levels expected within physical and social contexts	Individual	• Self-care activities • Play skills • Written communication • Leisure activities • Work-related tasks

Domain	Definitions	Level of Impact	Examples of Target Outcomes
			• Vocational training • Mobility
Societal limitations	Restrictions, attributable to social policy or barriers (structural or attitudinal) that limit fulfillment of roles or deny access to service opportunities that are associated with full participation in society	Society	• Attitudes • Beliefs • Accessible issues • Advocacy • Lived experiences • Fulfillment of social roles

Table 4-2 (Continued)

and wants of the client. As such, the ICF and NCMRR models provide a means for defining clear clinical outcomes. It is also imperative that the health care practitioner have a clear understanding of the scientific terminology regarding evidence-based practice and the use of statistics to measure desired outcomes.

MEASURING CLINICAL OUTCOMES

Measurement is essential to clinical research and practice as an integral part of the process of inquiry and evaluation. Measurement allows us to identify individuals most suited for particular types of interventions, to identify areas of focus for intervention, to adapt interventions to the specific needs and desires of clients, and to determine the outcome of the interventions. Advances in scientific inquiry and clinical practice are affected directly by advances in measurement; as measurements become more precise and more appropriate, research can become more sensitive and intervention can become more relevant and more individualized to the needs of specific clients.

Measurement refers to the assignment of numbers to aspects of events or behaviours according to a rule or convention. Typically, measurement is indirect (i.e., measurement is inferred from an indicator of the actual construct of interest). Consider, for example, the measurement of temperature. The indicator of temperature is the mercury in a thermometer, which expands and contracts in response to changes in temperature. Although the appropriateness of some indicators is well-established and justifiable, the appropriateness of others is less apparent. When considering the measurement of satisfaction with clinical treatment, determination of the appropriate indicators is challenging. The appropriateness of an indicator is determined, in large part, by the correspondence between the definition of the construct and the operationalization of the measurement.

When and How to Measure Clinical Outcomes

To evaluate clinical outcomes, data must be collected at various times throughout the process of intervention. This can be done either by taking measurements prior to and following intervention and evaluating the pre- to post-change or by taking a series of measurements prior to intervention, throughout the intervention process, and again following intervention. By taking measures before, during, and after intervention, the clinician is able to evaluate not only the change from pre to post, but also the rate or pattern of change. By focusing only on pre-post changes, important factors such as the point at which change is initiated and the point at which change reaches a maximum are not apparent. If change peaks and plateaus at about two-thirds of the way through the treatment process, it may be an indication that the length of treatment could be shortened. There are advantages to taking multiple measurements throughout the treatment process; however, this can be a costly and time-consuming procedure, which may not be feasible. Therefore, clinicians must consider a variety of measurement techniques that could be used to provide optimal opportunities to evaluate outcomes. For example, clinicians could obtain the following measurements, such as:

1. Pre and post scores using standardized assessments
2. Pre and post scores using specifically designed and developed rating scales or criteria lists
3. Scores using standardized assessments, specially designed rating scales, or criteria lists applied pre-, post-, and throughout the treatment process
4. Scores based on observations made pre-, post-, and throughout the treatment process

To maximize evaluation of outcome, combinations of these approaches can be used. For example, a clinician could use pre- and poststandardized assessment in combination with observational measurements made pre-, post-, and throughout treatment.

There are advantages to the use of each of these approaches. Standardized assessments allow for comparison across clients and allow the comparison of individuals to a normative group. When standardized assessments are used in a regular and consistent manner in a clinician's practice, data can be cumulated across clients, thereby facilitating the evaluation of outcomes for particular client groups. In addition, standardized assessments enable the performance of individuals to be compared to the results obtained in published, controlled studies.

Alternatively, customized ongoing measurements, whether rating scales, criteria lists, or observational measurements, allow for the identification of key points in the treatment process and provide the clinician and client with more immediate feedback on which to base changes in the treatment process. In addition, customized rating scales, criteria lists, and observational measures focus on the specific targets or goals of treatment. Because these targets are personal and unique to the client, they may not be readily captured by standardized assessments. By focusing on the target of the treatment, these measures facilitate the identification of personal and environmental factors that may have been otherwise overlooked.

Rating Scales

Rating scales can be developed relatively easily to quantify a wide variety of behaviours. They typically involve identifying the numerical value along a continuum that best reflects the rater's evaluation, judgment, or perception of a particular phenomenon or aspect of behaviour. Because rating scales can be used to measure an extremely wide variety of behaviours, there is great potential for their use in clinical measurement. For example, a rating scale can be used to quantify the quality of performance of a specific target motor task,

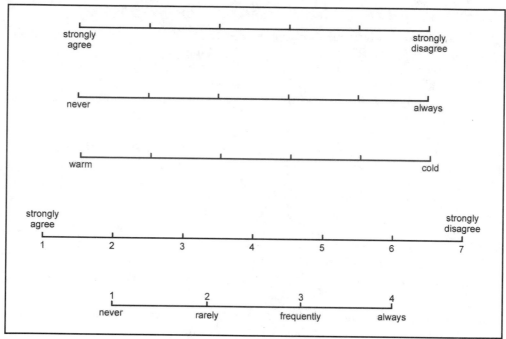

Figure 4-1. Examples of various graphic rating scales.

allowing the clinician to evaluate the change in performance quality prior to, during, and following treatment. A variety of scaling formats can be used. The common formats are based on graphic rating scales and visual analog scales.

Graphic Rating Scales

In these scales, a straight line is divided into equally spaced sections with numbers marking the notches along the line. The end points of the line are labeled with descriptors. The points in between may or may not be labeled with descriptors and/or numbers. See Figure 4-1 for examples of various graphic rating scales.

Visual Analog Scales

These scales comprise a straight line with a descriptive label, or anchor, at each end of the line but no divisions along the line. Rating scales provide a subjective quantification of the underlying construct and are reflective of the perceptual process of the rater. As such, their reliability across multiple raters may be questionable. In situations in which rating scales are to be used by multiple raters, it is necessary to establish inter-rater reliability.

Criteria List

A criteria list is comprised of a list of objectively observable behaviours or events, which are scored in terms of their presence or absence. Each behaviour on the list is recorded as either observed or not observed. To be clinically relevant, the behaviours included in the list should include the components, or sequential steps, necessitated in the performance of the target treatment goal. In many cases, listing the behaviours on the basis of a dynamic performance analysis (Polatajko, Mandich, & Martini, 2000) of the target task or goal is beneficial. Systematic observation of the performance of the target task, noting the presence or absence of each of the components or steps involved in the task, facilitates identification of performance barriers and allows for modification of intervention to address these barriers. As such, criteria lists may be particularly useful for the evaluation of specific multistep functional outcomes.

Observational Measures

Observational measures are obtained by measuring observable aspects of the individual's behaviour. The target behaviour to be observed must be defined with enough clarity to allow consistency and agreement in measurement across observers. A variety of characteristics of a target behaviour can be observed and measured; however, the appropriateness of each characteristic is dependent upon the nature of the target behaviour; certain characteristics are more appropriate than others for particular types of behaviours. The observable characteristics include the *frequency*, *duration*, and *latency* of a behaviour.

Frequency

When observing frequency, the observer counts each occurrence of the target behaviour within a fixed time interval. Frequency counts can be obtained during multiple intervention sessions and used to establish a pattern of performance change across intervention. Frequency counts are only appropriate for target behaviours that are discrete and relatively short in duration. In addition, they should be used only when the target behaviour could reasonably be expected to occur multiple times during each observation interval. An example of a target behaviour for which frequency could appropriately be observed is scoring baskets in basketball.

Duration

Duration is a measure of how long a behaviour lasts once it has been initiated, measuring the time from the onset of the behaviour to the completion of the behaviour. Durational measures can be obtained across treatment sessions, providing an illustration of any changes in duration across treatment. Duration is an appropriate measure only in cases in which the target behaviour has a clearly definable onset and completion. It is not appropriate for behaviours that occur so quickly that they cannot be timed accurately. If a client's treatment goal is to reduce dressing time, duration would be an appropriate measure.

Latency

Latency measures provide an indication of how long it takes for a target behaviour to be initiated once it has been prompted. Latency is measured as the time between the prompt, or cue, and the onset of the target behaviour. It is appropriate only when the goal of treatment is to achieve a consistent and quick initiation of the target behaviour in response to a particular prompt. This may be the case, for example, if the goal of an individual's treatment is to consistently and reliably turn off the teakettle when the whistle on the kettle begins to sound.

As with all forms of measurement, it is essential to consider the reliability and validity of the obtained measures. This necessitates demonstrating that the measures are accurate and replicable and that they address relevant and appropriate aspects of a client's intervention. For a more thorough discussion of reliability and validity, refer to Chapter 6.

Reporting and Interpreting Measurement with Statistics

In research, statistics are used for two purposes: to provide a description of the research sample and to perform statistical tests of significance on research hypotheses. *Descriptive statistics*, which are used to describe the research sample, make it possible to compare the samples used in different studies, thereby providing some insight into possible variations in the outcomes across studies. In addition, descriptive statistics enable practitioners to evaluate the relevance of a particular study by allowing comparison of the study sample to the practitioner's client, or client group, of interest. For example, a practitioner searching for research pertaining to the use of cognitive interventions for the treatment of motor skill deficits in children should refer to the descriptive statistics used to describe the sample in each relevant study, considering information such as the mean age of the children included in the study, the average level of motor performance of the children in the sample, the average performance of the study sample on the measures used to determine study eligibility, and the pattern of the sample on relevant demographic variables, such as gender. By comparing the descriptive statistics reported for a study sample with the client group of interest, the practitioner can determine the relevance and generalizability of the study to his or her own clinical practice. If the descriptive statistics indicate that the study sample was similar to the group of clients in which the practitioner is interested, then the study is of relevance and its finding could be considered as potentially generalizable to the practitioner's client, or client group.

Inferential statistics, which are used to perform tests of significance, allow the researcher to evaluate hypotheses. Inferential statistics provide an indication of the likelihood that the differences, changes, or relationships observed in a study are due to chance variations among the study participants. Typically, the larger the differences or changes, the smaller the likelihood that these differences or changes are due simply to chance variations. When differences cannot be attributed to chance, it is then assumed that they are due to a true treatment effect. For example, if the probability that the change from an average pretest score of 12 to an average post-test score of 20 is due to chance is less than 5/100, then it can be assumed that the pre to post change is due to a treatment effect. It is important to remember, however, that nonchance differences are not necessarily due to true treatment effects. Nonchance differences may be attributable to various confounds, such as maturation effects or testing effects. Therefore, it is imperative that the design of the study be evaluated carefully in order to determine the extent to which potential confounding factors were controlled. Nonchance differences can only be attributed to treatment under conditions in which all potential confounding factors have been adequately controlled.

Descriptive statistics are used to provide a description, or picture, of the research sample. Typically, descriptive statistics include *frequency distributions*, *measures of central tendency*, and *measures of variability*. These statistics illustrate the characteristics of the sample and allow comparison of the research sample to other clinical or research samples.

A *frequency distribution* is an arrangement of the scores of all participants in a research sample on a particular variable that provides a display of the range of scores and the frequency of occurrence of each score. A frequency distribution is created by arranging all the scores occurring within the sample from lowest to highest and by counting the number of times each score occurs within the sample. Frequency distributions can be created for quantitative variables and for categorical variables. As an illustration of a frequency distribution for a quantitative variable, consider the standardized Vineland Adaptive Behavior Composite Standardized Scores for a group of 26 children who participated in a study evaluating a treatment for developmental coordination disorder.

The frequency distribution presented in Table 4-3 illustrates the spread of scores from a low of 66 to a high of 115 and indicates the frequency of occurrence of scores observed for the 26 children in the study. Frequencies are typically presented as actual counts for each observed value and as percentages of the total sample who obtained each particular score. For example, two children obtained a score of 66, and these two children represent 7.7% of the total sample of 26 children. In addition, a cumulative frequency may be included to illustrate

Table 4-3			
FREQUENCY DISTRIBUTION OF VINELAND ADAPTIVE BEHAVIOR COMPOSITE STANDARDIZED SCORES			
Score	*Frequency*	*Valid Percent*	*Cumulative Percent*
66	2	7.7	7.7
68	1	3.8	11.5
69	1	3.8	15.4
70	1	3.8	19.4
76	1	3.8	23.1
78	1	3.8	26.9
80	2	7.7	34.6
82	1	3.8	38.5
83	1	3.8	42.3
84	2	7.7	50.0
85	1	3.8	53.8
88	1	3.8	57.7
92	1	3.8	61.5
96	2	7.7	69.2
98	2	7.7	76.9
100	2	7.7	84.6
102	1	3.8	88.5
104	1	3.8	92.3
113	1	3.8	96.2
115	1	3.8	100.0

the percentage of the sample who scored above and below particular values. For example, the cumulative frequency indicates that 50% of the study sample obtained a score of 84 or lower.

Frequency distributions can also be used to describe categorical variables. For example, a study of children referred for therapy services for problems associated with a learning disability included 43 children from kindergarten through grade 8. A frequency distribution for grade provides an illustration of the dispersion of study participants across the grades.

The frequency distribution presented in Table 4-4 indicates that the frequency of referrals across grades is not evenly distributed. Referrals occurred more frequently for students in grades 3 and 4 than in the lower or higher grades. In fact, 48.8% (27.9% + 20.9%) of the referrals were made for children in grades 3 and 4.

Frequency distributions can be presented in the form of tables, as illustrated in Tables 4-3 and 4-4, or in the form of graphs. For example, a *histogram* can be used to graphically illustrate the distribution of referrals across grades. The histogram presented in Figure 4-2 illustrates that grade 3 is the grade in which the most referrals were made, followed by grades 4 and 5, respectively.

Distributions of scores on variables are often assumed to take the form of a bell-shaped curve. The bell-shaped curve is referred to as a *normal distribution*. The normal distribution

| Table 4-4 |
| FREQUENCY DISTRIBUTION OF STUDENTS ACROSS GRADES |

Score	Frequency	Valid Percent	Cumulative Percent
K	1	2.3	2.3
1	2	4.7	7.0
2	5	11.6	18.6
3	12	27.9	46.5
4	9	20.9	67.4
5	7	16.3	83.7
6	4	9.3	93.0
7	2	4.7	97.7
8	1	2.3	100.0

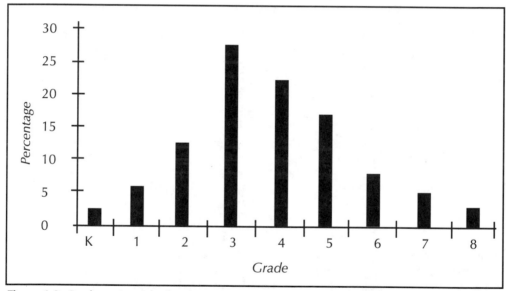

Figure 4-2. Grade at time of referral.

has several properties that make it valuable in the interpretation of descriptive statistics. Before discussing these properties, however, measures of central tendency and measures of variability should be addressed.

There are three *measures of central tendency*: the *mean*, the *median*, and the *mode*. The mean corresponds to the arithmetic average of a set of scores and is the most frequently used measure of central tendency. Because the mean is the arithmetic average of a set of scores, it will be affected by the inclusion of extreme scores or outliers, particularly when the total number of scores used to compute the mean is relatively small. The median is the score that divides the set of scores in half, with 50% of the sample scores falling below the median value and 50% falling above. The median value represents the 50th percentile of the set of scores. The median value is less affected than the mean by the presence of extreme scores.

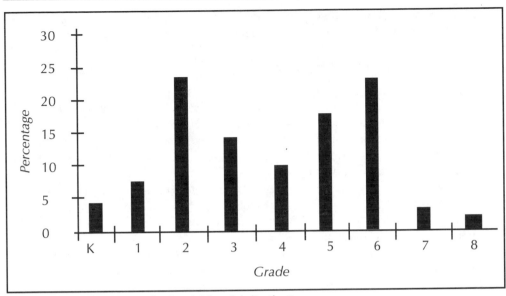

Figure 4-3. Grade at time of referral: bimodal distribution.

In samples that include outliers, the median value may provide a more valid measure of central tendency. The mode corresponds to the score that occurs most frequently within the sample. It is possible to have samples that are *bimodal* or even *multimodal*, indicating that two or more values are tied for being the most frequently occurring scores. The histogram presented in Figure 4-3 illustrates a sample bimodal distribution for referral across grades. As can be seen in this figure, grades 2 and 6 are tied for the modal, or most frequently occurring response, yielding an overall distribution that has two peaks. In samples that conform to the normal distribution, the mean, median, and mode all represent the same value.

The typical measures of variability are the *range*, the *variance*, and the *standard deviation*. The range is the difference, or spread, between the lowest and highest scores in the sample. Although easy to calculate, the range can be a misleading indication of variability. Because it represents the difference between the highest and lowest values obtained in the sample, it is easily affected by the presence of extreme scores, or outliers. As such, the range should not be presented as the only measure of variability. The variance provides an indication of the spread of scores around the sample mean. It is calculated as the sum of the squared differences of each observed sample value from the sample mean, weighted, or averaged, for the size of the sample. The standard deviation (SD), which is the most widely used measure of variability, is calculated by taking the square root of the variance. By evaluating how many SDs an individual's score falls from the sample mean, it is possible to interpret an individual's relative standing in the sample. For example, if the sample mean on a particular measure is 50 and the SD is 5, then an individual with a score of 40 is 2 SDs below the mean, whereas an individual with a score of 55 is 1 SD above the mean. The SD can be used to convert the observed scores for a sample to *standard scores* or *z-scores*. Z-scores, calculated by subtracting the mean from any particular score and dividing by the SD, allow each individual's score to be expressed as a deviation from the mean. Z-scores have specific properties that make them easily interpretable; z-scores for any given sample will have a mean of zero and an SD of 1.0. Therefore, an individual with a z-score of +1.5 is 1.5 SDs above the sample mean, whereas an individual with a z-score of -2.0 is 2 SDs below the mean. When interpreted in the context of the normal distribution, z-scores are particularly useful.

Standardization of Measures

The concepts of central tendency and variability are also applied in the calculation of the various types of scores reported in standardized assessments. Standardization of test scores assists in the interpretation of an individual's test performance. The interpretation of any individual's test score involves comparing that particular individual's performance to the performance of a larger, normative group. Ideally, the normative group comprises a large sample of individuals representative of the population to which the individual is assumed to belong. The descriptive statistics of the normative group provide the standard against which the individual is compared, allowing the individual's score to be interpreted in terms of its standing relative to the normative group. This method of interpreting test scores is referred to as *norm-referenced interpretation*.

Various types of scores can be derived using a norm-referenced approach. The most common types of scores include *percentiles*, *z-scores*, and *deviation scores*. Percentiles are ranks ranging from 1 to 99. They are based on the frequency distribution computed on the normative sample and indicate the percentage of individuals in the normative group who fall below a particular rank. For example, a percentile score of 75 indicates that 75% of the normative sample scored below this point. Z-scores, as discussed earlier, indicate the relative standing of a particular individual relative to the mean of the normative group. A z-score of -2 indicates performance that falls 2 SDs below the mean for the normative group. Deviation scores are a transformation of z-scores in which the mean and SD for the normative group have been converted to fixed values, typically values of 100 for the mean and 15 for the SD. Therefore, a score of 85 would indicate performance that is 1 SD below the mean of the normative group.

Normal Distribution

As stated previously, the normal distribution is depicted as a bell-shaped curve. Its properties make it an important model in the interpretation of scores. In the normal distribution, the mean, median, and mode represent the same value, and scores cluster around the mean, with an equal number of scores falling above and below the mean. Figure 4-4 provides an illustration of the normal distribution, highlighting the properties of the curve.

One of the most important properties of the normal distribution is the predictable nature of the spread of scores around the mean, which is represented as the peak in the curve. As can be seen, an equal number of individuals are expected to fall above and below the mean. Specifically, 68.26% of the population is expected to fall within the range from 1 SD below the mean to 1 SD above the mean, and 95.44% are expected to fall in the range from 2 SDs below the mean to 2 SDs above the mean. Only 2.27% of the population is expected to fall above 2 SDs above the mean and 2 SDs below the mean.

The various types of scores derived from standardized tests also adhere to the properties of the normal distribution. The 50th percentile, or median, falls at the mean of the distribution, and percentile scores are most densely distributed close to the mean. Moving away from the mean, either above or below, the distance between percentiles becomes larger. This lack of consistency in the spacing between percentile ranks may lead to difficulty in interpreting

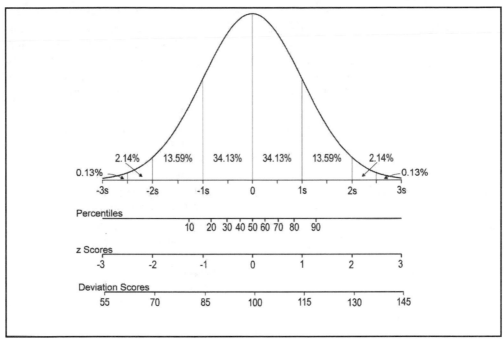

Figure 4-4. An example of normal distribution.

percentile scores. For example, the difference between percentile scores of 5 and 10 is not the same as the difference between percentile scores of 45 and 50. This leads to difficulty in the interpretation of differences or changes in percentile scores. Z-scores and deviation scores are not susceptible to this difficulty in interpreting differences or changes. The scalar units of z-scores and deviation scores are constant across the base of the normal distribution, allowing a meaningful interpretation of differences among scores. As can be seen in Figure 4-4, a z-score of 0 and a deviation score of 100 both correspond to the value of the population mean, and the distance between SD units is constant across both the z-score scale and the deviation score scale. For example, a z-score of -1 corresponds to a deviation score of 85, with both scores indicating performance that is 1 SD below the population mean.

The application of inferential statistics assumes that the scores obtained from research samples are normally distributed, adhering approximately to the properties of the normal curve. Violation of this assumption, particularly when extreme, can lead to erroneous and misleading interpretation of the results of the statistical analyses. Samples in which the distribution of scores above and below the mean is not equivalent are referred to as having *skewed distributions*.

INFERENTIAL STATISTICS AND CAUSATION

Inferential statistics are used for hypothesis testing. When interpreting inferential statistics, it is imperative to note that the statistic tests the *null hypothesis*, or the hypothesis of no difference or effect. A statistically significant statistic leads to rejection of the null hypothesis; however, rejection of the null hypothesis does not logically lead to confirmation of the researcher's hypothesis. Support for a research hypothesis comes only in part from a statistically significant statistic. To advocate support for a particular hypothesis, a researcher is required to present a reasoned and logical context for the expected finding and a sound, rational argument that rules out all potential competing explanations or hypotheses. For example, a researcher must be able to demonstrate that confounds, such as maturation, have been adequately controlled and do not affect the interpretation of the study's findings. Therefore, it is essential that a researcher provide the logical reasoning and rationale that enables a significant finding to be interpreted as support for the researcher's hypothesis.

There are a wide variety of inferential statistics used in research. Some statistics, such as correlation coefficients, are used to test the degree of association or relatedness among variables. Other statistics, such as the *t statistic* and the *F ratio*, are used to test differences across groups or treatment conditions. One common misinterpretation of such statistics relates to their application in the inference of causation. Often, the goal of research is to infer causation. For example, researchers may be interested in demonstrating that a particular approach to treating children with developmental coordination disorder leads to, or causes, improvements in functional performance.

Making sound causal inference, however, is not as straightforward as stating that a statistic is significant. Several conditions must be met in order to allow causal inference. These conditions relate to *measurement*, *covariation*, *temporal ordering*, and *theory*. The researcher must be able to reliably and validly measure both the outcome and the causal agent in order to argue for causation. This means that the treatment parameters must be well-defined and controlled and the outcome measured with accuracy and confidence. Covariation refers to the co-occurrence of the causal agent and the outcome. However, co-occurrence alone of two events does not substantiate causation. Consider the co-occurrence of thunder and lightening; although thunder and lightening co-occur, one does not cause the other. In fact, they co-occur because both are caused by a common underlying agent, an electrical discharge. The condition of temporal ordering requires that, in addition to co-occurrence, the causal agent precede the outcome. Theory provides the logical basis for causal interpretation. Notions of cause and effect are relevant and meaningful only when placed in the context of a theory explaining their relationship and when paired with a rationale eliminating competing explanations. Any causal inference is weakened by criticisms of its underlying theory. In order to draw sound causal inference from any research, all four of these conditions must be addressed and satisfied.

SUMMARY

Implementing an evidenced-based practice is a challenging task for practitioners. Current health care trends are demanding that practice be scientific and evidenced-based. In order to do this, practitioners can use the rehabilitation models to establish the outcome they will measure. As well, a clear understanding of measurement and statistics will provide a means of conceptualizing and measuring outcomes. The purpose of this chapter was to provide practitioners such knowledge and skill. A practice that is based on evidence will provide answers to the questions posed at the beginning of this chapter, ensure practice is evidence-based, and that consumers and stakeholders will understand the value of therapy in light of current health care.

Take-Home Messages

- Demand for evidence-based practice is increasing through the need to demonstrate value of the service to stakeholders and to strengthen the scientific foundation of a discipline.
- Evidence is established based on observable outcome and demands that practitioners understand terminology, data measurement and analysis, current research, and outcome measures that are valid and well-documented.
- Clinical research is based on outcomes that are specific, measurable, attainable, and time-limited.

Models of Rehabilitation
- Contemporary models are moving away from traditional concepts to acknowledging the contribution of physical, social, and psychological well-being and emphasizing the importance of the interaction between the individual and the environment.
- International Classification of Functioning and Disability (ICF) Model: Emphasis on environmental factors and their impact on body functions and structures; activities and participation.
- National Center for Medical Rehabilitation Research (NCMRR) Model: Individual is placed at centre of pathophysiology impairment, functional limitations, disability, and societal factors.

Measuring Clinical Outcomes
- Essential aspect of inquiry and evaluation of research.
- When to measure: Beneficial to take multiple measurements, more cost-effective to take only pre- and postmeasurements.
- How to measure: Use combinations of rating scales, criteria list, and observational measures (frequency, duration, and latency) to maximize evaluation.
- Essential to consider reliability and validity of the measures obtained.

Descriptive Statistics
- Describe research sample to compare cross-studies and evaluate relevance.
- Frequency distribution: Display of range of scores and frequency of occurrence of each score; histogram; normal distribution.
- Measure of central tendency: Mean; median; mode.
- Measure of variability: Range, variance, and standard deviation.
- Standardization of measures to compare individual's performance to larger normative group.
- Normal distribution gives a predictable nature to spread of scores and z-scores.

Inferential Statistics and Causation
- A statistically significant test leads to the rejection of a null hypothesis (hypothesis of no difference).
- Making sound causal inference demands that the researcher provide rational evidence that all other factors have been ruled out, as well as considering conditions related to measurement, covariation, temporal ordering, and theory.

WEB LINKS

International Classification of Functioning
www3.who.int/icf/icftemplate.cfm
This web site provides information about the new International Classification of Functioning developed by the World Health Organization.

Cochrane Library
www.updateusa.com/Cochrane/default.htm
This web site provides information and links to the Cochrane Library.

LEARNING AND EXPLORATION ACTIVITIES

The purpose of this chapter is to help establish some of the necessary skills of working toward evidence-based outcomes.
1. Following the models of Case Examples 1 and 2, construct a table describing the goal(s) of therapy, theoretical approach, examples of intervention strategies, and targeted outcomes. At what level(s) of the International Classification of Functioning is the intervention targeted?
2. Using a rehabilitation journal or assessment textbook, find an example of rating scales, criteria list, and observational measure. What are the key differences between these methods of measurement? Name a clinical example in which each type would be the preferable measurement method.

ADDITIONAL RESOURCES

Dubouloz, C. J., Egan, M., Vallerand, J., & von Zuweck, C. (1999). Occupational therapists' perception of evidence-based practice. *Am J Occup Ther, 53*, 445-453.

Hawkins, R. P., Mathews, J. R., & Hanndan, L. (1998). *Measuring behavioral health outcomes: A practical guide*. New York, NY: Kluwer Academic/Plenum Publishers.

Hayes, R., & McGrath, J. (1998). Evidence-based practice: The Cochrane Collaboration and occupational therapy. *Can J Occup Ther, 65*, 168-169.

Koes, B. W. (1997). Now is the time for evidence-based physiotherapy. *Physiother Res Int, 2*, iv-v.

Lincoln, Y. S., & Guba, E. G. (1985). *Naturalistic inquiry*. Beverly Hills, CA: Sage.

McDowell, I., & Newell, C. (1996). *Measuring health: A guide to rating scales and questionnaires*. New York, NY: Oxford University Press.

Portney, L. G., & Watkins, M. P. (2000). *Foundations of clinical research application to practice*. Upper Saddle River, NJ: Prentice-Hall, Inc.

REFERENCES

Altman, D. G. (1994). The scandal of poor medical research. *British Medical Journal, 308*, 283-284.

Bax, M. (1997). Quantitative or qualitative research? *Dev Med Child Neurol, 39*, 501.

Berg, B. (1998). *Qualitative research methods for the social sciences* (3rd ed.). Needham Heights, MA: Allyn & Bacon.

Estabrooks, C. A. (1999). Will evidence-based nursing practice make practice perfect? *Canadian Journal of Nursing Research, 30*, 273-294.

Evidence-Based Medicine Working Group. (1992). Evidence-based medicine: A new approach to teaching the practice of medicine. *Journal of the American Medical Association, 268*, 2420-2425.

Kamm, J., Thelen, E., & Jensen, J. (1990). A dynamical systems approach to motor development. *Phys Ther, 70*, 763-775.

Kitson, A. (1999). Research utilization: Current issues, questions, and debates. *Canadian Journal of Nursing, 31*, 13-22.

Law, M., & Baum, C. (1998). Evidence-based practice. *Can J Occup Ther, 65*, 131-135.

Law, M., Cooper, B., Strong, S., Stewart, D., Rigby, P., & Letts, L. (1996). The person-environment-occupation model: A transactive approach to occupational performance. *Can J Occup Ther, 63*, 9-23.

Nagi, S. (1965). Some conceptual issues in disability and rehabilitation. In M. Susman (Ed.), *Sociology and rehabilitation* (pp. 100-113). Washington, D.C.: American Sociological Association.

National Center for Medical Rehabilitation Research. (1993). *Research Plan for the National Center for Medical Rehabilitation Research* (NIH Publication No. 93-3509). Washington, D.C.: U.S. Government Printing Office.

Polatajko, H. J., Mandich, A., & Martini, R. (2000). Dynamic performance analysis: A framework for understanding occupational performance. *Am J Occup Ther, 54*, 65-72.

Sackett, D. L., Straus, S., Richardson, S., Rosenberg, W., & Haynes, R. B. (2000). *Evidence-based medicine: How to practice and teach EBM* (2nd ed.). London, England: Churchill Livingstone.

Shumway-Cook, A., & Woollacott, H. (2000). *Motor control theory and practical applications.* Baltimore, MD: Lippincott, Williams & Wilkins.

Taylor, M. C. (2000). *Evidence-based practice for occupational therapists.* Malden, MA: Blackwell Sciences.

Thelen, E. (1979). Rhythmical stereotypes in normal human infants. *Animal Behaviour, 27*, 699-715.

Wood, W. (1998). It is jump time for occupational therapy. *Am J Occup Ther, 52*, 403-411.

World Health Organization. (1980). *International Classification of Impairments, Disabilities, and Handicaps.* Geneva: Author.

World Health Organization. (2001). *ICIDH-2: International Classification of Functioning & Disability* (Pre-final draft). Geneva: Author.

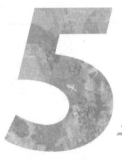

Searching for
the Evidence

Jennie Q. Lou, MD, MSc, OTR

LEARNING OBJECTIVES

After reading this chapter, the student/practitioner will be able to:
- Explain the origins of clinical research questions and identify the constituent elements of successful questions.
- Identify and understand the distinctions between various sources of evidence.
- Critically evaluate the value of web-based sources.
- Outline the key components and effective methods for a literature search.
- Describe different electronic databases and their various search mechanisms.

INTRODUCTION

In our daily clinical practice, questions about the best care for our clients arise frequently. As the current best evidence on a given topic changes at an unpredictable rate, even the most experienced clinician cannot assume that he or she knows the answer without looking into the most current literature. It has become increasingly obvious that the pace of development of new evidence from research is too quick for standard textbooks to be of dependable help. When questions do arise, it is unlikely that they will be answered by these textbooks accurately and quickly. Fortunately, the advent of better research, better information resources, and better information technology makes it possible for us to respond to these challenges by learning some basic literature search skills and acquiring access to key evidence resources in the hospital, clinic, or at home. Figure 5-1 illustrates the steps in acquiring the evidence. This chapter will describe some of the skills and resources for answering questions of relevance to the care of clients in occupational and physical therapy practice.

ASKING QUESTIONS

The first step in any evidence search is to formulate a "well-built question." This entails identifying a question that is important to the client's well-being, is interesting to you, and is likely to be encountered on a regular basis in your practice. For practical purposes, it is sometimes more efficient if you seek consultants for questions that you seldom address in your practice.

From Where Does the Question Come?

The most common origin of questions is *professional practice*. For example, you may have a client who has a specific visual perceptual problem, and you do not know how to treat him or her and none of your colleagues are able to help. You could develop a clinical question based on the clinical situation, such as, "What is the most appropriate intervention for your client?" Another common source for questions is *professional trends*. For example, in occupational therapy there is currently a push to understand the occupation in its entirety. From this knowledge, you could form a question to develop a better understanding of a particular occupation. You may also develop a question from the *existing published research*. For example, when you read an article in an occupational or physical therapy journal, it might raise more questions for you. You could use one of these questions to further explore the literature. Alternatively, you might read a body of literature, realize that there are gaps in knowledge, and develop a question to explore one of these gaps in more detail. *Existing theory* is another area in which questions can be developed. For example, you might use a particular model and frame of reference in practice and want to critically compare it to what happens in the real world. You could develop a question based on your own curiosity. For the purpose of this book, the following discussion will focus on questions that are generated from clinical practice.

How to Ask an Answerable Question

One of the benefits of careful and thoughtful question forming is that the search for evidence is easy. The well-built question makes it relatively straightforward to elicit and combine the appropriate terms needed in the query language. To be answerable, the question must

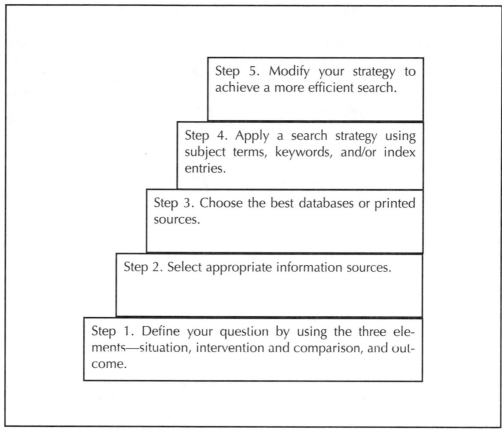

Figure 5-1. Steps for acquiring evidence.

be specified clearly so that it includes (a) a specific client group or population; (b) the assessment, treatment, or other clinical issues that you are addressing; and (c) the outcome in which you are interested. Basically, when you develop the question, you are preparing a checklist or writing a search strategy for your literature search. Essentially, you must convert a gap in your knowledge into a precise question so that you can then seek the best answer for it.

In practice, well-built clinical questions usually contain three elements: *client/population, intervention* or *exposure*, and *outcome*; a fourth element, *comparison*, is also often used in question building. This is a way of breaking down a clinical problem into a question that can be answered, which we sometimes refer to as the anatomy of a question. If you use this "anatomy," it will help you be more clear about the question you are trying to answer and facilitate the identification of elements that are of particular importance. Clinical Scenario 1 is used as an example to take you through the question-developing process.

Clinical Scenario 1

Recently, several elderly clients have suffered falls, leading to hospital admissions and surgery. The clients, although frail, had all been self-caring before their falls. Getting them back to their own homes was a slow process, and two have ended up in long-term institutional care. You wonder if there is a benefit in initiating a preventative program to stop elderly clients from having falls in the home.

Situation

The situation is what you are starting with. In evidence-based practice (EBP), this involves defining the client as a member of a population in terms of age, sex, ethnic group, etc. It could also deal with any aspect of health care delivery (e.g., how do we manage our appointments system?). Remember—when you search for articles, they should be explicit in describing the criteria used to select their subjects. In real life, however, you would be very lucky to find a study that selected exactly the sort of situation with which you are dealing. Therefore, you always need to keep this question in mind, "Are the subjects in this study so different from my situation that I cannot generalize its findings?"

Situation
Elderly clients who live independently at home

Intervention

Intervention is what you wish to do. This covers anything you plan to do. It also involves what you may be doing at present and wish to assess. This would be therapy (e.g., choice of specific intervention), assessments (e.g., which specific assessment tool is more appropriate to use for your client with visual perceptual deficits?), preventative measures (e.g., counseling on lifestyle or risk factors), and/or management (e.g., when to refer your client to a cardiac rehabilitation program). You may wish to look for a comparison of two or more interventions, particularly to see if some innovative intervention is "better" than your current practice or beats the accepted "gold standard."

Situation	*Intervention*
Elderly clients who live independently at home	Fall prevention program *Comparison*: Education on safety at home upon discharge from acute care

Outcomes

Outcomes are what you wish to achieve. This may also include possible adverse effects you wish to avoid or minimize. Prevention of disability; recovery of function; and saving of time, money, and effort are some examples of outcomes. Remember—outcomes should define something that is important to the client, such as recovery of function (e.g., combing hair), rather than merely of interest to the health care providers, such as controlling upper extremity spasticity.

Situation	*Intervention*	*Outcome*
Elderly clients who live independently at home	Fall prevention program *Comparison*: Education on safety at home upon discharge from acute care	Decreased incidence of falls at home

Once you have listed the three (or four) elements of the question, the question should be fairly straightforward.

Situation	Intervention	Outcome
Elderly clients who live independently at home	Fall prevention program *Comparison*: Education on safety at home upon discharge from acute care	Decreased incidence of falls at home

Question 1: Does a fall prevention program decrease the incidence of falls in elderly clients who live independently at home?

Or, if you use a comparison,

Question 2: Is a fall prevention program more effective than education upon discharge from an acute care center in decreasing the incidence of falls in elderly clients who live independently at home?

When preparing your question, remember that your question should be *relevant*, *direct* and *clear*, and *focused*. A common mistake that clinicians often make is to seek answers to questions about a whole process of care rather than a focused clinical issue. Searching for an answer to a generic question is often very difficult. Rather than asking, "What is the impact of a rehabilitation program on the quality of life for my clients?," the clinician may ask, "Can the incidence of falls be decreased by a fall prevention program?" Another example would be instead of asking, "Is occupational therapy effective in treating children with autism?," the clinician may ask, "Does sensory integration improve social behavior in children with autism?"

IDENTIFYING DIFFERENT SOURCES OF EVIDENCE

Now that you have developed the answerable question, you will need to identify different sources for your search. During your search, you must be able to organize and evaluate the information that you have obtained. A big part of this process is distinguishing relevant from irrelevant information and deciding which one contains the best and most credible information. For people who are relatively unfamiliar with scholarly publications, this can be a daunting task. The purpose of the following section is to help you identify different types of scholarly publications and to give you some guidelines for determining their relative merit.

Types of Scholarly Publications

There are three basic types of scholarly publications: books, nonpeer-reviewed journals and professional magazines, and peer-reviewed journals.

Books

Books can be focused on a single specialty topic (e.g., activity analysis) or they can be more general in nature (e.g., aging in Canadian society). Books may or may not be peer-reviewed. The credibility of books may be judged by the credentials of the author(s); the reputation of the publisher; the reputation of the author of the preface; the reviews of the book from other reputable sources; the targeted audience (general public versus specific professionals); and the quality, currency, and extent of the citations.

Nonpeer-Reviewed Journals and Professional Magazines

In nonpeer-reviewed publications, an author submits a paper and it may or may not be reviewed by the editor and/or the editorial staff of the publication. While many nonpeer-reviewed publications are of high quality, it is unwise to depend solely on these sources for the evidence in which you require an answer to your clinical question. Nonpeer-reviewed publications tend to have a faster turnover of papers (i.e., they get into print faster); therefore, they can be useful for learning about current trends and controversies in your field of interest. Remember that nonpeer-reviewed publications can be biased toward a targeted audience.

Peer-Reviewed Journals

Generally speaking, the articles published in peer-reviewed journals are considered more accurate and relevant. They are usually of a higher quality than those in nonpeer-reviewed publications. All of the articles, with the exception of editorials, have been scrutinized by experts in the field for accuracy of content, quality of research, and relevance to the field. There are five types of articles in peer-reviewed journals: short reports, editorials, systematic reviews, book and technology reviews, and research articles.

Short Reports

Short reports tend to describe new or developing programs, projects, or treatment techniques. They are also used to present results of research pilot studies and preliminary results from ongoing research. These reports tend to provide the latest advances in a particular area.

Editorials

In many peer-reviewed journals, editorials are papers written by invited experts in the field. They tend to raise important issues for the field, offer perspectives on controversial subjects, suggest gaps in current knowledge, or propose visionary directions for the future. Because editorials are usually written by an expert in the field, they tend to be useful when developing a background or rationale for proposals.

Systematic Reviews

Generally speaking, systematic reviews are full-length articles that undergo full peer-review. They can be critical reviews of the literature or meta-analyses of existing research. A systematic review is an overview of primary research studies that reaches specific standards in terms of methodology. This type of review should be explicit in describing the reviewers located in the studies and which exclusion and inclusion criteria they used. A meta-analysis is a mathematical synthesis of the results of two or more primary studies that addressed the same research question and that used comparable methodologies. Systematic reviews usually provide broad background information and pre-appraised material for your question. It can be very efficient and effective to use systematic reviews to find an answer to your clinical question; however, you need to be aware of the limitations of systemic reviews (e.g., reviewer's bias, missing evidence). When there is any chance it may be available, clinicians should seek a high-quality systematic review rather than the primary studies addressing their clinical question.

Book and Technology Reviews

Book and technology reviews are usually invited critiques of new, available resources. Generally speaking, the authors have some degree of expertise in the field specific to the content of the reviewed resource. These reviews provide information on the newest resource materials in a particular area.

Research Articles

There are many types of research articles, and many topologies to describe them. Please refer to the other chapters in this book for details on the format of research articles and how to evaluate their quality. These articles provide information on the newest scientific findings and advances in a particular area.

ELECTRONIC BIBLIOGRAPHIC DATABASES AND THE WORLD WIDE WEB

It is very important to distinguish between electronic bibliographic database searches and general searches on the World Wide Web! Electronic bibliographic databases are compilations of published research, scholarly articles, books, government reports, newspaper articles, etc. There are different databases, and each database has a particular focus. For example, MEDLINE is a compilation of medically and biomedically related publications, CINAHL focuses on publications from the allied health profession, ERIC focuses on materials from the field of education, AgeLine focuses on publications relating to older adults and aging, and SUMSearch provides a source of easy-to-read broad discussions of topics from multiple disciplines. It is important to know what databases are available to you and on what topics they focus. The information can usually be obtained from your local librarian or by reviewing the HELP section of the database. Most electronic bibliographic databases are international in scope and, as a result, will provide you with publications that are written in English as well as other languages.

In comparison to an electronic bibliographic database, the World Wide Web is made up of interconnected documents that are available through the Internet. The Internet contains a vast amount of information on just about any subject under the sun. Searching the World Wide Web will not limit you to published articles. Although you may find an article published on the web, you will also find program descriptions; personal opinions; government documents; information on businesses, organizations, and agencies; etc.

There are many different types of information available on the web, but most web pages can be categorized into types such as news and current events, business and marketing, informational, advocacy, or personal. Table 5-1 provides the function and examples of different types of web sites. Remember—web browsers such as Netscape and Internet Explorer simply go to web addresses, and search engines simply look for terms that you designate. It is crucial for you to understand that they do not evaluate the accuracy or value of the web sites, and there are sites that contain inaccurate, out-of-date, or false information. You are responsible for determining the usefulness of the sites. Figure 5-2 presents three steps for evaluating web sites. Many of the same criteria for judging library databases and resources can also be used for web sites. Relevancy has been important in judging other kinds of information sources, and the relevance of web sites accessed is also important when searching the Internet. Besides relevancy, you also need to evaluate the web site for its authority, accuracy, objectivity, currency, and commercialism. Table 5-2 provides a checklist of the questions you can ask yourself at each step as you evaluate a web page.

Table 5-1

TYPES OF WEB SITES AND THEIR FUNCTIONS

Type of Sites	Function and Examples
News and current events	<ul><li>Provides extremely up-to-date information</li><li>Includes news centers, newspapers, and other periodicals</li><li>Examples include CNN and *The New York Times*</li></ul>
Business/marketing	<ul><li>Usually are published by companies or other commercial enterprises</li><li>Primary purpose is to promote the company or to sell products</li><li>Often include a mixture of information, entertainment, and propaganda</li><li>For U.S.-based sites, the URL or web address usually ends in .com</li><li>Examples include Microsoft (www.msn.com) and Amazon (www.amazon.com)</li></ul>
Informational	<ul><li>Often provided by government (.gov) or educational institutions (.edu)</li><li>Provide factual information on a particular topic</li><li>May include reference materials, research reports, databases, calendars of events, statistics, etc.</li><li>Examples include the National Institutes of Health (www.nih.gov), National Library of Medicine (www.nlm.nih.gov), American Occupational Therapy Association (www.aota.org), and Harvard University (www.harvard.edu)</li></ul>
Advocacy	<ul><li>Usually are published by an organization with the purpose of influencing public opinion</li><li>Examples include National Abortion and Reproductive Rights Action League (www.naral.org) and National Right to Life Committee (www.nrlc.org)</li></ul>
Personal	<ul><li>Published by individuals who may or may not be part of a larger group or organization</li><li>May include almost any type of information including biographical data, information on work, hobbies, etc.</li><li>For U.S.-based sites, the URL often includes a tilde (~)</li><li>Examples include individual or family home pages, individual faculty or students at a university, and member pages from an Internet service provider</li></ul>
Others	<ul><li>Such as entertainment</li></ul>

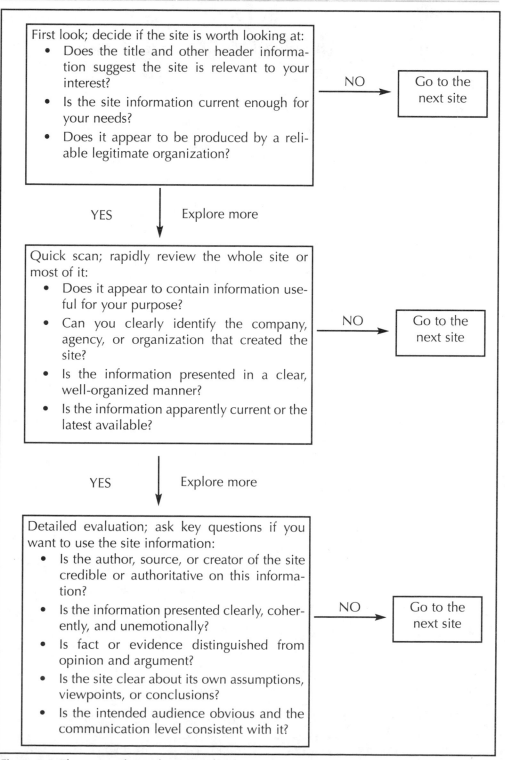

Figure 5-2. Three steps for evaluating web sites.

Table 5-2

CHECKLIST OF QUESTIONS YOU CAN ASK YOURSELF AT EACH STEP AS YOU EVALUATE A WEB PAGE

Authority

Check who is responsible for the page and their qualifications and associations:
- Who is sponsoring the site? Authors and creators of web sites should be clearly stated within the sites and means should be included for contacting them and/or the webmaster. Any commercial or organizational affiliations should also be included.
- What are the goals and/or values of the person/organization?
- What makes the author(s) an authority on this subject?
- Does the author(s) site his or her experience/credentials?
- Are they accredited or endorsed by a reputable organization?
- If the site contains articles, do they contain footnotes? If so, does material taken from other sources appear to be fully credited?

Accuracy

Try to determine the sources for the information at the site:
- Are the facts verifiable?
- Are the sources of information cited, and are individual articles signed and attributed?
- How is the information presented (fact, opinion, propaganda, etc.)? If presented as fact, is it accurate?

Objectivity

Look for the presence of bias and consider the impact of any stated affiliations on the possible attitudes toward the topic:
- What is the purpose of the site? Consider the six types of web pages listed in Table 5-1 and whether the page is trying to entertain, inform, persuade, or advertise.
- Is there a bias (cultural, political, religious, etc.)? If so, is the bias clearly stated?

Currency

Consider the age of the information:
- Is the date of the last revision posted anywhere on the page?
- What is the date of the last revision?
- How frequently is it updated?
- Is some of the information out of date?

Scope, Coverage, and Relevance

Consider the scope of the site and what it focuses on:
- What kind of information does it have and does this meet your needs? Who is the intended audience (general, specialized readership, scholars, etc.)?

Table 5-2 (Continued)

- What is the level of the material (basic, advanced, etc.)?
- What time period is covered?
- What geographical area is covered?
- Is this information a subset of a more comprehensive source?

Commercialism

- Is the presenter selling something—a product, a philosophy, him- or herself?
- Does the page have a corporate sponsor?
- Are there any hidden costs?
- Do you have to enter personal identification in order to proceed?

You probably have noticed that the greatest advantage of the Internet is that some portion of the world's literature has been made conveniently available to you. You also need to keep in mind that a major disadvantage is that quality control simply does not exist. There are two major problems with searching the World Wide Web as part of a literature review. The first problem is narrowing your search enough to find useful information, and the second problem is identifying those sites that are credible. Anyone can have a web site or a web page. Not all information that is taken off the World Wide Web can be considered credible, reliable, or even correct. As a result, it is important to have strict criteria for selecting sites to review. Generally speaking, it is a good idea to limit your searches initially to government, university, and professional association web sites.

CONDUCTING A LITERATURE SEARCH

Ways of Searching

Once you have identified your search sources, you should generate a search strategy that will allow you to first retrieve a list of references by providing a list of keywords and index terms, and then use a set of filters to help cut this down to a small list of relevant documents. Evidence searching is done primarily by using the following methods/tools:

- → Searching through electronic bibliographic databases (e.g., MEDLINE, CINAHL, Ovid, HEALTHSTAR, OTBibsys, OTDBASE, ERIC, SUMSearch, PsychLit, SocioFile, AgeLine, etc.)
- → Manually searching through specific journals (e.g., a journal that you know publishes material in your areas of interest, or newer journals that are not yet on the electronic system)
- → Retrieving articles listed in the reference lists of articles that you already have on your topic of interest
- → Searching the World Wide Web

Table 5-3

STRATEGIES FOR EFFECTIVELY SEARCHING ELECTRONIC DATABASES

Too many articles? You can increase *specificity* by narrowing or refining your search:
- Narrow your question
- Use more specific terms in a free text search
- Use a thesaurus/subject search rather than free text/keyword search
- Use more specific thesaurus/subject headings
- Select specific subheading with thesaurus/subject MeSH headings
- Add terms (using "and" to represent other aspects of the question
- Limit the article by language, human subject, publication types (e.g., randomized controlled trials, reviews, etc.), country, or year of publication

Too few articles? You can increase *sensitivity* by broadening your search
- Broaden your question
- Find more search terms from relevant records
- Try different combinations of terms
- Use truncation (* or $) or wildcard (?) in free text/keyword OR thesaurus/subject
- Add and combine terms of related meaning using "or"
- Use NEAR to retrieve items in the same sentence in either order
- Use a combination of free text/keyword and thesaurus/subject searches
- Use explosion feature of thesaurus searches
- Select ALL subheadings with thesaurus/subject MeSH terms
- Search further back in time
- Include all publication types

Don't forget to use the Help function from the database to increase your searching effectiveness!

A comprehensive literature search will probably use all of these methods/tools in an iterative fashion. There are two main goals to always keep in mind when you perform your searches:

1. Increase the likelihood of retrieving relevant items—sensitivity.
2. Increase the likelihood of excluding irrelevant items—specificity.

If you are doing a search and it yields an unmanageably large number of hits, you probably need to increase the specificity of your search. On the other hand, if you get too small a number of hits, you probably need to increase sensitivity. Table 5-3 provides some tips on increasing specificity and sensitivity in your searches. An effective evidence search is not an aimless and tangential hunt with the hopes of finding something that might be useful. *Systematic*, *explicit*, and *reproducible* are three key words!

An effective search is:

→ Guided by a specific answerable question or series of questions

→ Completed in a systematic and methodological manner

→ Documented explicitly

→ Reproducible on subsequent days or by other people

Different Databases

There are numerous electronic databases that can be used to conduct a search. All electronic databases are read-only, so you cannot damage the database by entering any "wrong" search terms. The worst thing that can happen is that you become stuck and have to exit and start again. Also, while searching the database, you cannot damage any material on your own files.

MEDLINE

What is MEDLINE?

MEDLINE is produced by the U.S. National Library of Medicine. It is widely recognized as the premier source for bibliographic and abstract coverage of a wide range of literature. MEDLINE encompasses information from Index Medicus, Index to Dental Literature, and International Nursing, as well as other sources of coverage in the areas of allied health. It also includes biological and physical sciences, humanities, and information science as they relate to medicine and health care, communication disorders, population biology, and reproductive biology. More than 9.5 million records from more than 3,900 journals are indexed, plus selected monographs of congresses and symposia (1976 to 1981). Abstracts are included for about 67% of the records. Although the majority of the records in MEDLINE relate to journal articles, the database also includes bibliographic details of systematic reviews, randomized controlled trials, and guidelines. Because the database is so large and comprehensive, MEDLINE is often a good place to start a search, as you will usually find something on your topic of interest.

MEDLINE can be found in most medical libraries, many of which have the full database dating back to 1966. There are also several free versions on the Internet. The U.S. National Library of Medicine provides free access to MEDLINE at www.ncbi.nlm.nih.gov/entrez/query. Because MEDLINE is sold to various software companies, you may find that the MEDLINE database looks different depending on where you use it, as different libraries choose to use different software. Generally speaking, the information is the same and it is only the interface (the way you interact with the database) that differs.

How to Search MEDLINE

There are basically two ways of searching databases like MEDLINE: free text or MeSH. Free text searching is a method of using words and phrases from the title, abstract, and keywords of references. There are some problems with this method of searching, as the database will search for exactly what you type in and does not automatically allow for different spelling, plurals, and so on. Free text searching is useful for broadening your search. A free text search means the database scans its records to see if any contain that exact term; therefore, if you enter the word "therapy," you will retrieve articles containing the word "therapy" but not "therapist" or "therapeutic."

Most databases have some form of indexing system. MEDLINE has one called *MeSH*, short for Medical Sub-Headings. This is a bit like the index at the back of a book. It also attempts to solve the problems of different authors using different terms to describe the same concept or process. MeSH contains almost 17,000 terms. Each of these terms, or keywords, represents a single concept appearing in the health care literature. As important new concepts appear, a new MeSH keyword is created. When a new reference is added to MEDLINE, indexers choose and add the appropriate MeSH keywords (usually 10 to 20) to represent the contents of the article. Although keyword searching using MeSH terms is a more precise way of searching, this may not always work for you. There may be times when there is no MeSH keyword for the subject you are searching. For example, until 1997, there was no MeSH keyword for "evidence-based medicine." In the absence of MeSH keywords, you need to search free text. In our Clinical Scenario 1, using MeSH keywords to search for fall prevention, you will not get any record because fall prevention is not a MeSH term. You will need to change your search to free text.

There is a very useful feature for obtaining comprehensive coverage of a subject area called *EXPLODE*. The keywords that make up MeSH are arranged into hierarchical structures called *trees*, starting with broad terms that branch off and become increasingly narrower with more specific terms. The tree structure of MeSH allows you to explode your search, which is less dangerous than it sounds! This means that you can simultaneously search for a keyword plus all its narrower terms. For example, if you wanted to run a comprehensive search for references relating to falls, you could explode the keyword *Fall* to pick up the following narrower terms:

→ Fall Prevention

→ Fall Risk Assessment Tool

→ Hendrich Fall Risk Model

→ Morse Fall Scale

→ Safety Behavior: Fall Prevention

How to Refine Your Search

Some MEDLINE searches are very precise and neat. You may have a very well-tuned MeSH term that retrieves a small and very well-focused set of about 20 articles through which you can scan. Most of the time, it is not that simple and you will have to plan and execute a search strategy. To show that MEDLINE can become overwhelming, do a search on Alzheimer's disease. Fill in this search as a major MeSH, and see how many articles come up! Now try something different. Before you run the search, scroll down to the line under the "retrieve" button. There are a number of "filters" here that allow you to restrict the document to those in English, those with an abstract, and those dealing with human subjects. To apply any of these, click on the small square box to the left so an X appears. Then click on the "retrieve" button. How many of the articles on Alzheimer's disease that are in English *and* contain an abstract *and* deal with human studies will now appear in a more specified way? You can also choose the years you wish to search. By default you get 1995 to 2000, but you can edit these boxes. Finally, you can restrict to certain age groups, journal sets, and article types. By adding the filters, you are narrowing your search to the ones that really fit into your question. You can also search for studies by asking for specific authors, journals, titles of articles, and words that you expect to be in the title and journals. Searching by specifics limits or narrows your search. This can be especially useful if you are not doing a comprehensive review. Other methods of narrowing the search include type of publication (e.g., review articles or randomized trials), age groups (e.g., infants, adolescents, adults), language, date, and whether the participants in the study are male or female. Table 5-3 (p. 82) provides some tips on how to narrow or broaden your search.

CINAHL

The Cumulative Index to Nursing & Allied Health (CINAHL) database, which is located at www.cinahl.com or through your university's subscription, provides authoritative coverage of the literature related to nursing and allied health. Virtually all English-language publications are indexed along with the publications of the American Nurses Association and the National League for Nursing. Primary journals are indexed from the following allied health fields: cardiopulmonary technology, occupational therapy, physical therapy, emergency service, physician assistant, health education, radiological technology, medical/laboratory, technology therapy, medical assistant, social service/health care, medical records, and surgical technology.

In total, more than 1,200 journals are regularly indexed. Online abstracts are available for more than 800 of these titles. There are more than 7,000 records with full text now included and 1,200 records with images. The database also provides access to health care books, nursing dissertations, selected conference proceedings, standards of professional practice, educational software, and audiovisual materials in nursing.

New documents are added to the CINAHL database every month. Using a limit to *Latest Update* will restrict your search to documents that were most recently added to the database. Approximately 70% of CINAHL headings also appear in MEDLINE. CINAHL supplements these headings with 2,000+ terms specifically designed for nursing and allied health. All explodable headings have been pre-exploded by Ovid.

When searching through CINAHL, you can use a limit to *Abstracts* to restrict retrieval to documents that include an author-written abstract. Abstracts have been included for a selected list of journals since 1986. Using a limit to *Full Text Available* restricts retrieval to records with links to Ovid's full text collections and to records containing CINAHL full text and PDF images.

Ovid

Ovid, which is located at http://gateway.ovid.com or through your university's subscription, is a database provider for a collection of health and medical subject databases. It often includes AARP (American Association of Retired Persons) AgeLine, AIDSLine (AIDS Information Online), BioethicsLine, CancerLit, CINAHL (Nursing & Allied Health), EBM Reviews—Cochrane Database of Systemic Reviews, EBM Reviews—Best Evidence, EMBASE Drugs & Pharmacology, Health and Psychosocial Instruments (HAPI), HealthSTAR, International Pharmaceutical Abstracts, Journals@Ovid Full Text, MEDLINE, and SPORTDiscus.

When using Ovid, you may select more than one database at a time. This would allow you to simultaneously search up to five databases. It is a very efficient way to search different databases at the same time. A step-by-step search for information for the question developed from Clinical Scenario 1 through Ovid is provided later in the chapter.

The Cochrane Library

The Cochrane Library, located at www.update-software.com/cochrane/cochrane-frame.html, is a primary source for clinical effectiveness information. It contains four databases and several other useful sources of information.

Cochrane Database of Systematic Reviews

The Cochrane database of systematic reviews (CDSR) contains the full text of systematic reviews undertaken by the Cochrane Collaboration, an international network of individuals and institutions committed to preparing, maintaining, and disseminating systematic reviews of the effects of health care. All reviews are updated as new studies are identified. CDSR contains completed reviews and protocols of reviews in progress.

Database of Abstracts of Reviews of Effectiveness

Database of Abstracts of Reviews of Effectiveness (DARE) is produced by the NHS Centre for Reviews and Dissemination (CRD) at York, UK. The database includes structured abstracts of reviews identified and appraised by the CRD. DARE is also available on the World Wide Web, along with the CRD's NHS Economic Evaluations Database (NHSEED), at http://nhscrd.york.ac.uk.

Cochrane Controlled Trials Register

The Cochrane Controlled Trials Register (CCTR) contains references on tens of thousands of controlled trials identified by the Cochrane Collaboration and includes reports published in conference proceedings and trials found by hand-searching journals. It is now the greatest single source of clinical trials, exceeding even the number of trials found on MEDLINE.

Cochrane Review Methodology Database

This database contains references to articles and books on carrying out systematic reviews.

Other Useful Sources Of Information

The Cochrane Library includes additional information relevant to clinical effectiveness and evidence-based practice:

→ About the Cochrane Collaboration

From here, you can access a range of information about the Cochrane Collaboration, including details of their Collaborative Review Groups, Methods Working Groups, networks, and centres.

→ Netting the Evidence at www.health.usyd.edu.au/ebm/netting.htm

This is a guide to sources of evidence on the Internet compiled by Andrew Booth, who is the director of information resources at the School of Health and Related Research (ScHARR) at the University of Sheffield, UK.

→ International Network of Agencies for Health Technology Assessment

These are abstracts of technology assessments undertaken by members of the International Network of Agencies for Health Technology Assessment (INAHTA). This information is also available from the NHSCRD web site.

OTDBASE

OTDBASE, located at www.otdbase.com, is an occupational therapy journal literature search service that is accessible to individuals or schools/institutions on an annual subscription basis. There are 17 international occupational therapy journals' abstracts in the database dating back to 1970.

OT Bibsys

OT Bibsys, located at http://otbibsys.aota.org/index.asp, is an occupational therapy bibliographic system hosted by the American Occupational Therapy Foundation and American Occupational Therapy Association. This bibliographic database covers literature in occupational therapy and related subject areas, such as rehabilitation, education, psychiatry or psychology, and health care delivery or administration. Author abstracts are included when available.

All About Outcomes CD-ROMs

Developed at McMaster University in Hamilton, Ontario, Canada, *All About Outcomes* are computerized, multimedia software programs for practitioners working in rehabilitation with pediatrics, adults, and seniors. These two CD-ROMs enable the user to select the most appropriate outcome measure to use for an individual, client, service, and/or program evaluation. These programs guide you through a protocol for making decisions about outcomes developed using a modified version of the International Classification of Impairment, Disability, and Handicap (ICIDH) framework. These software programs are linked to a database of critically appraised outcome measures. Users can select desired measurement criteria and psychometric information (e.g., reliability, validity, sensitivity) on appropriate outcome measures will be provided. The interactive nature of these programs allows you to choose measures for specific clinical situations and compare decision-making measures. There are over 139 outcome measures in pediatrics, over 200 outcome measures in adults, and over 1,000 literature sources are included in *All About Outcomes*. The CD-ROMs are available from SLACK Incorporated.

SUMSearch

SUMSearch, located at http://SUMSearch.uthscsa.edu, is a very user-friendly site that allows you to search for easy-to-read broad discussions of topics from multiple disciplines.

Combined Health Information Database

The Combined Health Information Database (CHID), located at www.chid.nih.gov, is a bibliographic database produced by health-related agencies of the U.S. federal government. This database provides titles, abstracts, education resources, health promotion, and program descriptions that are not indexed elsewhere.

Best Evidence

Best Evidence, which is located at http://hiru.mcmaster.ca/acpjc/acpod.htm, contains the full text of the *ACP Journal Club* and *Evidence-Based Medicine*, providing structured abstract and commentaries of selected articles.

EMB Review

Evidence-Based Medicine Reviews, from Ovid Technologies, provide content from two premier sources: the Cochrane Database of Systematic Reviews and Best Evidence, and it can be searched through Ovid.

Other Resources

Some other very useful resources are Evidence-Based Practice Internet Resources at www-hsl.mcmaster.ca/ebm; PEDro: The Physiotherapy Evidence Database at http://ptwww.cchs.usyd.edu.au/pedro; and the Canadian Centres for Health Evidence at www.cche.net.

STEP-BY-STEP SEARCHING FOR EVIDENCE

First, there are some questions you need to ask yourself at the beginning of your search:
- → How far back in the literature do I wish to go?
- → Which journals do I wish to review?
- → Do I want only those available in my local library?
- → What sort of articles will be useful: recent research, overviews, systematic reviews?

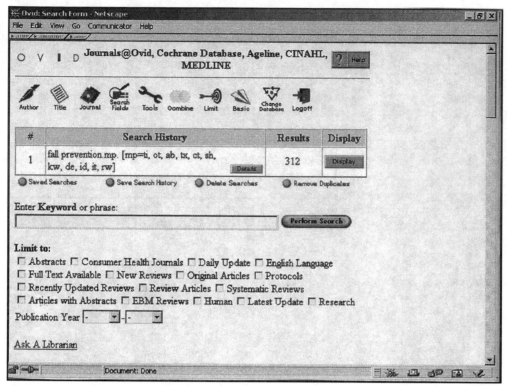

Figure 5-3. Step-by-step searching.

→ Are there any languages beyond my own that I would consider retrieving?

→ Do I only want articles that have an online abstract?

Through Ovid, five databases (Journals@Ovid, Cochrane Database, AgeLine, CINAHL, and MEDLINE) are chosen for the search on fall prevention. When using fall prevention as the keyword, we have 312 articles (Figure 5-3). This is obviously too many to retrieve or review.

Now, we will narrow our search on fall prevention to English language articles with abstracts, human only, and articles published within the last 10 years. We still have 289 articles on the search results (Figure 5-4).

Now we limit our search to older adults with the same filters (English-language articles with abstracts, and human only). This time we have 1599 articles (Figure 5-5).

Next, we combine the search for fall prevention and older adults. Now we have 14 articles (Figure 5-6). This is a manageable amount of evidence with which to start. We now have 14 articles that may answer the original clinical question. The next step is selecting the relevant articles from the search.

Selecting the Relevant Articles from the Literature Search

Once you have retrieved details of an article and obtained a copy, you will want to see whether it is suitable for answering your question. You will want to judge its validity, reliability, and, most important of all, applicability. Here are the questions you need to ask yourself:

→ Are the results of the article valid (validity)?

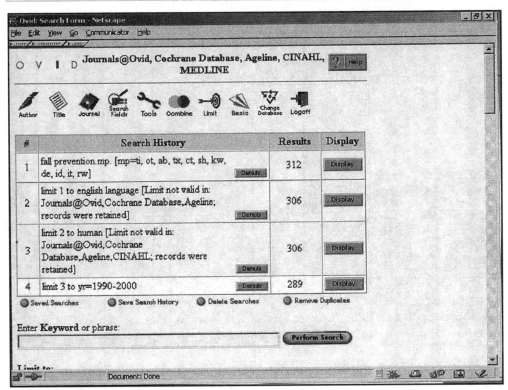

Figure 5-4. Step-by-step searching.

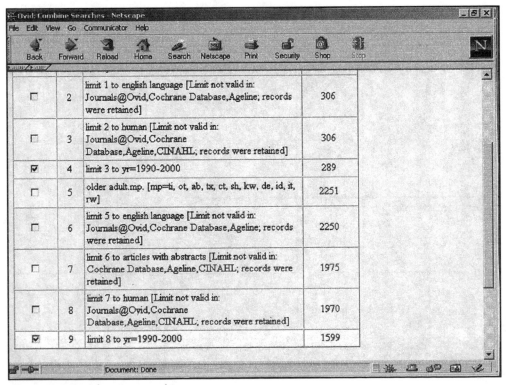

Figure 5-5. Step-by-step searching.

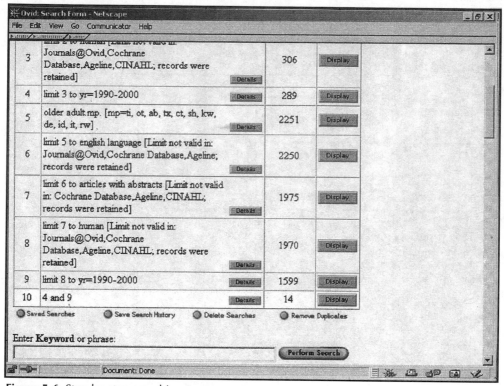

Figure 5-6. Step-by-step searching.

→ What are the results (reliability)?

→ Will the results help me in caring for my clients (applicability)?

You may find it helpful to use a checklist to assess whether it meets these three conditions.

Take-Home Messages

Asking Questions
- A well-built question originates from professional practice, professional trends, existing published research, or existing theory.
- Answerable questions should include the following:
  - specific client, group, or population
  - intervention (assessment, treatment, or other clinical issues)
  - outcome in which you are interested
  - comparison
- Good questions are relevant, direct, clear, and focused.

Different Sources of Evidence
- Books—Important to judge their credibility.
- Nonpeer-reviewed journals or professional magazines—Good for learning about current trends, but do not carry absolute credibility.
- Peer-reviewed journals—Considered more accurate and relevant; usually of a higher quality.

Electronic Bibliographic Databases and the World Wide Web
- Electronic bibliographic databases are compilations of published research, scholarly articles, books, etc., each with a different focus (e.g., MEDLINE, CINAHL, Ovid).
- World wide web—Researcher is responsible for judging relevancy, authority, accuracy, objectivity, currency, and commercialism. It is difficult to narrow search parameters to the degree needed to find relevant and useful information.

Conducting a Literature Search
- Adjust search parameters in accordance with sensitivity (to increase the likelihood of retrieving relevant items) and specificity (to increase the likelihood of excluding irrelevant items).
- All effective literature searches should be:
  - systematic
  - explicit
  - reproducible

LEARNING AND EXPLORATION ACTIVITIES

The purpose of this chapter is to outline some key aspects of undertaking research, including the methods for developing an appropriate question and the process for searching various resources. It is essential for students to recognize that the best way to become skilled at evidence searching is through practice. The format presented here serves as a good template for students to use in order to develop their future research questions.

1. Developing an Answerable Question

Your Clinical Scenario

Write down a clinical scenario that you have encountered in your own experience.

Step 1: Identify the situation you are in.

Situation

Step 2: List the intervention (and comparison, if any)—What do you wish to do?

Situation	Intervention

Step 3: Identify the outcome you wish to achieve.

Situation	Intervention	Outcome

Step 4: Now write out the question using the three (or four) key elements.

Situation	Intervention	Outcome

Question:

Congratulations! You should have an answerable question now. Remember—your question should always be *relevant*, *direct*, *clear*, and *focused*!

2. Searching for Evidence

List the key words in the question you developed from question 1. Developing an Answerable Question.

1. _____

2. _____

3. _____

Select databases (remember to first use the ones you can access easily). Narrow or broaden your search by using some of the strategies in Table 5-3 (p. 82). Set a screen criteria to pick out the articles that are relevant to your original question.

BIBLIOGRAPHY

Barber, G. (1995). Searching the therapy and rehabilitation literature. *British Journal of Therapeutic Rehabilitation, 2*, 203-208.

Booth, A. (1996). In search of the evidence: Informing effective practice. *Journal of Clinical Effect, 1*, 25-29.

Finlayson, M., & Lou, J. Q. (1999). *Practical steps to critical appraisal: A foundation for evidence-based practice*. Ft. Lauderdale, FL: Nova Southeastern University.

Guyatt, G. H., & Rennie, D. (1993). Users' guides to the medical literature [Editorial]. *JAMA, 270*, 2096-2097.

Hunt, D. L., Jaeschke, R., & McKibbon, K. A. (2000). Users' guides to the medical literature, XXI: Using electronic health information resources in evidence-based practice. *JAMA, 283*, 1875-1879.

Oxman, A. D., Sackett, D. L., & Guyatt, G. H. (1993). Users' guides to the medical literature, I: How to get started. *JAMA, 270*, 2093-2095.

Richardson, W. S., Wilson, M. C., & Nishikawa, J. (1995). The well-built clinical question: A key to evidence-based decisions. *ACP J Club, 123*, A12-A13.

Zemke, R., & Clark, F. (1996). *Occupational science: An evolving discipline*. Philadelphia, PA: F. A. Davis.

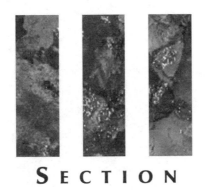

SECTION

Assessing the Evidence

Evaluating the Evidence

Mary Law, PhD, OT(C) and Ian Philp, BASc

LEARNING OBJECTIVES

After reading this chapter, the practitioner/student will be able to:

- Critically evaluate evidence by assessing the significance of different study designs, both quantitative and qualitative.
- Critically evaluate assessment tools used in quantitative research.
- Define the various types of evidence and recognize the benefits and limitations of various evidence-ranking systems.
- Understand the differences in design and application of quantitative and qualitative methodologies.

INTRODUCTION

Evaluating evidence is the meat-and-potatoes of evidence-based practice, and developing the ability to do it competently is important in becoming a successful evidence-based practitioner. After identifying a clinical question, formulating and completing a search of the literature, and reviewing the articles retrieved, the next step in the evidence-based practice process is evaluating the evidence. There are literally tens of millions of published articles in the current health care archives; however, not all are of the same quality. Evaluating the evidence means sifting through the articles and studies you have found in order to decide which are valid and clinically useful.

Because of evidence-based practice's need for substantiated, high-quality research work to function correctly, there are systems for ranking clinical and research evidence. As with other aspects of evidence-based practice, there are many different ways to specifically define the "levels of evidence" one should use. Various study designs have different levels of rigor built into them. Using quantitative methods, the "gold standard" of evidence (i.e., a randomized double-blinded controlled clinical trial) is considered the least susceptible to error because of the rigorous steps it requires researchers to follow. The caveat to this statement is that any study is still susceptible to unforeseen problems and contamination by bias. All things considered, a "gold standard" study is almost certainly more scientifically reliable and applicable than informally collected data or anecdotes. Ultimately, no evidence classification is absolutely "right" or "wrong," but the systems described here are guides that are useful rules of thumb. For qualitative research, the fit of design and methods to the research question being addressed is more important than the use of one particular design. This chapter will present several different categorization schemes to give you an understanding of the generally accepted evaluations of different types of evidence. We will discuss research using quantitative methods first.

LEVELS OF EVIDENCE IN
RESEARCH USING QUANTITATIVE METHODS

Trisha Greenhalgh (1997a-j) has written a series of very useful papers about the critical evaluation of research. The first and most comprehensive approach to defining the levels of evidence, which appears here, has been adapted from Trisha Greenhalgh's *How to Read a Paper: The Basics of Evidence-Based Medicine* (1997a). Greenhalgh's evidence rating is as follows (1997a, p. 49), in order of most to least rigorous:

1. Systematic reviews and meta-analyses
2. Randomized controlled trials with definitive results
3. Randomized controlled trials with nondefinitive results
4. Cohort studies
5. Case control studies
6. Cross-sectional surveys
7. Case reports

Depending upon which point you are at in your clinical training, you may or may not know these different terms. Some of them, such as systematic reviews and meta-analysis, will be expanded upon in Chapter 7; however, a short summary of each has been given here. The following descriptions of study designs focus on the level of evidence provided by each.

These descriptions can assist in the important process of critically appraising the study methods and analyses. A critical review form and guidelines to enable such an appraisal are provided in Appendices A and B.

Systematic Reviews and Meta-Analyses

Systematic reviews are based on a comprehensive review of the literature and provide an overview of the validity of the research methods and of results for a particular topic. Meta-analysis is a systematic review in which a statistical summary is used. Streiner (1991) says, "Meta-analysis is a technique for summarizing the results of many studies which can allow reviewers in a particular field to arrive at a synthesis of the various findings in a more objective manner than relying on expert opinion..." (p. 357).

While the overall aim of a meta-analysis is to provide an unbiased summary of effectiveness, there can be bias present in these reviews. For example, the reviewers may not search comprehensively enough to find all relevant articles. If studies are flawed in their design or sampling, the quality of the meta-analysis is affected. In reviewing a meta-analysis, it is important that the authors use and clearly describe the specific criteria employed for inclusion of a study in the meta-analysis. Currently, there are fewer systematic reviews and meta-analyses in rehabilitation than in other medical fields.

Randomized Controlled Trials with Definitive Results

A randomized controlled trial (RCT) is a study in which the participants are randomly assigned to either the experimental group or a control group. In this way, if a large number of participants are involved (or a large number of RCTs are done about the same treatment), on average the composition of the experimental and control groups were the same. Any differences in the outcome resulted from the treatment of interest and not individual differences within the participants. RCTs are placed below systematic reviews simply because a RCT represents one study, while a systematic review represents the amalgamated results of many such studies.

The "gold standard" of evidence mentioned earlier—a randomized double-blinded controlled clinical trial—is a distinction made when the study is being carried out. All RCTs are by their nature "single blind" (i.e., the participants do not know whether or not they are in the experimental or control groups). A double-blinded trial further heightens the credibility of the study by ensuring that the experimenters also do not know which group the person is in. Although this may sound strange, cases have been documented in which researchers treat subjects in the control group differently than those subjects in the experimental group, thus biasing the results.

Greenhalgh (1997e) mentions that "a randomized controlled trial with definitive results" specifies only RCTs in which the 95% confidence interval for the change scores do not cross zero. What does this mean? RCTs, just like any other type of statistical study, try to make generalizations about the population at large by looking at a *representative sample*. What can be said about the population by looking at a sample? Any value measured within the sample is an estimate of that same value for the whole population. However, because the sample is only an approximation of the population, the statistic itself is also approximate because using different members of the population in your sample would produce a slightly different value.

To explain how confidence intervals work, we turn to the extremely helpful and easy-to-understand statistics web site, "A New View of Statistics," compiled by William Hopkins (n.d.). As Hopkins says of confidence intervals, "...it is possible to use your sample to calculate a range within which the population value is likely to fall. 'Likely' is usually taken to be '95% of the time,' and the range is called the 95% confidence interval..."

Knowing now what a 95% confidence interval is, what does Greenhalgh (1997e) mean by "the 95% confidence interval for the results *does not cross zero*?" To understand this, remember that the 95% confidence interval is the *likely range of the true value* and the numbers it specifies indicate the helpfulness of the treatment. Thus, a 95% confidence interval that runs from 0.5 to 1.5 means that a 95% chance exists that the treatment in question helps patients by at least 0.5 "points." Understanding exactly what 0.5 points means is much less important than recognizing the difference between positive and negative numbers in the confidence interval. If the confidence interval ran from -0.5 to 0.5 instead of running from 0.5 to 1.5, that would mean that there was a chance that the net effect of the treatment was not helpful to the client. When a confidence interval crosses zero, it is more difficult for us to say with confidence that the treatment it measures will likely benefit the client.

Randomized Controlled Trials with Nondefinitive Results

RCTs with definitive results are, within the confines of a study, more useful for practice than RCTs with nondefinitive results. However, that does not mean that RCTs with nondefinitive results are "wrong." We know that RCTs must have a 95% confidence interval that does not cross zero to be considered "definitive," but how do we evaluate RCTs with confidence intervals that dip slightly underneath zero, especially those whose confidence interval dips only slightly below zero while maintaining a large part of their confidence interval in the positive figures? RCTs with nondefinitive confidence intervals simply show that the treatment in question is likely to have a positive impact on the outcome of some patients or is equivalent to the other treatment provided in the study.

Cohort Studies

A cohort study is a study that follows one or more group(s), or cohort(s), of participants for a defined amount of time. Cohort studies are often completed with persons in the population who don't have the condition in question and who may or may not develop it. For example, this type of study is used for conditions such as certain forms of cancer, which take decades to develop, and are organized by setting up two cohorts—one that is exposed to a risk factor in question (e.g., smoking) and another that is not exposed. By examining the long-term difference in outcome between the two cohorts, the extra risk that a factor represents for developing the condition in question can be identified. The effect of interventions can also be studied using a cohort design. For example, the effectiveness of the provision of activity programs in different nursing home settings can be evaluated by comparing the results of each nursing home cohort. Cohort studies are not randomized, so the groups being studied may not be similar in all characteristics. Because of this, cohort designs are not as strong as RCTs or systematic reviews.

Case Control Studies

Case control studies are very similar to cohort studies but are retrospective in time. In a case control study, similar individuals (one with a condition, one without) are matched and then the presence or absence of the condition or event of interest in the past is examined. For example, some of the initial studies about smoking and lung cancer examined similar individuals who had or did not have lung cancer and analyzed differences in their rates of smoking. Both cohort studies and case control studies identify possible causative events and make predictions, but they do not prove causality. Therefore, both types of evidence are inferior to studies such as RCTs.

Cross-Sectional Studies

Moving further down the evidence hierarchy, cross-sectional studies are surveys or study designs with a specific focus distributed to a large number of participants, asking about a certain fact or issue at one point in time. Researchers attempt to make the survey group a cross-section of the population they're studying and take the resultant data as representative of the larger group. However, cross-sectional studies only take into account the surveys that participants have returned, and this can introduce a possible bias into the results. Because all variables are measured at the same time, causality is not inferred in the relationship between any of the measured variables.

Case Reports

Moving down from systematic reviews of RCTs, the last rung on the evidence ladder is case reports. It should be noted that despite the fact that case reports are the lowest level of the evidence ladder, this in no way means that they can not convey important clinical information. Designed to be a written summary of a clinical suspicion or possibility, case reports are the basis for future work and the starting point for investigations of clinical possibilities using the higher levels of evidence available.

In Appendices A and B, we outline a critical review form and guidelines that can be used to appraise studies using quantitative methods. Copies of this form can be downloaded from the School of Rehabilitation Science web site at McMaster University at www.fhs.mcmaster.ca/rehab/ebp.

LEVELS OF EVIDENCE CLASSIFICATION SYSTEMS

The breakdown of levels of evidence given by Greenhalgh (1997d) is exhaustive and covers a great deal of possible types of evidence that are included in studies. A second example of evidence classification comes from the Steering Committee on Clinical Practice Guidelines for the Care and Treatment of Breast Cancer (1998). The levels of evidence that they lay out are as follows:

Level I: Evidence is based on RCTs (or meta-analysis of such trials) of adequate size to ensure a low risk of incorporating false-positive or false-negative results.

Level II: Evidence is based on RCTs that are too small to provide level I evidence. These may show either positive trends that are not statistically significant or no trends and are associated with a high risk of false-negative results.

Level III: Evidence is based on nonrandomized, controlled, or cohort studies; case series; case-controlled or cross-sectional studies.

Level IV: Evidence is based on the opinion of respected authorities or that of expert committees as indicated in published consensus conferences or guidelines.

Level V: Evidence expresses the opinion of those individuals who have written and reviewed these guidelines based on their experience, knowledge of the relevant literature, and discussion with their peers.

This classification is similar to that given by Greenhalgh (1997d), although less precise. One important feature of the Steering Committee classification, which Greenhalgh does not touch upon, is the mention of false-positive and false-negative results. False-positives (called *Type I error in statistics*) and false-negatives (called *Type II error*) are important complications with which the evidence-based practitioner must deal, and they will be touched upon in the chapter on meta-analysis.

A third breakdown of the levels of evidence comes from the National Health Service (NHS) (n.d.) in the United Kingdom. The NHS system is similar to the first two, although it sets up its classification somewhat differently:

1++   High-quality meta-analyses, systematic reviews of RCTs, or RCTs with a very low risk of bias.

1+   Well-conducted meta-analyses, systematic reviews of RCTs, or RCTs with a low risk of bias.

1 -   Meta-analyses, systematic reviews of RCTs, or RCTs with a high risk of bias.

2++   High-quality systematic reviews of case-control or cohort studies; high-quality case-control or cohort studies with a very low risk of confounding, bias, or chance, and a high probability that the relationship is causal.

2+   Well-conducted case control or cohort studies with a low risk of confounding, bias, or chance, and a moderate probability that the relationship is causal.

2 -   Case control or cohort studies with a high risk of confounding, bias, or chance, and a significant risk that the relationship is not causal.

3   Nonanalytic studies (e.g., case reports, case series).

4   Expert opinion.

Here, evidence is grouped in yet another way, and the judgment of individual practitioners is incorporated into it. The difference between a "low risk of bias" and a "very low risk of bias" is left to the practitioner's judgment, and it is something that practitioners must take seriously. As you use evidence-based practice more and more, your skill at correctly identifying the biases and deficiencies of evidence will greatly improve.

Comparing the three classification systems presented, there are, and should be, many similarities between evidence-ranking systems. In general, evidence rankings should have the same theme (i.e., moving from systematic reviews down to individual assessments). If evidence ranking seems counterintuitive and difficult to remember, attempt to think of it as moving from structures that are the most to the least resistant to unconscious human bias. Systematic reviews and RCTs have a lot of built-in barriers to bias—they are double-blinded, they are randomized, and so on. If done properly, it is very difficult to contaminate an RCT with erroneous assumptions about the outcome, the participant, or the treatment. With a case report, the evidence is coming from a single practitioner who is subject to all the biases his or her clinical training may have given him or her. The evidence ranking does not attempt to discredit the efforts of individual researchers but realizes the limitations which they face. Opponents of evidence-based practice cite this as one more affirmation of the fact that evidence-based practice does not "trust" practitioners. On the contrary, evidence-based practice is an acknowledgment that each practitioner is limited to the knowledge of his or her surroundings, but together evidence can be gathered and conclusions made that impact everyone. Knowledge in any profession is built piece by piece, often beginning with a case report and proceeding to further and larger studies. Each piece in the puzzle of the development of rehabilitation evidence is important.

MEASUREMENT ISSUES

Within all quantitative studies, measurement of specific variables is completed. These measures can vary from range of motion or strength to activities of daily living to participation in play or work. The assessment tools that are used in quantitative studies can also be critically reviewed to determine their clinical utility, standardization, reliability, and validity. Appendices C and D include a critical review form and guidelines for the appraisal of the assessment tools used in quantitative studies. These can be downloaded from the CanChild Centre for Childhood Disability Research at McMaster University web site at www.fhs.mcmaster.ca/canchild.

LEARNING BIOSTATISTICS

In order to comprehend, analyze, and put into practice evidence from clinical journals and other sources, one will need to have a working knowledge of biostatistics. The *Canadian Medical Association Journal* has published a series of "basic statistics for clinicians" articles that are helpful when reviewing research articles (Guyatt et al., 1995a, 1995b, 1995c, 1995d).

THE CRITICAL REVIEW OF RESEARCH USING QUALITATIVE METHODS

In research, there often exists a perceived hierarchy of research design and methods that quantitative methods are of higher quality than qualitative methods. In fact, the generation of knowledge from both types of designs is important. The most appropriate design to be used in a specific study depends more on the research question and the knowledge required than on prior ideas of best methods. For example, the final testing of a drug is best accomplished using a RCT because one wants to ensure that the results are causal in nature and applicable to the broad population. Equally, the experience of living in the community with a newly acquired disability is best studied using qualitative methods such as ethnography or biography. The use of qualitative methods in rehabilitation research is increasing and has generated much knowledge about the experience of illness and disability as well as other issues important to persons involved in rehabilitation.

Criteria being used for this appraisal should suit qualitative methods, as the application of quantitative methods criteria to studies using qualitative methods is not appropriate. The development of appraisal criteria for qualitative methods is relatively new, and the criteria are not as precise as the criteria for quantitative methods. Such differences reflect the methodology of qualitative research, as illustrated by increased comfort with ambiguity and less perceived need for the "right" answer. Issues to pay particular attention to when evaluating qualitative research follow.

Study Design

In constructing qualitative research, there are many different types of research approaches or designs. Creswell (1998) has outlined five major approaches, or designs, used in qualitative research. These approaches include biography, ethnography, phenomenology, grounded theory, and case study. Of these approaches, ethnography, phenomenology, and grounded theory are most often seen in the rehabilitation literature and will be discussed in more detail here.

Ethnography

Ethnography is a qualitative research approach that traces its history to development in the field of anthropology. In this research design, the purpose is to study a particular culture or group of people to identify their daily life patterns, meanings, and beliefs. Ethnography has been used to study cultural groups as well as groups of people with health problems or disabilities.

Phenomenology

A research study using this approach or design focuses on the lived experience of the person or a group of people. The purpose of this research is to understand lived experience, interpret that experience, and thus provide information that can be shared with and used by others.

Grounded Theory

Grounded theory design is very common in rehabilitation and nursing research literature. The primary purpose of this approach is theory construction and verification. Using grounded theory, researchers seek to understand and identify theoretical processes in the real world. Themes that emerge from research are used to develop an understanding and theoretical explanation of the social world of the people being studied.

Methods

There are a variety of methods used by qualitative researchers, including participant observation, interviews, focus groups, and review of documents or other material. The methods chosen for particular study should be the most appropriate in collecting research data for that study. Commonly, qualitative researchers use multiple methods to enhance the trustworthiness of their findings. The use of multiple methods is one type of triangulation, a group of strategies used to ensure the rigor of a qualitative research study.

Sampling

The purpose of sampling in qualitative research is quite different from quantitative methods. In qualitative research, participants are selected for a specific purpose. Random selection is not used. For example, participants may be chosen because they are of a certain age or culture or have experienced specific events better important to the study. The sampling strategies used in a study should be well described and justified by the authors. A sample size of qualitative studies is generally smaller than quantitative studies, and there are no specific formulae to calculate appropriate sample size. Rather, sampling in a qualitative study is continued until sampling redundancy or theoretical saturation of the data is achieved.

Data Collection

Achieving descriptive clarity is a very important characteristic for a qualitative research study. Authors of qualitative studies should include clear descriptive information about the participants, the study site, and the researcher so that readers develop an excellent understanding of the context of the research. All data collection procedures should be explicitly described, including specific methods, training of data gatherers, the length of time for the study, and the data collected. Procedures to enhance the rigor of the study, such as triangulation, member checking, and consistency of coding themes, should be described.

Appendices E and F outline the critical review guidelines and form to be used for the appraisal of research using qualitative methods. The appraisal criteria in these tables should be viewed as a "work in progress" and a "guide" to examining research using qualitative methods.

Take-Home Messages

Evaluating the Evidence
- Evidence-based practice requires the researcher to search through the evidence and evaluate different study designs and different levels of reliability.
- Different levels of evidence include RCTs, cohort studies, case control studies, cross-sectional studies, and case reports.
- It is important to recognize the hierarchy of evidence in evaluating quantitative research.
- Critical review of qualitative studies must be done using criteria specific for that type of methodology.
- The most appropriate design for a specific study depends on the nature of the research question and the type of knowledge that is needed.

WEB LINKS

Randomized Controlled Trials: A User's Guide
www.bmjpg.com/rct/contents.html
This is the online version of Alejandro Jadad's book (1998), which takes readers through the very basics of RCTs all the way to meta-analysis in an easy-to-read format. This book is highly recommended for beginners and perhaps even worth buying the print copy.

The Consolidated Standards of Reporting Trials (CONSORT) Statement
www.ama-assn.org/sci-pubs/journals/archive/jama/vol_276/no_8/sc6048x.htm (Article)
www.consort-statement.org (Homepage)
The CONSORT statement lays out a number of guidelines for conducting good RCTs, which are essential for sound systematic reviews. The article is a link to the original *Journal of the American Medical Association* publication of the idea; the homepage has more detailed information and updates on current work.

Centre for Evidence-Based Medicine Levels of Evidence Classification
http://cebm.jr2.ox.ac.uk/docs/levels.html
This "levels of evidence" system was prepared by the UK-based Centre for Evidence-Based Medicine (CEBM). This system is even more detailed than the levels discussed in the chapter, breaking evidence up into letter grades and subcategories.

University of Illinois at Chicago—Is All Evidence Created Equal?
www.uic.edu/depts/lib/lhsp/resources/levels.shtml
This site, compiled by the University of Chicago Library, takes an open-ended approach
to the topic. Students will likely find the bottom of the page the most useful, as it discusses
the characteristics of specific types of evidence and where to find them.

A New View of Statistics
www.sportsci.org/resource/stats/index.html
An excellent primer or refresher to many aspects of statistics, complied and created by
New Zealander William Hopkins.

LEARNING AND EXPLORATION ACTIVITIES

The purpose of this chapter is to introduce students to various types of evidence and the
different means of classifying this evidence. The following practical exercises are intended
to allow the student to become comfortable with the different means of evaluating the evidence:

1. Decide upon a treatment of interest (perhaps one you have been studying in class), and
   perform a search of the literature for articles or studies relating to that treatment. When
   you find one, attempt to place it in one of the "levels of evidence" system cited in this
   chapter. What are the greatest strengths of the study? The greatest weaknesses? Why
   did you place it where you did in the hierarchy? Justify your answers.

2. Obtain the following article from the library: Friedman, R., & Tappen, R. M. (1991).
   The effect of planned walking on communication in Alzheimer's disease. *Journal of
   American Geriatrics Society, 39*, 650-654. Using the Quantitative Critical Review
   Form and Guidelines (Appendices C and D), critically review this study and complete
   the review form. Use this as a basis for discussion of the rigor of this study with your
   fellow students.

3. Select a rehabilitation outcome measure that you are currently studying or are interested in learning. Perform a literature review to identify research on the measure. Obtain
   the measure's manual if it exists. Using Appendices A and B, complete a critical review
   of this measure. Some suggested measures to review include the Functional
   Independence Measure (FIM), Barthel Index, Medical Outcomes Study (MOS) SF-36,
   and Oswestry Low Back Pain Disability Questionnaire.

4. Obtain the following article from the library: Borell, L., Gustavsson, A., Sandman, P.
   O., & Kielhofner, G. (1994). Occupational programming in a day hospital for patients
   with dementia. *Occupational Therapy Journal of Research, 14*(4), 219-238. Using the
   Qualitative Critical Review Form and Guidelines (Appendices E and F), critically
   review this study and complete the review form. Use this as a basis for discussion of
   the rigor of this study with your fellow students.

5. Choose a quantitative and/or qualitative article that focuses on a rehabilitation intervention of your choice. Use Appendices C, D, E, and F to critically review these articles.

REFERENCES

Cresswell, J. W. (1998). Qualitative inquiry and research design. Thousand Oaks, CA: Sage Publications.

Greenhalgh, T. (1997a). *How to read a paper: The basics of evidence-based medicine*. London: BMJ Publishing Group.

Greenhalgh, T. (1997b). The Medline database. *British Medical Journal, 315*(7101), 180-183.

Greenhalgh, T. (1997c). Getting your bearings (deciding what the paper is about). *British Medical Journal, 315*(7102), 243-246.

Greenhalgh, T. (1997d). Assessing the methodological quality of published papers. *British Medical Journal, 315*(7103), 305-308.

Greenhalgh, T. (1997e). Statistics for the non-statistician. I: Different types of data need different statistical tests. *British Medical Journal, 315*(7104), 364-366.

Greenhalgh, T. (1997f). Statistics for the non-statistician. II: "Significant" relations and their pitfalls. *British Medical Journal, 315*(7105), 422-425.

Greenhalgh, T. (1997g). Papers that report drug trials. *British Medical Journal, 315*(7106), 480-483.

Greenhalgh, T. (1997h). Papers that report diagnostic or screening tests. *British Medical Journal, 315*(7107), 540-543.

Greenhalgh, T. (1997i). Papers that tell you what things cost (economic analyses). *British Medical Journal, 315*(7108), 596-599.

Greenhalgh, T. (1997j). Papers that summarise other papers (systematic reviews and meta-analyses). *British Medical Journal, 315*(7109), 672-675.

Guyatt, G., Jaeschke, R., Heddle, N., Cook, D., Shannon, H., & Walter, S. (1995a). Basic statistics for clinicians. 1. Hypothesis testing. *Canadian Medical Association Journal, 152*, 27-32.

Guyatt, G., Jaeschke, R., Heddle, N., Cook, D., Shannon, H., & Walter, S. (1995b). Basic statistics for clinicians. 2. Interpreting study results: Confidence intervals. *Canadian Medical Association Journal, 152*, 169-173.

Guyatt, G., Jaeschke, R., Heddle, N., Cook, D., Shannon, H., & Walter, S. (1995c). Basic statistics for clinicians. 3. Assessing the effects of treatment: Measures of association. *Canadian Medical Association Journal, 152*, 351-357.

Guyatt, G., Jaeschke, R., Heddle, N., Cook, D., Shannon, H., & Walter, S. (1995d). Basic statistics for clinicians. 4. Correlation and regression. *Canadian Medical Association Journal, 152*, 497-504.

Hopkins, W. (n.d.). *A new view of statistics*. Retrieved January 10, 2002, from http://www.sportsci.org/resource/stats/index.html.

Jadad, A. R. (1998). *Randomized controlled trials*. London: BMJ Publishing Group.

National Health Service. (n.d.). *Levels of evidence and grader of recommendation*. Retrieved January 10, 2002, from http://www.show.scot.nhs.uk.

Steering Committee on Clinical Practice Guidelines for the Care and Treatment of Breast Cancer. (1998). Clinical practice guidelines for the care and treatment of breast cancer. *Canadian Medical Association Journal, 158*(3). Retrieved January 10, 2002, from http://www.cma.ca/cmaj/vol-158/issue-3/breastcpg/0002.htm.

Streiner, D. L. (1991). Using meta-analysis in psychiatric research. *Can J Psychiatry, 36*, 357-362.

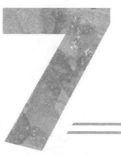

Systematically Reviewing the Evidence

Mary Law, PhD, OT(C) and Ian Philp, BASc

LEARNING OBJECTIVES

After reading this chapter, the practitioner/student will be able to:
- Understand the various methodologies for preparing a systematic review.
- Interpret the findings of meta-analysis.
- Illustrate the role of the Cochrane Collaboration in evidence-based practice.

SYSTEMATIC REVIEWS

Introduction

Systematic reviews are essentially the heart of evidence-based practice. Evidence-based concepts such as critically appraised topics (CATS) (discussed in Chapter 9) allow for the critical evaluation of one article pertaining to your clinical question. However, CATs are both inadequate and very limited in a larger sense because they contain no critical evaluation of the complete current knowledge on a question and can present results which are actually biased with respect to the overall literature. In order to ensure that an evidence-based tool is not biased, one must evaluate evidence in an ordered and logical way; in other words, systematically. From this idea, systematic reviews were born.

Why do we need systematic reviews? The Thomas C. Chalmers Centre for Systematic Reviews (n.d.a) explains that "systematic reviews provide summaries of the results of evidence-based health care, which can be made available to clinicians, policy decision makers, and patients."

Systematic reviews are a logical, ordered way to deal with the information glut that has come with advances in rehabilitation. They are a way to ensure that the self-directed learning of practitioners is done in an efficient manner and proves both sound and beneficial for their clients.

How are systematic reviews defined? In their article in the *Annals of Internal Medicine*, Cook, Mulrow, and Haynes (1997) offer an excellent definition of systematic reviews. They state, "A systematic review involves the application of scientific strategies, in ways that limit bias, to the assembly, critical appraisal, and synthesis of all relevant studies that address a specific clinical question."

Cook et al. (1997) are right that systematic reviews use *scientific strategies*; in fact, using the correct method is one of the most important parts of constructing a good systematic review. Because of this fact, there are major differences between a regular review of the literature (sometimes called a *narrative review*) and a systematic review. Cook et al. list several of the important differences in Table 7-1.

Different schools of thought on systematic reviews have produced different methodologies for conducting them. Several will be presented here in order to compare and contrast their important elements. We begin with the large and comprehensive methodology presented by the University of York's National Health Service Centre for Reviews and Dissemination (2001). The process it defines is as follows:

Planning the Review
- Phase 0—Identification of the need for the review
- Phase 1—Preparation of a proposal for a systematic review
- Phase 2—Development of a review protocol

Conducting the Review
- Phase 3—Identification of the literature
- Phase 4—Selection of studies
- Phase 5—Study quality assessment
- Phase 6—Data extraction and monitoring progress
- Phase 7—Data synthesis

Table 7-1

DIFFERENCES BETWEEN
NARRATIVE REVIEWS AND SYSTEMATIC REVIEWS

Feature	Narrative Review	Systematic Review
Question	Often broad in scope	Often a focused clinical question
Sources and search	Not usually specified, potentially biased	Comprehensive sources and explicit search strategy
Selection	Not usually specified, potentially biased	Criterion-based selection, uniformly applied
Appraisal	Variable	Rigorous critical appraisal
Synthesis	Often a qualitative summary	Quantitative summary*
Inferences	Sometimes evidence-based	Usually evidence-based

*A quantitative summary that includes a statistical synthesis is a meta-analysis.

Reprinted from Cook, M. D., Mulrow, C. D., & Haynes, R. B. (1997). Systematic reviews: Synthesis of best evidence for clinical decisions. *Ann Intern Med, 126*(5), 376-380 with permission of BMJ Publishing Group.

Reporting and Dissemination

→ Phase 8—The report and recommendations

→ Phase 9—Getting evidence into practice

This is only a brief summary of their methods; the entire detailed methodology is laid out in an approximately 100-page-long document, which can be downloaded in parts from their web site, www.york.ac.uk/inst/crd/report4.htm. The NHS methodology document is beyond the scope of this book but is available for consultation.

A second, slightly less detailed systematic review procedure comes from the University of Leicester and the British National Health Service's Systematic Reviews of Trials and Other Studies (SROTOS) Project (n.d.). The steps given here have been distilled from a longer text but encompass the basic ideas of the report:

1. Compile through systematic review methods of as comprehensive a set as possible of reports of relevant studies.

2. Identify a common set of definitions of outcome, explanatory, and confounding variables, which are, as far as possible, compatible with those in each of the primary studies.

3. Extract estimates of outcome measures and of study and subject characteristics in a standardized way and with due checks on extractor bias.

4. Where warranted by the scope and characteristics of the data compiled, meta-analysis using methods and models appropriate to explore and allow for all important sources of variation, including those related to the characteristics of the subjects, the nature of the intervention/exposure, and the quality of the study.

5. Explore the sensitivity of the results of the meta-analysis to the choices and assumptions made in all of the above stages.

6. Present key aspects of all of the above stages in the study report clearly.

The SROTOS report mentions meta-analysis more than the others discussed, which will be touched on later in this chapter. Meta-analysis is used primarily for quantitative reviews, while qualitative reviews focus more on language and non-numerically-measurable outcomes.

Finally, the last methodology to be discussed comes from the Cochrane Collaboration. The Cochrane Collaboration is a clearinghouse for the collection of systematic reviews worldwide and is discussed in more depth later in this chapter. In such a position, the Cochrane Collaboration has the ability to set the standards for reviews and their composition. The following methodology is from the *Cochrane Reviewer's Handbook* (Cochrane Collaboration, n.d.):

1. Conceiving, designing, and coordinating the review.

2. Data collection for the review.

3. Developing search strategy, undertaking searches, screening search results.

4. Screening retrieved papers against inclusion criteria, appraising quality of papers.

5. Abstracting data from papers.

6. Analysis and interpretation of data.

7. Writing the review.

All three of the methodologies presented are good guidelines for conducting a systematic review, but they are quite complicated and may seem rather abstract. By comparing two further methodologies found in the literature, students will gain a greater understanding of the steps of a systematic review.

The first of the two methodologies from the literature is from Trisha Greenhalgh's article series and book, *How to Read a Paper* (1997a, 1997b). She claims that systematic reviews are defined by two points: (1) they must both "contain an explicit statement of objectives, materials, and methods and (2) they must have been conducted according to explicit and reproducible methodology" (1997a, p. 111). The "explicit and reproducible methodology" of which Greenhalgh speaks is outlined in a flowchart (1997b, p. 672) (Figure 7-1). Greenhalgh's process is compared and contrasted with a second process, suggested by Joseph Lau and colleagues in the 1997 article, "Quantitative Synthesis in Systematic Reviews" (Lau, Ioannidis, & Schmid, 1997). Lau et al.'s process consists of only six steps, as opposed to Greenhalgh's eight. Lau et al.'s steps are as follows:

1. Define and decide on what data is to be combined.

2. Evaluate the statistical heterogeneity of the data.

3. Estimate a common effect.

4. Explore and explain heterogeneity.

5. Assess the potential for bias.

6. Present the results.

This chapter uses information from the processes of both Greenhalgh (1997a, 1997b) and Lau et al. (1997) to develop three broad "stages" that are undertaken in the systematic review process.

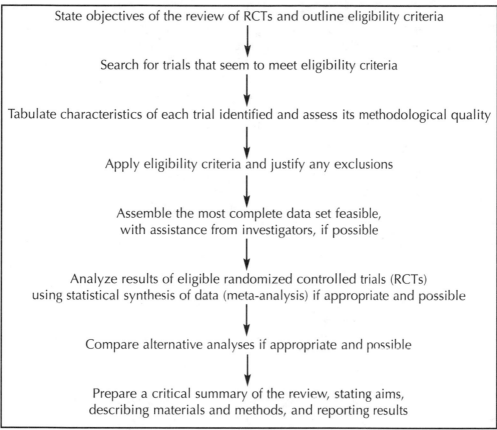

Figure 7-1. A flowchart for systematic review (reprinted with permission from Greenhalgh, T. [1997]. *How to read a paper: Papers that summarise other papers (systematic reviews and meta-analyses)*. British Medical Journal, 315, 672-675).

Stage 1. Preparing to Do Your Systematic Review

Greenhalgh	• State the objectives of the review of RCTs and outline eligibility criteria • Search for trials that seem to meet eligibility criteria • Tabulate characteristics of each trial identified and assess its methodological quality • Apply eligibility criteria and justify any exclusions
Lau et al.	• Define and decide on what data is to be combined

In the first stage of making a systematic review, the final product is but a distant goal on the horizon, and the business of properly constructing its foundations is at hand. Both Greenhalgh (1997a, 1997b) and Lau et al. (1997) acknowledge that the proper selection of RCTs in this stage is critical to the successful completion of a good quantitative systematic review. Before plunging into systematic reviews, you should have a good working knowledge of RCTs. If you are unsure about them, Alejandro Jadad's book *Randomised Controlled Trials: A User's Guide* (1998) is excellent and will be more than sufficient to give you a background (look in the Web Links section for more information). It should be noted that systematic reviews can be done on articles that do not describe RCTs; however, the results will not be as authoritative.

When attempting to choose studies to use in your systematic review, it will quickly become clear that no two researchers will have done their study in the same way. Even if, for example, you are looking at two RCTs that both claim to gauge the effect of the same drug on similar populations, the data will have been presented differently, and different variables may have been measured and charted. This leads to a critical point for systematic reviews; much of their strength lies in the precise definition of what studies are to be included, or the systematic review's "eligibility criteria." Do not simply say that you wish, for example, to look at RCTs on "stroke rehabilitation"—you must closely define the age values, medical histories, and states of the patient samples from which you want to draw RCTs. As your training in clinical diagnosis and differentiation increases, the process of creating good eligibility criteria for systematic reviews will become much easier as you learn this important skill.

After defining the eligibility criteria of the studies for which you are looking, begin the search for them. Usually, this is done within the health literature by using MEDLINE or another comparable database. If you are attempting to conduct a large systematic review, however, you can contact specialists in the field and ask them if they have done any studies or RCTs that haven't been published but that are useful and valid all the same. Gathering studies, sorting through them, and deciding whether or not they are worthy of inclusion can be a time-consuming and monotonous job, but it is absolutely crucial to a good outcome in a systematic review.

The final part of the first stage involves tabulating the trial's characteristics and looking at its methodological quality. If the systematic review only includes RCTs, the normal "levels of evidence" hierarchy does not apply. However, within the field of RCTs, there can be major differences. Not all researchers are completely exacting or precise in their research methods, and as we look closely at individual RCTs, errors in methodology become apparent. Many RCTs do not randomize their patient samples properly; others fail to correctly blind the study groups or the researchers to the results, and there are other commonly committed errors that can be present in RCTs in even the most rigorous journals. Errors in RCTs are easy to commit and easy to unwittingly hide because often the improper methodology is not discussed, and assumptions are made that the researchers did the study correctly. Only by looking in close detail at the internal workings of studies is it possible to assess the methodological quality of each researcher's report.

As the process of completing an RCT is quite complex and involves a great number of steps and processes, the majority of RCTs have at least one error in them, no matter how small. Overlooking small errors in RCTs is acceptable because by setting your standards at perfection you will effectively eliminate all data from your systematic review. Those studies with serious flaws, however, should be rejected from consideration, and those that remain should be readied to pass into the next stage.

Some work has been done on improving the standards of RCTs, which will make the sorting process much easier. The most significant advancement is the CONSORT statement, which was published in the *Journal of the American Medical Association* in 1996 and is available on-line (see Web Links at the end of this chapter). CONSORT consists of checklists and flowcharts that help researchers report RCTs in a standardized way, regardless of each study's internal complexities. The standardization of RCTs guards against methodological error, makes them easier to evaluate, and makes them easier to combine in a systematic review. The authors of the CONSORT statement intended it to give systematic reviewers the "ability to make informed judgments regarding the internal and external validity of the trial" (Begg et al., 1996). This statement will go a long way toward making systematic reviews easier and more authoritative.

Stage 2. Analyzing and Quantifying the Accepted Data

Greenhalgh	• Assemble the most complete data set feasible, with assistance from investigators, if possible
	• Analyze results of eligible RCTs by using statistical synthesis of data (meta-analysis) if appropriate and possible
Lau et al.	• Evaluate the statistical heterogeneity of the data
	• Estimate a common effect
	• Explore and explain heterogeneity

Having cleared the first hurdle of finding the data to systematically review, the next step is to move on to the actual business of combining and reviewing. First, all of the remaining articles to be analyzed must be judged for their overall quality. Greenhalgh suggests analyzing RCTs based on three considerations: methodological quality, precision, and external validity (1997a, p. 117). Methodological quality was already covered in Chapter 6, indicating that RCTs are generally of higher quality and should be regarded more seriously than other study designs. Precision refers to the likelihood of random errors in the result. A study that predicts that an outcome will be within a moderately wide range with a high degree of certainty is much more useful than one that predicts a narrow band of outcome with no great confidence. Finally, external validity refers to the generalizability of the study—how applicable are the results of the RCT to the population on which the systematic review is focused? In this light, a very precise trial focusing on an improper age group may be of the same value or even less than one that is less precise focusing on the correctly-aged population of interest.

The actual analysis of quantified results through meta-analysis will be touched on later in this chapter, but when the results of the review are analyzed, a common effect will or will not be apparent. After the analysis is done, attempt to find explanations for the heterogeneity or nonheterogeneity of the data. Why would the results have looked the same (other than that it was caused by the treatment)? What other factors may have biased or otherwise altered the treatments? The examination of possible sources of bias or error is important in the next stage of the process.

Stage 3. Presenting and Reporting Your Findings

Greenhalgh	• Compare alternative analyses, if appropriate and possible • Prepare a critical summary of the review, stating aims, describing materials and methods, and reporting results
Lau et al.	• Assess the potential for bias • Present the results

In this step, all of the work that has been put into the systematic review comes to fruition. The entire process—not just the end result—must be written up. All of the variables and choices made along the way affect how the final outcome emerges. Cite any and all possibilities for bias that could have existed both in the original RCTs and in the secondary work of the systematic review. For an example of a completed systematic review, see Chapter 8 in this text.

One final comment on publishing should be made. Once a systematic review is done, it should be published or at least made public on the Internet, no matter what its findings. Many people think that a systematic review finding no significant results from a group of RCTs is not useful. The truth could not be more to the contrary. Many clinical misjudgments are made daily because of the negative publication bias or the tendency for journals to only publish results that are positive. If practitioners knew about the negative results coming from some RCTs and systematic reviews, they would change their practice habits. However, negative results aren't as "interesting" as positive ones; therefore, they get less coverage. Publishing both positive and negative RCTs and systematic reviews is the only way in which a more complete knowledge of which interventions or treatments are beneficial can be garnered. Through the publication of all research, the health sciences and rehabilitation community can find out which currently fashionable treatments deserve to be abandoned.

Other Sources of Information

This chapter has only scratched the surface of the information that could be written about systematic reviews. Some practitioners have spent careers studying systematic reviews and still have difficulties at times. This chapter is intended to give the reader an introduction to the topic and the scope to learn more on his or her own. For those wishing to learn more about systematic reviews, an excellent series of articles was recently published in the *Annals of Internal Medicine* that introduces systematic reviews in an easy-to-understand format. The citation data for the series is listed below; while most are available online, some are only in print.

1. Cook, D. J., Mulrow, C. D., & Haynes, R. B. (1997). Systematic reviews: Synthesis of best evidence for clinical decisions. *Ann Intern Med, 126*, 376-380. Retrieved January 10, 2002, from http://www.acponline.org/journals/annals/01mar97/bestevid.htm.

2. Hunt, D. L., & McKibbon, K. A. (1997). Locating and appraising systematic reviews. *Ann Intern Med, 126*, 532-538. Retrieved January 10, 2002, from http://www.acponline.org/journals/annals/01apr97/systemat.htm.

3. McQuay, H. J., & Moore, R. A. (1997). Using numerical results from systematic reviews in clinical practice. *Ann Intern Med, 126*, 712-720. Retrieved January 10, 2002, from http://www.acponline.org/journals/annals/01may97/numeric.htm.

4. Badgett, R. G., O'Keefe, M., & Henderson, M. C. (1997). Using systematic reviews in clinical education. *Ann Intern Med, 126*, 886-891. Retrieved January 10, 2002, from http://www.acponline.org/journals/annals/01jun97/clineduc.htm.

5. Bero, L. A., & Jadad, A. R. (1997). How consumers and policy makers can use systematic reviews for decision making. *Ann Intern Med, 127*, 37-42. Retrieved January 10, 2002, from http://www.acponline.org/journals/annals/01jul97/consumer.htm.

6. Cook, D. J., Greengold, N. L., Ellrodt, A. G., & Weingarten, S. R. (1997). The relation between systematic reviews and practice guidelines. *Ann Intern Med, 127*, 210-216. Retrieved January 10, 2002, from http://www.acponline.org/journals/annals/01aug97/systrev.htm.

7. Counsell, C. (1997). Formulating questions and locating primary studies for inclusion in systematic reviews. *Ann Intern Med, 127*(5), 380-387.

8. Meade, M. O., & Richardson, W. S. (1997). Selecting and appraising studies for a systematic review. *Ann Intern Med, 127*, 531-537.

9. Lau, J., Ioannidis, J. P. A., & Schmid, C. H. (1997). Quantitative synthesis in systematic reviews. *Ann Intern Med, 127*, 820-826. Retrieved January 10, 2002, from http://www.acponline.org/journals/annals/01nov97/quantsyn.htm.

10. Mulrow, C., Langhorne, P., & Grimshaw, J. (1997). Integrating heterogeneous pieces of evidence in systematic reviews. *Ann Intern Med, 127*, 989-995. Retrieved January 10, 2002, from http://www.acponline.org/journals/annals/01dec97/evidence.htm.

Final Thoughts on Systematic Reviews

One final issue to heed when considering systematic reviews is that there may be more than one systematic review published on a specific topic, and the results reported by the systematic reviews differ. One researcher's systematic review could report that a specific course of treatment has a positive effect, while other systematic reviews found the course of treatment to be deleterious. In this unusual case, look closely at the systematic reviews themselves and examine how they were made. Jadad, Cook, and Browman's article on interpreting discordant systematic reviews (1997) provides a useful guide for weighing the systematic reviews against each other and finding which is better. Hopefully, with tools such as CONSORT, this problem with systematic reviews will be minimized, but there always exists a danger of human error, which can never be completely eradicated.

In closing, completing systematic reviews, like many concepts in EBP, is an acquired skill and requires a lot of practice to do and understand correctly. This guide aims to give you a brief introduction to them, but more knowledge will come with time and practice. In order to gain a stronger understanding of systematic reviews, one can examine meta-analysis as the process through which systematic reviews are completed.

META-ANALYSIS

As previously mentioned, meta-analyses are a specific subset of systematic reviews that statistically combine data from many studies in order to find a "common effect." The idea of a systematic review was introduced in 1976 by the researcher Gene V. Glass in his article "Primary, Secondary, and Meta-Analysis" (1976). Glass opened the discussion on meta-analysis and offered this definition, "Meta-analysis refers to the analysis of analyses... the statistical analysis of a large collection of analysis results from individual studies for the purpose of integrating the findings" (p. 3). Dr. Glass works today at the University of Arizona, continuing his work on meta-analysis. More of his work is available online at http://glass.ed.asu.edu/gene. Glass' definition has remained in use since it was first published in 1976; however, other, more informative definitions have been constructed. Such a definition is offered by Dr. Alejandro Jadad in his book *Randomised Controlled Trials: A User's Guide* (1998). Dr. Jadad states, "Meta-analysis is a name that is given to any review article in which the results of several independent studies are combined statistically to produce a single estimate of the effect of a particular intervention or health care situation."

There are other definitions of meta-analysis that have been offered, but the essence is that a meta-analysis' power comes from its ability to statistically digest many different studies and emerge with a final assessment of their common effect.

At this point, the reader may know that meta-analysis involves statistically combining study results, but he or she may be wondering what actual statistical process is undertaken. The statistical methods and procedures of this process go beyond the scope of this summary and are usually taught in advanced statistics classes or classes for meta-analysts. However, a description of the process is as follows: in principle, it uses general formulae that have been developed to combine two or more sets of data. Those interested in some of the more in-depth statistical methods used in meta-analysis can find them outlined in journal articles, such as Hasselblad and McCrory's "Meta-Analytic Tools for Medical Decision Making: A Practical Guide" (1995) or medical statistics textbooks. Because of the technical skill required for meta-analysis, however, many researchers will work with a meta-analyst.

Without charging into the details of meta-analysis, several major points of reference will be mentioned. When doing a meta-analysis, the meta-analyst will first examine the data to determine which data variable is both present in all of the studies and is a good indicator for the study. This is known as *selecting a proper outcome measure*.

Next, the meta-analyst will manipulate the data from the studies to align the data in a unified way. For example, if some studies report the 1 week mortality rate, others the bimonthly rate, and others the rate every day, the meta-analyst will need to choose a standard of measure and format all of the data so it fits within it. At this stage, contacting the authors of studies for additional data becomes useful, for outcome data that was not included in a journal article may still have been collected and will likely be available upon request from the researcher.

The end product of all of this work is truly astounding: a simple diagram that presents the overarching results of the meta-analysis at one glance. This type of diagram (usually referred to as a *forest plot*) is well known in the EBP world, most notably as the logo of the Cochrane Collaboration (Figure 7-2). The Cochrane Collaboration itself will be discussed in further detail later in this chapter. What does a forest plot tell us?

Ignoring the C's on the outside, a forest plot is, quite simply, a vertical line with a number of horizontal lines running across it. During meta-analysis, each study involved is distilled down to a *confidence interval* (as previously discussed), which states with 95% certainty the effects of that study. As the Cochrane Collaboration (2001a) web site explains, "the Cochrane Collaboration logo illustrates a systematic review of data from seven randomized controlled trials... each horizontal line represents the results of one trial (the shorter the line, the more certain the result); and the diamond represents their combined results."

Thus, a forest plot represents the pooled odds ratios of all the studies in the review. If a (horizontal) confidence interval of a result crosses the (vertical) line of no effect, then either a significant difference does not exist between the treatment and the control or the sample size was too small to allow us to be confident where the true result lies. The diamond repre-

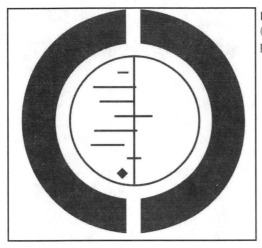

Figure 7-2. The Cochrane Collaboration logo (this logo has been reproduced with the kind permission of The Cochrane Collaboration).

sents the pooled data from all the studies in question, and since the diamond is to the left of the line of no effect, we can say that this meta-analysis has allowed us to show that the treatment in question has had an effect. For an example of a forest plot related to a rehabilitation intervention, see Chapter 8 of this text.

Heterogeneity

An important factor to remember when thinking of meta-analysis is heterogeneity. This is touched on by Trisha Greenhalgh in her *How to Read a Paper* series (1997b). Greenhalgh states,

> *In the language of meta-analysis, homogeneity means that the results of each individual trial are mathematically compatible with the results of any of the others. Conversely, [if the horizontal lines do not overlap], these trials could be said to be heterogeneous.*

Testing for heterogeneity takes more than just "eyeballing" whether or not all of the study confidence intervals overlap; a statistical technique called a *chi square test* is used to be certain. Homogeneity is very important when interpreting the results of a meta-analysis. If the studies are *heterogeneous*, no common effect can be drawn from them. Heterogeneity can sometimes be corrected by limiting the data in the studies (e.g., considering the effect of a treatment on only a certain age range instead of looking at the population at large). Some researchers still remain critical of meta-analyses because of the very potential for heterogeneity. Greenhalgh cites Professor Hans Eysenck as one of the foremost amongst the critics, telling us that "it offends his sense of the qualitative and the particular to combine the results of studies which were done on different populations in different places at different times and for different reasons."

There are also others who criticize meta-analysis. Meta-analysis, while a rigorous statistical tool, is not perfect. As the British NHS SROTOS report (n.d.) explains:

> *...Two potentially serious ones [with meta-analysis] are publication bias and missing data. Methods for detecting/adjusting for publication bias exist, and others are currently being developed. Dealing with missing data within a meta-analysis has not been considered to the same extent.*

Table 7-2

ADVANTAGES AND DISADVANTAGES OF META-ANALYSIS

Advantages

- Produces a single, precise estimate of benefit and harm
- Can be applied (with caution) to cohort and case control studies as well as RCTs

Disadvantages

- The "numerical bottom line" can be distracting and overlook important sources of bias and diversity between individual trials
- Conclusions expressed as recommendations for the "average" or "typical" patient may be unhelpful in practice
- Few interventions have been adequately addressed by meta-analysis, and the method, while theoretically sound, "often fails in ways that are invisible to the analyst"

Adapted from http://www.ucl.ac.uk/primcare-popsci/uebpp/table31.htm.

Publication bias is when researchers want to put forward for publication or journals only those studies that have positive outcomes. This is understandable in that no practitioner wishes to be seen continuously publishing research with negative results, but it hurts the health care community at large if only positive or successful studies are available for consideration. Does this mean that all meta-analyses are inherently biased toward the positive because of the pool of RCTs that are available? The jury is still out; nonetheless, this is an important question that EBP must face. The second criticism, missing data, arises when RCTs or meta-analyses are done incorrectly or cannot be done because researchers have not adequately completed their studies.

Along the same lines as SROTOS, the University College London has compiled a list of advantages and disadvantages of meta-analysis (Table 7-2).

Finally, a further and more detailed critique of meta-analysis comes from Dr. John C. Bailar in his 1997 editorial, "The Promise and Problems of Meta-Analysis" in the *New England Journal of Medicine*. In it, Dr. Bailar assesses the strengths and weaknesses of meta-analysis and comes down negatively on the final stage—the distillation of all of the studies down to the diamond, the single "combined estimate" of effect. Bailar argues that "there are often biologic reasons, statistical evidence, or both showing that the studies included in the meta-analysis have in fact measured somewhat different things, so that a combined estimate cannot be meaningful unless additional, doubtful assumptions are made."

Bailar (1997) goes on to speak of the other problems that have plagued meta-analysis, such as "failure of the investigator performing the meta-analysis to understand the basic issues, carelessness in abstracting and summarizing appropriate papers, failure to consider important covariates, bias on the part of the meta-analyst, and, perhaps most often, overstatements of the strength and precision of the results." In fact, Bailar claims that "it is not uncommon to find that two or more meta-analyses done at about the same time by investigators with the same access to the literature reach incompatible or even contradictory conclusions." These limitations, Bailar claims, restrict the ability of meta-analyses to summarize research data accurately.

In the face of Bailar (1997) and others' criticisms (Felson, 1992), researchers have been working to improve meta-analysis and restore some of its credibility. One example of such an initiative is the QUOROM statement. The QUOROM (Quality of Reporting of Meta-analyses) statement is very similar to the CONSORT statement, in that it aims to "improve the quality of reporting of meta-analyses of RCTs" and is directed at meta-analysts (Thomas C. Chalmers Centre, n.d.b).

Another heartening fact is that much of meta-analysis today is done on a computer (rather than by hand), limiting the potential for error. There are a number of computer programs that will do meta-analysis for you; web links to some of the more popular ones have been listed here. Readers can download the following samples and become familiar with them, and how they work:

→ *Review Manager (RevMan) 4.1*

www.cochrane.org/cochrane/revman.htm

→*Metaxis*

www.update-software.com/metaxis/metaxis-frame.html

→*EasyMA*

www.spc.univ-lyon1.fr/~mcu/easyma/index.htm

→*META (Meta-analysis Easy To Answer)*

http://nw3.nai.net/~dakenny/meta.htm

→Other Software Packages

www.prw.le.ac.uk/epidemio/personal/ajs22/meta/6pack.html

Conclusion

In conclusion, meta-analysis is without a doubt a powerful tool and at the heart of evidence-based practice. However, as has been discussed, it must be used with care, for it presents significant risks as well. Dr. Bailar (1997) concludes his editorial by writing, "we never know as much as we think we know," which seems a good warning to heed. We must be cautious as we proceed, but we must also recognize that meta-analysis is one of the best clinical tools we possess for confidently assessing clinical results.

THE COCHRANE COLLABORATION

Once systematic reviews and meta-analyses have been completed, what should practitioners do with them? Of course each practitioner will hold on to the studies he or she completes, but that number represents only a fraction of the number he or she will require to serve his or her clients well. Could the results of systematic reviews and meta-analyses from around the world somehow be brought together?

It was this question that inspired the creation of the Cochrane Collaboration. The collaboration is named after the British epidemiologist Archie Cochrane, who strongly advocated for the widespread use of systematic reviews to guide practice. It was Dr. Cochrane's belief that we need to change the way we provide health care because of the outpouring of health care information created each year. To resolve this problem, Dr. Cochrane proposed creating an organization that would conduct systematic reviews in all aspects of health care, and would act as a clearinghouse, distributing them worldwide.

Unfortunately, Dr. Cochrane died in 1988, 5 years before the creation of the collaboration that would take his name. At the founding of the Collaboration, inspiration was taken from Dr. Cochrane's words, when he wrote that, "it is surely a great criticism of our profession that we have not organized a critical summary, by specialty or subspecialty, adapted periodically, of all relevant RCTs" (University of Maryland, n.d.). The creation of the Cochrane Collaboration was also spurred on by the realization of a medical failure. Systematic reviews can help change health care practice. For example, the use of a corticosteroid drug for women having a premature birth can reduce the baby's complications by over 30%. This information was only put into practice after there had been multiple trials that were summarized in a systematic review. It was not until the systematic review that the effectiveness of this treatment became so apparent.

As such, the collaboration itself is based around the following 10 founding principles (Cochrane Collaboration, 2001b), which all members attempt to uphold in their work:

1. Collaboration
2. Building on the enthusiasm of individuals
3. Avoiding duplication
4. Minimizing bias
5. Keeping up to date
6. Ensuring relevance
7. Ensuring access
8. Continually improving the quality of its work
9. Continuity
10. Enabling wide participation

There are a number of tasks that the Cochrane Collaboration undertakes, but the main output of the Cochrane Collaboration is systematic reviews. In order to be able to speak competently in various specialties, the collaboration has created *Collaborative Review Groups* (CRGs). As the collaboration states, "the members of these groups—researchers, health care professionals, consumers, and others—share an interest in generating reliable, up-to-date evidence relevant to the prevention, treatment, and rehabilitation of particular health problems or groups of problems" (Cochrane Collaboration, 2001c). The CRGs are, in turn, advised by the *Methods Groups*, specialists in systematic reviews and meta-analyses who attempt to structure the reviews in an optimal way, through the creation of software such as RevMan (see Chapter 5). Furthermore, *Cochrane Fields/Networks* are groups that concentrate on broad dimensions of health care, not specific diagnoses, that may be relevant to the Cochrane Collaboration's work. Finally, the Cochrane Collaboration's presence is maintained worldwide through *Cochrane Centres* (there are currently 15), which fulfill a number of tasks, from raising awareness to conducting seminars and workshops, as well as serving as a local clearinghouse for the Cochrane Library.

The Cochrane Library itself is the mainstay of the Cochrane Collaboration and is comprised of a number of parts. First, the *Cochrane Controlled Trials Register (CCTR)* contains a collection of nearly 160,000 RCTs, which supply high quality evidence for systematic reviews. A second part of the library is the *Cochrane Database of Systematic Reviews (CDSR)*, which lists the Cochrane Collaboration's completed reviews and outlines of its reviews in progress (over 600 have been completed to date). The *Database of Abstracts of Reviews of Effectiveness (DARE)* also lists systematic reviews, but those which were undertaken and published outside of the Cochrane Collaboration. Finally, the *Cochrane Review*

Methodology Database (CRMD) provides information on the procedures, methods, and processes of EBP.

The Cochrane Library is available from a variety of sources, both online and on CD-ROM. Update Software publishes both the online and the software version of the library, and more information can be found at www.update-software.com/cochrane.

To find the Cochrane Centre in your area, consult the list of regional Cochrane Centre web sites at www.cochrane.org/cochrane/crgs.htm#CENTRES. The Cochrane Collaboration Brochure, from which much of the above information was found, is also on-line at www.cochrane.org/cochrane/cc-broch.htm. Finally, more information about the collaboration's structure and its goals for the future can be found in Alex Robinson's article in the *Canadian Medical Association Journal* (1995).

The Cochrane Collaboration represents a vast worldwide effort toward evidence-based practice, which will become more and more necessary as the volume of health care information grows while budgets shrink. The collaboration itself is the first step toward creating a more integrated, evidence-based network for drawing on the vast resources of the entire medical profession to serve clients.

The need to critically evaluate the available evidence constitutes an integral aspect to evidence-based practice. Through an understanding of the details of different types of studies and the corresponding factors, one can better address the search for evidence to incorporate into practice. This comprehension allows the evidence-based practitioner to better evaluate the evidence available in order to incorporate it into practice.

Take-Home Messages

Systematic Reviews
- Use scientific strategies to incorporate clinical trials done by different researchers on the same topic.
- There are various methodologies for preparing systematic reviews.
- Analyze RCTs with respect to methodological quality, precision, and external validity.
- All RCTs within the study will have some small error, but those studies with significant errors should be rejected.
- The CONSORT statement consists of checklists and flowcharts to help standardize the researcher report RCTs and to guard against methodological error.
- Systematic reviews should still be published even if there are no positive results.

Meta-Analysis
- Analysis of analyses; integrates findings from a large variety of individual studies to achieve a systematic review.
- Result portrayed in a "forest plot" diagram using confidence intervals.
- Meta-analysis often critiqued for publication bias and missing data.
- QUOROM statement attempts to improve the quality of reporting.
- Meta-analysis using computer analysis can greatly reduce the potential for error.

Cochrane Collaboration
- Database of systematic reviews and meta-analyses from around the world.
- Main output is systematic reviews; groups and databases address different practice areas.
- Represents an integrated evidence-based network that is accessible both on the Internet and CD-ROM.

Web Links

Update Software—The Cochrane Library
www.update-software.com/cochrane
Update Software publishes the Cochrane Library on CD-ROM, as well as maintaining a link to it from their site.

The Canadian Cochrane Centre
http://hiru.mcmaster.ca/cochrane/centres/Canadian
The Canadian Cochrane Centre is based at McMaster University in Hamilton, Ontario, and has a number of resources and contacts that will be of interest to Canadian practitioners.

Meta-analysis in Educational Research—An Overview
www.ericae.net/faqs/meta-analysis/meta-analysis.htm
A large file put together by the Educational Resources Information Center (ERIC), this page has links to a number of resources that cover many aspects of meta-analysis.

The CONSORT Statement
www.ama-assn.org/sci-pubs/journals/archive/jama/vol_276/no_8/sc6048x.htm (Article)
www.consort-statement.org (Homepage)
As mentioned in the chapter, the CONSORT statement lays out a number of guidelines for conducting good RCTs, which are essential for sound systematic reviews. The article is a link to the original *Journal of the American Medical Association* publication of the idea; the homepage has more detailed information and updates on current work.

Centre for Evidence-Based Medicine Levels of Evidence Classification
http://cebm.jr2.ox.ac.uk/docs/levels.html
This "levels of evidence" system was prepared by the UK-based Centre for Evidence-based Medicine. This system is even more detailed than those discussed in the chapter, breaking evidence up into letter grades and subcategories.

Randomised Controlled Trials
www.bmjpg.com/rct/contents.html
This web site includes information and the contents of Jadad's book, *Randomised Controlled Trials: A User's Guide.*

LEARNING AND EXPLORATION ACTIVITIES

The purpose of this chapter is to introduce students to different methods for systematically reviewing the evidence as well as demonstrating some of the appropriate tools with which to perform these evaluations.

1. Systematic Reviews
   a. Read through the systematic review methodologies listed, and explore them until you feel you have a good sense of the commonalties between all of them. Now, write a simple methodology in your own words. Compare this with those your fellow students have prepared. Where do they differ? Where are they similar? If possible, attempt as a group to merge all of your individual methodologies by consensus and produce a methodological statement that is distinctly your own. This will be helpful in understanding why reviews are structured as they are.
   b. Look briefly at the CONSORT statement (listed in Web Links). What are the important factors that a RCT must have? What makes a good RCT? What makes a poor RCT? Write a short paragraph answering these questions. Now, search for RCTs on a topic of interest (your best bet is to use MEDLINE) and find two or more. Examine each and assess its strengths and weaknesses. Which of the two is better? Why? Justify your answer.

2. Meta-Analysis
   a. Search on MEDLINE for meta-analysis on a topic of your choosing. Attempt to find more than one, and compare the results. Did they both reach the same conclusion? Why? Why not? What does this say about meta-analysis?

3. The Cochrane Collaboration
   a. Go online and find your local Cochrane Centre. Browse through the page and become familiar with its layout. Go to your local Health Sciences library and find out how to log onto the Cochrane Library from their computers. Search for systematic reviews on a topic of interest, and find out how to retrieve them. Continue working until you understand how the software functions and you are comfortable with its features.

REFERENCES

Bailar, J. C. (1997). The promise and problems of meta-analysis [Editorial]. *N Eng J Med, 337*(8), 559-561.

Begg, C., Cho, M., Eastwood, S., Horton, R., Moher, D., Olkin, I., et al. (1996). Improving the quality of reporting of randomized controlled trials: The CONSORT statement. *JAMA, 276*(8), 637-639.

British National Health Service. (n.d.). *Systematic reviews of trials and other studies.* Retrieved January 10, 2002, from http://www.prw.le.ac.uk/epidemio/personal/kral/srotos.html.

Cochrane Collaboration. (n.d.). *Guide to the format of a Cochrane review.* Retrieved January 10, 2002, from http://www.cochrane.uk/cochrane/handbook/hbookAPPENDIX_2A_GUIDE_TO_THE_FORMAT_.htm.

Cochrane Collaboration. (2001a). *Cochrane brochure.* Retrieved January 10, 2002, from http://www.cochrane.org/cochrane/cc-broch.htm.

Cochrane Collaboration. (2001b). *The ten principles of the Cochrane Collaboration.* Retrieved January 10, 2002, from http://www.cochrane.org/cochrane/cc-broch.htm#PRINCIPLES.

Cochrane Collaboration. (2001c). *Collaborative review groups.* Retrieved January 10, 2002, from http://www.cochrane.org/cochrane/cc-broch.htm#CRG.

Cook, M. D., Mulrow, C. D., & Haynes, R. B. (1997). Systematic reviews: Synthesis of best evidence for clinical decisions. *Ann Intern Med, 126*(5), 376-380.

Felson, D. T. (1992). Bias in meta-analytic research. *J Clin Epidemiol, 45*, 885-892.

Glass, G. V. (1976). Primary, secondary, and meta-analysis. *Educational Researcher, 5*(10), 3-8.

Greenhalgh, T. (1997a). *How to read a paper: The basics of evidence-based medicine.* London: BMJ Publishing Group.

Greenhalgh, T. (1997b). How to read a paper: Papers that summarize other papers. Systematic reviews and meta-analyses. *British Medical Journal, 315*(7109), 672-675. Retrieved January 10, 2002, from http://www.bmg.com/archive/7109/7109ed2.htm.

Hasselblad, V., & McCrory, D. C. (1995). Meta-analytic tools for medical decision making: A practical guide. *Med Decis Making, 15*, 81-96.

Jadad, A. R. (1998). *Randomised controlled trials: A user's guide.* London: BMJ Publishing Group.

Jadad, A. R., Cook, D. J., & Browman, G. P. (1997). A guide to interpreting discordant systematic reviews. *Canadian Medical Association Journal, 156*(10),1411-1416.

Lau, J., Ioannidis, J. P. A., & Schmid, C. H. (1997). Quantitative synthesis in systematic reviews. *Ann Intern Med, 127*(9), 820-826.

Robinson, A. (1995). Research, practice, and the Cochrane Collaboration. *Canadian Medical Association Journal, 152*(6), 883-889.

Thomas C. Chalmers Centre for Systematic Reviews. (n.d.a). *Why systematic reviews?* Retrieved January 10, 2002, from http://www.cheori.org/tcc/syst.htm.

Thomas C. Chalmers Centre for Systematic Reviews. (n.d.b). *QUOROM: Improving the quality of reporting of meta-analyses.* Retrieved January 10, 2002, from http://www.cheori.org/tcc/view-points/quorom.htm.

University of Maryland Complimentary Medicine Program. (n.d.). *The Cochrane Collaboration.* Retrieved January 10, 2002, from http://www.compmed.ummc.umaryland.edu/compmed/cochrane/collaboration/cochrane.htm.

University of York National Health Service Centre for Reviews and Dissemination. (2001). *Undertaking systematic reviews of research on effectiveness: CRD's guidance for those carrying out or commissioning reviews.* Retrieved January 10, 2002, from http://www.york.ac.uk/inst/crd/report.htm.

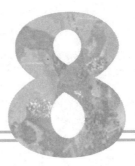

The Effectiveness of Cognitive-Behavioral Interventions with People with Chronic Pain

An Example of a Critical Review of the Literature

Debra Stewart, MSc, OT(C); Mary Law, PhD, OT(C);
Nancy Pollock, MSc, OT(C); Lori Letts, MA, OT(C);
Jackie Bosch, MSc, OT(C); Muriel Westmorland, MHSc;
and Angela Everett, BHSc(OT)

LEARNING OBJECTIVES

After reading this chapter, the student/practitioner will be able to:
- Understand the method for performing a critical review of the literature on a certain topic.
- Gain insight into the literature concerning cognitive-behaviour interventions for people with chronic pain.
- Understand how to critically analyze and validate the quality of a study.

BACKGROUND

A cognitive-behavioural approach is used widely in interdisciplinary settings with people with chronic pain (Keefe, Dunsmore, & Burnett, 1992; Turner & Chapman, 1982). Occupational therapists are usually part of the interdisciplinary team, and they are interested in evaluating the outcomes of their interventions. Increased emphasis on evidence-based practice in health care makes it essential for occupational therapists and other service providers to base their practice on best evidence.

Literature describing a cognitive-behavioural approach for people with chronic pain has grown in the past decade. It focuses on both behavioural and cognitive components of chronic pain, teaching people with chronic pain about the relation of pain to cognitive, affective, and physiological issues in order to help them reconceptualize their own ability to control pain. Cognitive-behavioural strategies teach skills that change the way people cope with pain on a daily basis. The approach is multimodal and usually includes treatment methods such as relaxation training, visual imagery, pacing, assertiveness training, and goal-setting, as well as practice and consolidation of coping skills through role-playing and other behavioural techniques (Kerns, Turk, & Holzman, 1983).

Research on the effectiveness of cognitive-behavioural intervention for people with chronic pain has increased as this approach has been incorporated into health care practice. Articles published in the early 1980s reported on laboratory pain studies and the evaluation of new multidisciplinary treatment programmes that included a cognitive-behavioural approach (Kerns et al., 1983; Turner & Chapman, 1982). In the past 10 years, outcome studies have compared the effectiveness of a cognitive-behavioural approach with other well-known treatments for people with chronic pain (Basler, 1993; Keefe et al., 1992; Scheer, Watanabe, & Radack, 1997). Two review articles published in the 1990s examined cognitive-behavioural interventions for patients with chronic pain from different perspectives. Basler (1993) analyzed treatment effects of a cognitive-behavioural group programme for people with different forms of rheumatic disease and found that pain reduction was greatest in patients with low back pain and least in ankylosing spondylitis. Scheer et al. (1997) reviewed 12 studies utilizing nonsurgical interventions for industrial low back pain, including cognitive-behavioural strategies, multidisciplinary pain clinics, exercise, and others. They concluded that most of the studies had methodological limitations and called for more rigorous research. Linssen and Spinhoven (1992) found similar methodological problems in their review of existing studies on the multimodal treatment of chronic pain.

Keefe et al. (1992) conducted an exploration of research advances and future directions in the area of behavioural and cognitive-behavioural interventions for chronic pain. They found that most outcome studies focused on comparing cognitive and behavioural interventions with control conditions or testing the relative efficacy of two treatment methods. They found that no one treatment approach had a consistent advantage over the other, and they suggested that further research is needed with larger populations and different chronic pain conditions.

No specific review of the effectiveness of cognitive-behavioural interventions alone for people with chronic pain was found in the literature. The need to critically review the research literature on the effectiveness of a cognitive-behavioural approach to chronic pain was thus identified.

OBJECTIVES

A critical review of the published literature was undertaken to determine the effectiveness of cognitive-behavioural interventions with people with chronic pain. Specifically, we were interested in the reported effectiveness of cognitive-behavioural interventions in improving outcomes of interest to therapists, namely occupational performance and/or performance components. Our primary question was:

→ What is the effectiveness of cognitive-behavioural interventions in improving occupational performance (function) for people with chronic pain?

A secondary question was:

→ What is the effectiveness of cognitive-behavioural interventions in improving performance components, environmental components, and/or pain-related outcomes for people with chronic pain?

MATERIALS AND METHODS

Criteria for Considering Studies for This Review

Types of Studies

The systematic review selected randomized and quasi-randomized clinical trials that involved cognitive-behavioural approaches and adults with chronic pain. Studies have been published in the literature since 1982 (when cognitive-behavioural approaches were first described in the literature).

The descriptive critical review (see Summary of Descriptive Review on p. 131) included all articles that reported a study of the effect of cognitive-behavioural approaches with adults with chronic pain. The study designs included randomized controlled trials, cohort, before-after, single case, cross-sectional, case control, and case study.

Types of Participants

→ Adults (ages 18 years and older)

→ Inpatient and outpatient

→ Chronic pain condition of at least 3 months' duration, usually identified by physician or rehabilitation team

→ Location of chronic pain can be in back, neck, upper or lower extremity, or as a result of a condition such as fibromyalgia, rheumatic disease (e.g., rheumatoid arthritis [RA]), whiplash, or headache

→ Participants with acute, subacute, or chronic pain due to cancer are not included

Types of Intervention

Cognitive-behavioural interventions are multimodal in nature and include at least three of the following modalities:

→ Relaxation

→ Stress management

→ Goal-setting/contracting

→ Self-monitoring/self-talking

→ Assertiveness training

→ Modeling

→ Imagery

→ Pacing

→ Family training

Intervention can be either inpatient or outpatient.

Unimodal interventions, or approaches that are behavioural or cognitive only (not combined) are not included. Biofeedback, hypnosis, or other physical modalities on their own are also not included. Articles that did not fully describe the treatment approach are not included.

Types of Outcomes

Outcomes should be clinically relevant to occupational therapists working with people with chronic pain. These outcomes include:

1. Occupational performance outcomes
   - → In general, such as participation in daily activities
   - → In specific areas of self-care, productivity, and/or leisure
2. Performance component areas
   - → Physical components
   - → Psychological components
   - → Cognitive components
   - → Pain-related behaviours and perceptions
3. Environmental component areas, including family/caregiver perspectives

Search Strategy for Identification of Studies

Search strategies followed recommended procedures in the *Cochrane Collaboration Handbook* (Mulrow & Oxman, 1997).

1. Computer search (e.g., electronic databases)
   - → Search of published literature using MEDLINE, CINAHL, abstracts, PsychLit, Social Sciences Index, or HealthStar for years 1966 to the present
   - → Review of Cochrane Library
2. Hand searching
   - → Review of bibliographies and databases on cognitive-behavioural approaches and chronic pain supplied by field experts
3. Citation review
   - → Review of all reference lists of retrieved articles
   - → Science citations review of all primary authors and studies included in this review from 1995 to present.

The search involved combining keywords related to cognitive-behavioural interventions with different conditions and chronic pain. Key words included the following:
- → Cognitive-behavioural therapy/intervention
- → Cognitive therapy/intervention
- → Behaviour therapy/intervention
- → Multimodal programs
- → Occupational therapy
- → Rehabilitation
- → Psychological factors
- → Chronic pain, pain
- → Back pain, neck pain, fibromyalgia, rheumatic disease

A final combination was done with the following text words:
- → Effectiveness, treatment outcomes, validity, reliability

SUMMARY OF DESCRIPTIVE REVIEW OF COGNITIVE-BEHAVIOURAL INTERVENTIONS WITH PEOPLE WITH CHRONIC PAIN

Altmaier, Lehmann, Russell, Weinstein, & Kao, 1992

Purpose

- To evaluate the effectiveness of a psychological intervention versus placebo control (physiology only) for patients with chronic low back pain

Design and Sample

- Randomized control trial (RCT) design, with patients randomly assigned to one of the programs. Evaluations conducted pretreatment, on discharge, and at 6-month follow-up
- N = 45 outpatients admitted to a low back pain inpatient rehabilitation program

Outcomes and Intervention

- Multiple outcomes evaluated, including "process" variables such as exercise endurance and confidence, and program outcomes on three levels: disability, self-reported pain, and life interference
- Inpatients assigned to either a placebo physiological regime (2x/day) or placebo plus operant conditioning, relaxation training, group and individual cognitive-behavioural (CB) training for 3 weeks duration

Results

- All patients showed improvements in outcome measures over time, but no statistically significant differences were found regarding improvements in functioning, return to work, or pain interference in either group. Sixty percent of patients in both groups returned to some form of employment
- Multiple outcomes were taken into account in the analysis

Conclusions and Implications

- Both interventions were found to be somewhat effective in improving patient functioning; however, no significant differences were found between physiological only and physiological plus CB strategies
- Short time period (3 weeks) may have influenced lack of significant results
- These findings were supported in other studies that found no significant differences in outcomes between different forms of treatment for chronic pain

Applebaum, Blanchard, Hickling, & Alfonso, 1988

Purpose

- To compare the relative efficacy of CB pain management with a symptom-monitoring control group for veterans with rheumatoid arthritis (RA)

Design and Sample

- RCT design, random assignment to either active treatment group or control group
- Evaluations conducted pre- and post-treatment and at 18-month follow-up
- N = 18 outpatients with RA, ranging from 1 to 39 years in duration

Outcomes and Interventions

- Outcomes included psychological function measured with a variety of standardized tools, pain intensity, arthritis symptoms, sleep patterns, and daily activities
- Outpatient programme for 6 weeks; 10 trials of progressive relaxation, 10 trials of biofeedback and CB pain management strategies, including self-monitoring, and problem solving. Symptom control group contacted once in 6 weeks

Results

- Statistically significant improvements noted in treated group in pain perception, control, coping, weekly pain ratings, total pain activity, and joint range of motion
- Only 10 of 18 subjects were assessed at the 18-month follow-up. No statistically significant differences were found between the groups

Conclusions and Implications

- Results found significant short-term improvements in pain perception and control, coping, and range of movement (ROM) in a group of people with severe RA. These findings were similar to other studies
- Limitations such as small sample size, multiple analyses, and large number of dropouts at follow-up make it difficult for therapists to have confidence in these findings

Basler, Jakle, & Kroner-Herwig, 1997

Purpose

- To evaluate the effect of cognitive-behavioral therapy (CBT) and medical care versus medical care only in patients with chronic low back pain

Design and Sample

- RCT design comparing two treatments
- Evaluations conducted pre- and post-treatment for both groups, and 6-month follow-up for CB group
- N = 76 patients with diagnosis of chronic low back pain; average duration of pain is 10 years

Outcomes and Interventions

- Outcomes included pain control, use of medication, coping, extent of disability, and loss of work days
- Patients in both groups received medical treatment, transcutaneous electrical nerve stimulation (TENS), and physical therapy. Patients in the CB group received additional education, relaxation, and CB strategies such as modifying thoughts and postural training. Treatment was provided for 12 sessions, in group format, 2.5 hours weekly

Results

- Statistically significant changes in pre-and post-treatment scores found in outcomes of pain intensity, control over pain, avoidance behaviour, pleasant activities, catastrophizing, social roles, physical functions, and mental performance
- Gains made in the CB group post-treatment were maintained at 6-month follow-up
- Number of work days lost decreased in the CB group at 6-month follow-up, but this could not be confirmed due to drop-outs

Conclusions and Implications

- Results indicate that a package of medical and CB treatments is more effective than medical treatment alone, particularly in areas of pain control, coping ability, and decreased disability
- Limitations existed in large number of drop-outs and inability to mask patients to treatment allocation
- Results are relevant for practitioners using CB approaches in combination with traditional medical treatment

Bradley et al., 1987

Purpose

- To evaluate the impact of one form of biofeedback-assisted CBT versus social support for people with RA

Design and Sample

- RCT design, pre-and post-treatment and 6-month follow-up evaluation of three treatment groups: two forms of group therapy and a control group receiving no adjunct treatment
- N = 53 (out of an initial 68) outpatients with RA with average duration of 11.5 years

Outcomes and Interventions

- Outcomes of anxiety, depression, pain intensity and pain behaviours, health locus of control, and physiological variables were assessed using a variety of self-report, behavioural, and physiologic measures
- Interventions were 15 sessions each: CB group therapy with biofeedback or structured social support group therapy

Results

- CBT group displayed significantly less pain behaviour, decreased pain intensity and unpleasantness, and decreased anxiety levels post-treatment. Anxiety reduction was maintained at 6-month follow-up
- Relaxation seemed to be the most important part of CBT clinically

Conclusions and Implications

- Short-term benefits of CBT demonstrated in areas of pain behaviour, intensity, and anxiety
- Identification of relaxation as most helpful strategy is important
- Questions raised regarding long-term benefits based on lack of maintenance of benefits on follow-up evaluation

Cinciripini & Floreen, 1982

Purpose

- To report on the outcomes of an inpatient behavioural program for the management of chronic pain

Design and Sample

- Before-after design; no control group
- Pre- and post-treatment and follow-up evaluations at 6 and 12 months postdischarge
- N = 121 inpatients of Pain Control Centre, variety of pain sites, at least 1 year's duration of pain

Outcomes and Intervention

- Several measures of verbal/nonverbal pain behaviour, use of medication, and physical functioning obtained through observation pre- and post-treatment and self-report at follow-up
- 4 week in-patient program included medication reduction, physiology, behavioural therapy, biofeedback, relaxation, self-monitoring, contracting, and family training

Results

- Over 90% of patients were free of all medication post-treatment. This reduced to 65% and 55% at 6- and 12-month follow-up, respectively
- Statistically significant differences found post-treatment in observations of verbal and nonverbal pain behaviours, physical fitness, exertion, and mobility
- Follow-up reports indicated that changes made in the desired direction were maintained

Conclusions and Implications

- Results are favourable for inpatient behavioural group program, but they are not conclusive due to lack of control group

- Multiple components of this treatment program make it difficult to determine which aspects may have resulted in the most benefit
- Lack of functional outcomes limits the applicability of study findings to OT practice

Cohen, Heinrich, Naliboff, Collins, & Bonebakker, 1983

Purpose
- To compare two outpatient group treatment methods for chronic low back pain

Design and Sample
- Before-after design, treatment-outcome study comparing two groups, no random assignment, no control group
- N = 25 outpatients with chronic low back pain of at least 6 months duration
- Evaluations pre- and post-treatment, no follow-up

Outcomes and Intervention
- Four domains of pain experience evaluated: physical abilities, physical functioning, psychological and psychosocial functioning, and pain intensity and perception
- Two group interventions compared: physical therapy (PT) treatment and behaviour therapy, which included relaxation, guided imagery, goal setting, activity management, problem solving, and assertiveness training. Each group had 10 sessions

Results
- Significant improvements found in both treatment groups in terms of less pain, less activity limitations from pain, less psychological distress, and satisfaction with treatment
- PT group demonstrated improved low back control but not generalization to daily activities. There was also a significant decrease in overall depression scores
- Behavioural group demonstrated a trend toward increasing social and physical activities, but it was not statistically significant

Conclusions and Implications
- Weak support found for the hypotheses that group treatment would have similar outcomes in four domains of pain experience; differential effects for each type of treatment were minimal in this study
- Methodological flaws weaken strength of conclusions; in particular, no control group and small sample size
- Limited application to practice due to methodological weaknesses

Corey, Etlin, & Miller, 1987

Purpose
- To evaluate a CB treatment program for people with chronic pain, conducted in their homes

Design and Sample

- Before-after design, program evaluation, no control group
- N = 72 subjects referred to one clinic; variety of diagnoses. All had not worked due to pain for a mean of 28 months
- Evaluations conducted before and immediately after treatment, and one follow-up, average 18 months after discharge

Outcomes and Intervention

- Outcomes focused on work status; pain reduction, functioning level, and coping ability were reported subjectively by subjects post-treatment and on follow-up
- CB programme included education about pain management, coping skills, stress management, exercise and lifestyle restructuring, behavioural techniques, medication reduction, and sleep scheduling techniques. In-home visits averaged 2x/week initially to 1x/month for 5 months

Results

- Seventy percent of subjects had returned to some form of work or retraining immediately after treatment and on follow-up
- Subjective reports of pain reduction indicated that subjects who returned to some form of work reported a mean percent of pain reduction of 32% to 79%, as well as a range of 27% to 77% increase in functioning and 27% to 82% increase in coping ability. In comparison, those subjects not working reported a range of 2.5% to 11% pain reduction, 3% to 7% functioning increase, and 6% to 8% increase in coping

Conclusions and Implications

- Outcomes indicate positive benefits of a CB programme for people with chronic pain
- Results are not conclusive due to weak methodology and no control group
- Self-report measures were found to be highly associated with a more objective measure of functioning-work status
- Strengths of programme are worthy of therapists attention: home setting, involvement of families, individualized treatment, and focus on activity

Edelson & Fitzpatrick, 1989

Purpose

- To examine the effectiveness of CBT and hypnosis versus attention control for people with chronic pain

Design and Sample

- Weak RCT design: assignment to three treatment groups was done sequentially as patients were referred
- Evaluations were conducted pre- and post-treatment and 1 month after treatment
- N = 27 males with chronic pain (minimum 6 months) at multiple sites: 24 outpatients, three inpatients

Outcomes and Intervention

- Outcomes focused on two categories of pain behaviour: overt motor behaviour (activities) and cognitive-verbal behaviour
- CBT included self-instruction, education, imagery, and self-talk. Hypnosis presented same information after a standard hypnotic induction. Control group received attention through nondirective therapy
- Both groups lasted 2 weeks for a total of four sessions

Results

- Statistically significant differences were found in two areas: amount of walking/standing and amount of sitting for subjects in the CB group. Differences were sustained at 1-month follow-up
- No statistically significant differences were found in pain intensity or pain rating in treatment groups, but trends favoured the CB group for pain intensity and the hypnosis group for pain rating

Conclusions and Implications

- Results show weak support for CBT improving activity levels of people with chronic pain
- Small sample size may have limited power to detect change in more subjective pain behaviours
- Limited application to therapists as we are not involved with hypnosis

Flor & Birbaumer, 1993

Purpose

- To compare three types of treatments for chronic musculoskeletal pain (low back pain and temporomandibular [TMJ] joint pain)

Design and Sample

- Before-after design comparing efficacy of three different treatments
- N = 78 outpatients with chronic (more than 6 months duration) low back pain or TMJ pain assigned to one of three treatment groups
- Evaluations conducted pre- and post-treatment and 6- and 24-month follow-up

Outcomes and Intervention

- Outcome measures were organized into three main areas: verbal-subjective, behavioural, and psychophysiological outcomes
- Three types of treatment:
  1. Electromyogram (EMG) biofeedback: eight 60 minute sessions with homework exercises
  2. CBT sessions, same number as EMG, including pain and stress management, relaxation, problem solving, and coping skills

3. Medical (MED) intervention of variable duration, including medication, chiro-
   practy, nerve blocks, etc.

Results

- Statistically significant improvements noted post-treatment in verbal-subjective areas
  of pain severity, catastrophizing pain, and activity interference for the EMG group
  compared to subjects in CBT or MED groups; follow-up scores at 6 and 24 months
  showed improvements were more pronounced in pain severity and activity interference in EMG group. Coping skills and life control scores were significantly lower in
  the EMG group. Number of health care visits was significantly lower for subjects in
  the EMG group only at 24 months follow-up

Conclusions and Implications

- Results demonstrated that EMG biofeedback may be a superior treatment for people
  with mild chronic musculoskeletal pain. EMG treatment included a stress management component in this study, which may have influenced outcome. CBT treatment
  was found to be only marginally efficacious, which could be related to the short duration of treatment. Limitations included large number of outcome measures and the
  fact that assessors were not masked
- Most noticeable treatment effects were found at 6- and 24-month follow-ups, which
  support the evaluation of long-term benefits

Heinrich, Cohen, Naliboff, Collins, & Bonebakker, 1985

Purpose

- To study the impact of behaviour and PT on different components of chronic low
  back pain

Design and Sample

- Before-after design, treatment-outcome study comparing two types of treatment. No
  control group
- Evaluations completed pre- and post-treatment and follow-up times of 6 months and
  1 year
- N = 33 patients with chronic low back pain (duration of 6 months or more) referred
  to clinic assigned to treatment group by order of entry

Outcomes and Intervention

- Outcomes focused on four areas of functioning: physical abilities, current physical
  functioning, psychological and psychosocial functioning, and pain intensity and pain
  perception
- Treatments conducted in group outpatient setting for 10 weekly sessions. Behaviour
  therapy utilized education and training in self-responsibility, personal effectiveness,
  pain control, goal setting, and activity management

Results

- Statistically significant improvements found in both treatment groups in pain ratings, depression, and anxiety at post-treatment and 6-month evaluations. Overall ratings of improvement on the post-treatment interview were similar for the two groups
- PT group improved in low back control on post-treatment and 6-month evaluations and in back protection manouevre at post-treatment time only

Conclusions and Implications

- Results indicate that PT increases low back control and back protection techniques. No advantage was found in behaviour therapy over physical therapy on psychosocial measures, as both groups showed improvements. Group format may have had a positive influence
- Results not conclusive due to lack of control group and small sample size. Limited application to practice

Jensen, Dahlquist, Nygren, Royen, & Stenberg, 1997

Purpose

- To evaluate whether a CB treatment designed specifically for women with chronic spinal pain is more effective than a regular CB approach

Design and Sample

- RCT design comparing two treatment groups
- Evaluations conducted pretreatment, immediate post-treatment, and 6- and 18-month follow-up
- N = 54 women with nonspecific spinal pain that is chronic in nature

Outcomes and Intervention

- Variety of outcomes including sick leave, pain intensity/anxiety, depression, perceived helplessness, coping strategies, and disability rating
- Regular multimodal cognitive-behavioural treatment (MMCBT) using a team approach included exercise, education, problem solving, relaxation, goal setting, and self-efficacy training. Gender-specific program had added component of psychologist-led group sessions focusing on gender-specific behaviour. Both treatments were inpatient, 5 weeks in duration, 8 hours per day

Results

- The only statistically significant difference between the groups was in the level of disability, with the experimental group showing a decrease compared with regular treatment. Some significant differences were seen in depression at the 6-month follow-up only. These gains were not maintained at 18-months, and there were no significant differences in sick leave or overall health and well-being

Conclusions and Implications

- Results were inconclusive due to low power of study and small sample size
- Results did not support the development of a gender-specific MMCBT programme
- No OT was involved in the team approach; therefore, direct implications for are limited

Kerns, 1986

Purpose

- To investigate the clinical efficacy of behavioural and CB treatments for outpatients with chronic pain

Design and Sample

- RCT design with two treatment conditions and one waiting list control condition
- Evaluations conducted pre- and post-treatment and at 3- and 6-month follow-ups
- N = 28 outpatients with different types of chronic pain of at least 6 months duration

Outcomes and Intervention

- Multidimensional outcomes of pain experience, including pain intensity, impact of activities, depression, anxiety, health locus of control, as well as use of health care system and individualized treatment goals
- Subjects randomized to one of three groups: CBT, behavioural treatment, or waiting list control. Each group lasted 10 weeks

Results

- Statistically significant improvement found in the CB group for all four components of pain measures: affective distress, pain severity, activities, and dependency, as well as an overall improvement in this group at post-treatment and 3-month follow-up. Marginal improvement maintained at 6-month follow-up. No significant effect found for behavioural group at any time

Conclusions and Implications

- Improvements demonstrated in outpatients receiving CBT on a set of multidimensional variables relevant to pain, including severity, affective state, activities, and dependency. These improvements were maintained over a short term (3 months)
- Generalizability of results are limited due to small sample size and drop-outs
- Results are applicable to therapists working with people with chronic pain

Newton-John, Spence, & Schotte, 1995

Purpose

- To determine the efficacy of CBT versus EMG biofeedback in the treatment of chronic low back pain

Design and Sample

- Before-after design; subjects assigned to either CBT or EMG biofeedback
- N = 44 convenience sample, chronic low back pain of more than 6 months duration

Outcomes and Intervention

- Multiple outcomes organized into two main areas: pain-related outcomes and mood-related outcomes. Seven different measures were used
- Group treatment for both forms of intervention, eight 1-hour sessions twice a week. CBT included education, goal setting, activity scheduling, relaxation, and cognitive restructuring techniques. Wait list control group

Results

- Statistically significant improvements found for both types of treatment (vs. wait list control) in outcomes of pain intensity, perceived level of disability, and depression immediately after treatment and at 6-month follow-up. Decreased anxiety and increased coping skills noted but not statistically significant. No differences were found between the two types of treatment

Conclusions and Implications

- Results indicate both forms of treatment (CBT and EMG biofeedback) can be efficacious in reducing pain intensity, perceived level of disability, and depression
- Results are not generalizable to other populations due to small sample size

Nicholas, Wilson, & Goyen, 1991

Purpose

- To examine the relative efficacy of operant-behavioural versus CB group treatments, with and without relaxation, compared with two control conditions

Design and Sample

- RCT design: assignment to one of six experimental conditions—four treatment groups and two control groups
- Six conditions x four trials
- Repeated measurements at pre- and post-treatment and 6- and 12-months
- N = 58 patients from pain clinic, chronic back pain at least 6 months

Outcomes and Intervention

- Outcomes included pain rating, anxiety and depression, pain beliefs, coping strategy, health status, medication intake, and follow-up evaluation of treatments
- Four treatment groups (5 weeks each): CB with and without relaxation, operant-behavioural with and without relaxation. Two control conditions: with and without attention (discussion group). All groups received physiology

Results

- Statistically significant improvements in all treatment groups on measures of affective distress, functional health status, medication use, pain-related dysfunction, and coping were maintained at 6- and 12-month follow-ups
- Operant-behavioural group improved more on self-reported Sickness Impact Profile, but this was not maintained at 6- and 12-month follow-ups
- Relaxation added little to overall benefit

Conclusions and Implications

- Results lend support to the use of both types of treatment with relaxation for patients with chronic low back pain. Similar findings to other studies using the Sickness Impact Profile as outcome measure
- Problems with drop-outs limit confidence in findings
- Interesting results for therapists using a variety of CB treatment modalities

Nielson, Walker, & McCain, 1992

Purpose

- To evaluate the efficacy of inpatient CB treatment for persons with fibromyalgia syndrome (duration not specified)

Design and Sample

- Before-after design, "quasi-experimental" programme evaluation
- Subjects acted as own wait list controls; assessed at two time intervals before entering treatment, 5 months apart, then post-treatment
- N = 25 patients consecutively selected from outpatient department

Outcomes and Intervention

- Multidimensional outcome measures of pain and psychosocial functioning were divided into "target" (expected to change with treatment) and "nontarget" (not expected to change) to assess potential demand characteristics
- In-patient CB programme ran for 3 weeks and included relaxation training, cognitive techniques, exercises, pacing, and family education

Results

- No changes were found in either the target or nontarget response measures during the 5-month wait list period
- Comparison of pre- and post-test scores indicated that the target variables, but not the nontarget variables, changed in the expected direction (statistical significance achieved). Target variables were pain severity, perceived interference with life, sense of control over pain, emotional distress, and pain behaviours

Conclusions and Implications

- Encouraging results demonstrated significant improvement in targeted pain behaviours and psychosocial function for people receiving CBT on an inpatient basis
- Limited generalizability due to small sample size and short time frame
- Findings relevant to therapists working on inpatient programmes

O'Leary, Shoor, Lorig, & Holman, 1988

Purpose

- To evaluate the effects of a CB treatment on pain, physical function, other arthritis outcome variables, and immune function for people with RA

Design and Sample

- RCT design treatment group and control group
- Evaluations conducted pre- and post-treatment, no follow-up
- N = 30 female patients with RA (average duration 8 years) matched in pairs by pain level and medication and randomly assigned to treatment or control group

Outcomes and Intervention

- Multiple outcome measures used to evaluate arthritis outcomes; self-efficacy to manage pain, psychological functioning, and immunological assays
- CB treatment took place in groups for 5 weeks. Treatment included pain-management strategies and goal setting, with self-reward to increase activity. Both groups received a copy of *The Arthritis Handbook*

Results

- Statistically significant improvements found in the treatment group in pain intensity, joint impairment, self-efficacy to manage pain, and other effects of arthritis. Treatment group also reported less depression and increased coping but not statistically significant. Immunological rates did not change
- Significant relationships found between higher levels of perceived self-efficacy and pain reduction, increased coping, and reduced joint impairment

Conclusions and Implications

- Significant improvements in pain perception and perceived self-efficacy to manage pain and other arthritis symptoms were achieved in a CB treatment programme
- Inter-relationships found between self-efficacy, pain levels, psychosocial functioning, and joint impairment
- Large number of measures reduces confidence in results
- Results, in particular information about perceived self-efficacy, of interest to OTs

Parker et al., 1988

Purpose

- To examine the effectiveness of a CB pain management programme for people (veterans) with RA

Design and Sample

- RCT design, random assignment to one of three groups: CB treatment, attention-placebo group, and control group
- Measurements at baseline, 6- and 12-months post-treatment
- N = 83 patients of a veterans hospital with RA

Outcomes and Intervention

- Variety of outcomes included pain perception, coping, depression, and other affective variables; arthritis status; impact; and helplessness
- Treatment was 1 week hospital stay with education, information, coping strategies, problem solving, relaxation, attention diversion; outpatient support programme with visits every 1 to 3 months for 1 year
- Attention-placebo group received basic education program on in- and outpatient basis for 1 year

Results

- The group receiving the CB programme improved significantly in pain coping scores at 6-month follow-up, in particular, diverting attention from pain, catastrophizing pain less, increased control over pain, and ability to decrease pain. Improvements showed greater statistical significance at 12-month follow-up
- No other measures showed statistical significance

Conclusions and Implications

- For this sample of people with RA, a CB programme demonstrated significant improvements (maintained over the long-term) in pain coping variables, but not in psychosocial variables
- Subjects with high adherence to programme regime demonstrated the most significant improvements, which is important information

Philips, 1987

Purpose

- To evaluate the impact of an outpatient behavioural treatment program on people with diverse chronic pain problems

Design and Sample

- RCT design, treatment group and wait list control group, evaluated pre- and post-treatment and at 2- and 12-month follow-up points

- N = 40 outpatients with diverse chronic pain problems of duration between 2 and 30 years

Outcomes and Intervention

- Outcomes focused on pain behaviour and impact of pain on daily functioning (subjective experience), plus patient and therapist perceptions of treatment effects
- Behavioural therapy conducted in groups of five to seven people for 9 weeks. Strategies included relaxation, graded increase in exercise and physical fitness, graded reduction of medications, increased control over pain episodes, activity pacing, anxiety management, and mood control

Results

- Statistically significant changes in all measures except behavioural complaint in the treatment group, with no changes found in the control group at post-treatment. Strongest effects occurred in affective components, depression, and reduction in avoidance behaviour. Improvements were sustained at 2-month follow-up and more pronounced at 12 months
- Medication use was significantly reduced immediately post-treatment, but this was not maintained at follow-up

Conclusions and Implications

- Self-designed study demonstrated significant improvements in self-efficacy and control over pain for people involved in an outpatient behavioural therapy group. The nature of improvements was analyzed in terms of affective reaction to pain, reduced depression, and avoidance behaviour. These changes appear to influence long-term attitudes toward pain
- Findings important for therapists working with people with chronic pain

Richardson, Richardson, Williams, Featherstone, & Harding, 1994

Purpose

- To examine the effectiveness of CB pain management course on employment status and quality of work

Design and Sample

- Before-after design, program evaluation
- Measurements at pre- and post-treatment and at 6- and 12-month follow-up
- N = 109 patients with chronic pain, average 10 years duration, variety of pain sites
- Classified as workers (26% at beginning of study) and nonworkers (74%)

Outcomes and Intervention

- Employment outcomes included changes in work status and quality of work. Other measures included Sickness Impact Profile, Depression Inventory, State-Trait Anxiety Inventory, Pain Self-Efficacy Questionnaire, and Pain Inventory and Rating Scale
- Inpatient programme, 4 weeks, using CB strategies, exercises, and relaxation

Results

- Significant improvement found in depression, confidence, pain-related distress, and overall impact of pain in "workers" group. No significant change noted in anxiety, pain intensity, or walking
- Work status fluctuated, but there was a trend (32% increase overall) toward employment

Conclusions and Implications

- Findings support benefits of one programme in terms of affective state, pain distress, and impact on activities; however, impact on work status was variable
- Positive changes were noted in most measures of impairment from pre- to post-treatment, but results must be interpreted with caution as there was no control group and multiple outcomes

Skinner et al., 1990

Purpose

- To investigate the efficacy of an inpatient CB program for patients with chronic pain

Design and Sample

- Before-after design, program evaluation
- One-group repeated measures: twice pretreatment, immediate post-treatment, and 1-month follow-up
- N = 34 outpatients with a variety of chronic pain conditions of minimum 1 year duration

Outcomes and Intervention

- Variety of outcomes including depression, anxiety, pain responsibility, pain response, locus of control, and medication use
- Outpatient program, 7 weeks, included coping skills, goal setting, relaxation, and exercises

Results

- Significant changes after treatment found in measures of medication use, anxiety, depression, physical disability, and coping skills. No changes noted in pain intensity
- Patients showed no significant change during baseline pretreatment period, supporting the treatment programme's effects

Conclusions and Implications

- Study supports benefits of an outpatient programme on affective state and coping skills for people with chronic pain. Similar findings to inpatient programme studies, demonstrating that outpatient services may be equally effective
- Lack of control group limits confidence in findings

Spence, 1989

Purpose

- To investigate the effectiveness of group versus individual CBT for people with chronic, work-related upper limb pain

Design and Sample

- RCT design: subjects allocated to one of three groups: individual CBT, group CBT, or wait list control group
- Repeated measures evaluation pre- and post-treatment and 6-month follow-up
- N = 45 outpatients with chronic pain (more than 6 months) in the upper limb; 44/45 females; work-related injuries

Outcomes and Intervention

- Variety of pain-related and psychological outcomes including depression, anxiety, coping strategies, pain ratings, and sickness impact
- Nine-week programme, either group or individual sessions each 1.5 hours per week. Major components were goal setting, cognitive restructuring, coping skills and pain management, assertion skills training, and relaxation

Results

- Subjects in both group and individual CBT showed statistically significant improvements on all outcome measures, with little difference between the three types of treatment. Wait list controls showed no improvement. Therapy gains were maintained at 6-month follow-up, with no statistically significant differences between the types of treatment
- Client evaluation ratings favoured individual CBT treatment

Conclusions and Implications

- Results indicate that CBT intervention is better than no intervention for people with chronic work-related upper limb pain in psychological and pain-related outcomes
- Individual treatment was preferred by clients, but benefits of individual treatment versus group treatment were the same statistically in outcome measures

Spence, 1991

Purpose

- 2-year follow-up study to previous research comparing the effectiveness of group versus individual CBT for chronic, work-related upper limb pain

Design and Sample

- Same RCT design and sample as previous study
- 2-year follow-up evaluation
- N = 19 of the original 45 subjects involved in first study

Outcomes and Intervention

- Same outcome measures as previous study
- Follow-up evaluation of group versus individual CBT versus wait list control

Results

- Statistically significant improvements in depression, coping, sickness impact, pain index, and distress. Some relapse was found from post-treatment levels in scores of positive coping strategies
- Minimal differences were found between individual and group CBT: group CBT showed continued improvement in self-reported pain and activity interference, but individual CBT did not

Conclusions and Implications

- Long-term benefits of CBT found for people with chronic, work-related upper limb pain, as psychopathology was reduced and coping abilities enhanced. Very few subjects reported being pain-free
- Group CBT was found to be as effective as individual CBT and more cost-effective

Turner, 1982

Purpose

- To evaluate the effectiveness of group progressive-relaxation versus CB group therapy for people with chronic low back pain

Design and Sample

- RCT design, assignment to one of three conditions: relaxation group alone, relaxation with CB group therapy, or control group
- Measurements pre- and post-treatment and at 1-month and 2-year follow-up by mail
- N = 34 outpatients with chronic low back pain, 6 months or more duration

Outcomes and Intervention

- Outcomes included physical and psychosocial dysfunction, medication use, depression, pain severity, self-ratings of improvement. Two-year follow-up by mail focused on work status, health services use, medication, and pain severity
- Five weekly sessions with five to seven patients per group:
  1. Progressive-relaxation alone
  2. Relaxation with CB strategies
  3. Wait list control with weekly phone call

Results

- Both treatment groups showed statistically significant improvement in depression, physical and psychological functioning, and pain rating. CB group also improved significantly on daily pain ratings and pain tolerance and showed continued improvement on all measures at 1-month follow-up
- Decreased health care use in both groups at 2-year follow-up

Conclusions and Implications

- Evidence provided that both types of treatment result in improvement in physical and psychological function, depression, and perception of pain. CB treatment demonstrates long-term benefits for people with mild, chronic low back pain
- Study supports use of CB and relaxation therapy in an outpatient group format, although sample size was small

Turner & Clancy, 1988

Purpose

- To evaluate and compare operant-behavioural and CB approaches for the treatment of chronic low back pain

Design and Sample

- RCT design, assignment to one of two treatment groups or a control group
- Repeated measures pre- and post-treatment and at 6- and 12-month follow-up
- N = 81 subjects with chronic low back pain for more than 6 months duration

Outcomes and Intervention

- Outcome measures included Pain Questionnaire, videotapes of pain behaviours, pain behaviour checklist, Sickness Impact Profile, and Cognitive Errors Questionnaire
- Outpatient treatment groups run 1x/week for 8 weeks: operant-behavioural or CB approaches. Control group on wait list

Results

- Statistically significant improvements on Sickness Impact Profile, cognitive errors, and pain behaviours in both treatment groups. Improvement was greater in operant-behavioural group immediately post-treatment, but CB group continued to improve at 6- and 12-month follow-up to even out. CB group was more satisfied with treatment

Conclusions and Implications

- Both types of behavioural treatment resulted in short and long-term improvement in multiple aspects of chronic pain
- Patterns of improvement varied with operant-behavioural treatment, showing immediate improvement, and CB, showing steady improvement over time
- Well-designed study supports both types of treatment for people with mild low back pain

Turner & Jensen, 1993

Purpose

- To study the effects of outpatient group cognitive therapy, relaxation training, and combined cognitive and relaxation therapy for people with chronic low back pain

Design and Sample

- RCT design of three treatment conditions (relaxation alone, cognitive alone, combined relaxation and cognitive therapies) and one control (wait list) condition
- Repeated measures pre- and post-treatment and at 6- and 12-month follow-up
- N = 102 outpatients with low back pain of more than 6 months duration

Outcomes and Intervention

- Four main outcomes: pain intensity, sickness impact (physical and psychological functioning), depression, cognitive errors; and one process measure using videotapes of pain behaviours
- Group treatments weekly for 6 weeks, Five to 10 patients per group:
  1. Relaxation training group
  2. Cognitive therapy
  3. Combined cognitive/relaxation training. Control group on wait list

Results

- Subjects in all three treatment groups improved significantly in self-reported pain intensity and showed decreases in cognitive errors. These improvements were maintained at 6- and 12-month follow-up. Other outcome measures did not show any statistically significant differences

Conclusions and Implications

- Results provide some evidence that cognitive therapy and relaxation training are equally effective in reducing pain
- Insufficient power in this study may have resulted in lack of detection of differences in other outcomes
- Results support group treatment format for therapists working with patients with chronic pain

White & Nielson, 1995

Purpose

- Follow-up study to previous research on short-term effects of CB treatment with persons with fibromyalgia (see Nielson, Walker, & McCain, 1992)

Design and Sample

- Quasi-experimental design, repeat of earlier study with 25 inpatients with fibromyalgia
- Follow-up evaluation at a mean of 30 months after discharge

Outcomes and Intervention

- Same "target" and "nontarget" outcomes as first study. Target outcomes (variables that the program addressed) included pain severity, control, activity interference, emotional/affective status, and observed pain behaviour
- Same treatment programme as previous study

Results

- Three out of 10 target variables remained statistically different from pretreatment: worry, observed pain behaviour, and control over pain. All other target variables changed in the direction of improvement but were not statistically significant
- Nontarget variables did not show any significant difference, as expected

Conclusions and Implications

- Improvements found at follow-up support a CB approach for people with fibromyalgia
- Limitations included small sample size, no control group, and cointervention of medication use. Results are not generalizable based on these limitations, but they do show promise

Williams et al., 1993

Purpose

- To evaluate an inpatient CB programme for patients with chronic pain

Design and Sample

- Prospective, longitudinal study using a before-after design
- Evaluation conducted pretreatment and 1 and 6 months after treatment
- N = 212 inpatients with a variety of chronic pain conditions, mean duration 10.5 years

Outcomes and Intervention

- Outcome measures included pain rating scale, pain self-efficacy scale, Sickness Impact Profile, Beck Depression Inventory, mobility activities, and medication use log
- Inpatient programme run for 4 weeks. Components included teaching behavioural and cognitive skills, goal setting and pacing, relaxation, exercise, and medication reduction

Results

- Statistically significant improvements found at 1- and 6-month follow-up times in mean scores of psychological dysfunction, depression, fitness, pain self-efficacy, and pain distress. No significant change in pain intensity. High percentage of subjects reduced medication use

Conclusions and Implications

- Improvements found in physical and psychological functions after an inpatient CB programme
- No definite conclusions can be made due to lack of control group, but findings are positive and similar to other studies
- Findings are relevant to therapists working with people with chronic pain on an inpatient basis

Young, Bradley, & Turner, 1995

Purpose

- To report on the efficacy of a CB intervention in reducing the number of RA-related clinic visits and days hospitalized over an 18-month period

Design and Sample

- Follow-up to an earlier study (see Bradley et al., 1987) that compared CB treatment with social support (SS) group treatment or no treatment (control). RCT design used in original study
- N = 53 patients with RA involved in original study; unclear if there were any drop-outs for this follow-up part

Outcomes and Intervention

- Health care resource utilization was evaluated through a review of financial records from the local hospital and outpatient clinic. Measures included duration of inpatient admission for RA, charges associated with hospitalization, number of outpatient visits related to RA, and clinic charges associated with each clinic visit. The unit of time was 6 months before treatment, 6 months immediately following treatment, and 7 to 12 months after treatment

Results

- Patients in the CB group had 13.1% fewer clinic visits than patients in either the social support or control groups. Clinic charges were reduced by 16.9% in the CB group compared with a 2.0% reduction in the SS group and a 17.5% increase in the control group
- Relative reductions in inpatient hospital days were also found in the CB group (-72.3%) compared with the SS (-28.3%) or control (+3.9%) groups. CB group inpatient charges declined progressively over the 12-month follow-up

Conclusions and Implications

- This follow-up study indicates that participation in a CB intervention is associated with reduction in health care resource utilization, and costs. These results are clinically significant, however statistical significance was not established
- Cost-benefit analysis of CB treatment demonstrated economic benefits of this approach

Methods of the Reviews

Article Selection

Lists of articles from the literature search were reviewed by two researchers for possible inclusion. Abstracts of articles were reviewed using the inclusion and exclusion criteria (above).

Data Abstraction

Those articles that met the inclusion criteria were reviewed using forms and guidelines developed by the McMaster University Occupational Therapy Evidence-Based Practice Research Group for critical appraisal of quantitative literature (Law et al., 1998). Data were descriptive and narrative in nature and focused on the clinical relevance and quality of the study.

Six researchers reviewed articles in the initial phase, using the forms and guidelines, until they were in 75% agreement. After this, one researcher completed the review. A systematic review of articles that were experimental (RCT or quasi-experimental) in design was then conducted using guidelines for the preparation of a systematic review from the Cochrane Collaboration. A data collection form was developed specifically for this review to ensure that the data were extracted accurately from each article. Agreement of 75% was reached between two researchers for this form, with one researcher completing the data collection after the agreement was reached.

Data Analysis

1. The descriptive review of the studies was outlined in table form and summarizes the important clinical and methodological issues for occupational therapists (see Summary of Descriptive Review).
2. The data from the systematic review was entered into RevMan (Review Manager) software (Cochrane Collaboration, 1998). This software summarized the results of the individual articles into two main tables:
   - → A description of the key characteristics of the included studies (see Characteristics of Included Studies on p. 154)
   - → A table of comparisons of the key outcomes of the studies (Table 8-1 on p. 162)

Description of Studies

Studies included in this systematic review were randomized controlled trials or quasi-experimental in design. Sufficient data were reported in the article for RevMan analysis. Of the 29 potential articles from the descriptive critical review, 10 were selected for this systematic review.

Methodological Quality of Included Studies

Study quality was assessed using a quality scale developed by Jadad et al. (1996). The main components of the quality scale were the following:
- → Allocation concealment, which was judged as adequate, possibly adequate, and inadequate
- → Study design, which was randomized or nonrandomized
- → Masking of subject, assessor, and provider
- → Drop-outs/withdrawals reported

An overall quality score was assigned for each article selected for the systematic review.

Results

Literature Search

The first round of searching using electronic databases found over 1,500 titles with the main key words related to interventions and conditions used. Application of the inclusion and

CHARACTERISTICS OF INCLUDED STUDIES OF THE EFFECTIVENESS OF COGNITIVE-BEHAVIORAL INTERVENTIONS WITH PEOPLE WITH CHRONIC PAIN

Altmaier et al., 1992

Method

- Randomized controlled trial (RCT)
- Allocation concealment not described
- Subjects and providers not masked to group assignment
- Assessor masking unclear
- Drop-outs were reported

Participants

- N = 45 adults
- Age range was 25 to 58 years; mean age = 40 years
- 33 males and 12 females
- Inpatients of one rehabilitation program
- Low back pain with duration ranging from 3 to 30 months
- Two groups were equivalent on initial outcome measure scores and demographics using chi square and t-tests

Interventions

- Standard inpatient program included physiotherapy, fitness training, education, and vocational rehabilitation
- Additional psychological program included cognitive-behavioral interventions of operant conditioning, relaxation, biofeedback, and coping strategies
- Individual and group formats
- Three-week inpatient program, daily treatment

Outcomes

- Pre- and post-treatment and 6-month follow-up
- Pain intensity measured by the McGill Pain Questionnaire (MPQ) (PPI part)
- Pain perception measured by the MPQ (PPI part)
- Control measured by the self-control subscale of the West Haven Yale Multidimensional Pain Inventory (WHYMPI)
- Activity level measured by the WHYMPI
- Physical abilities measured the Low Back Pain (LBP) Rating Scale
- Return to full- or part-time employment measured by the self-report

Notes

- 45 out of the 47 subjects completed the study. No control group was available for follow-up evaluation

Applebaum et al., 1988

Method

- RCT
- Allocation concealment not described
- Subjects and providers not masked
- Assessor masking was unclear
- Drop-outs were reported

Participants

- N = 18 participants
- Age range was 43 to 76 years
- 16 male and 2 female
- Outpatients of a veterans hospital with stages II and III rheumatoid arthritis (RA) with a duration of 1 to 39 years
- Two groups were equivalent on demographics except treatment group had longer duration of RA (mean = 20 years vs. 9.3 years for control group)

Interventions

- Active treatment included cognitive pain management strategies, relaxation training, and biofeedback
- Individual treatment format with homework
- Symptom monitoring used diary
- Six week duration; 10 trials for active treatment

Outcomes

- Pre- and post-treatment and 18-month follow-up
- Pain intensity measured by a weekly diary, rating scale
- Pain behaviors and perception measured by the MPQ
- Anxiety measured by the State-Trait Anxiety Inventory
- Depression measured by the Beck Depression Inventory
- Activity level measured by the Daily Activities Questionnaire
- Control measured by the Response to Arthritis and Pain Questionnaire
- Physical abilities measured by the PT Assessment
- Sleep measured by sleep indices

Notes

- Only 10 out of the 18 subjects were available for follow-up (six treatment and four control). There were insufficient data (no standard deviation scores) at follow-up for analysis

Basler, Jakle, & Kroner-Herwig, 1997

Method

- RCT
- Allocation concealment not described
- Masking unclear
- Drop-outs were reported

Participants

- N = 76
- Outpatients with chronic low back pain
- 25% were male; mean age = 49.3 years

Interventions

- Cognitive-behavioral group treatment
- Twelve sessions included education, relaxation, modifying thoughts, and activity scheduling
- Control is usual medical care

Outcomes

- Pre- and post-treatment and 6-month follow-up
- Disability rating
- Days lost at work
- Coping
- Pain intensity
- Control
- Medication use

Bradley et al., 1987

Method

- Randomized trial
- Allocation concealment unclear
- Subjects and assessor not masked
- Drop-outs reported

Participants

- N = 53 subjects; 10 male and 43 female
- Mean age = 50.09 years
- Pain duration of 11.49 years average
- RA—5 in class 1, 28 in class 2, and 20 in class 3

Interventions

- Group and individual sessions; mixed outpatient basis
- 15 sessions in total for each condition
- CB treatment with education, relaxation, goal setting, self-rewards, and individual biofeedback training
- Structured social support in small groups with family included education and coping strategies
- Control group—"no adjunct therapy"

Outcomes

- Pre- and post-treatment and 6-month follow-up
- Trait form of State-Trait Anxiety Inventory
- Depression Adjective Checklist
- Health Locus of Control
- Arthritis Helplessness Scale
- Videorecording of pain bchavior
- Physiological tests of skin temperature, grip strength, RA factor titers, and sedimentation rates

Notes

- Fifteen drop-outs reported; reasons were reported, but it is unclear if they analyzed if the drop-outs were different in any way
- Follow-up study conducted by Young et al. (1995) on health care utilization

Edelson & Fitzpatrick, 1989

Method

- Quasi-experimental design (not randomized)
- Allocation concealment inadequate
- Subjects and assessor not masked
- Unclear about drop-outs

Participants

- N = 27 subjects at the start of the study
- Mix of inpatients (three) and outpatients; all were male
- Multiple pain sites, including back (seven); pain duration mean = 9 years

Interventions

- CB sessions included verbalization, alteration of thoughts, self-instruction, and imagery
- CB plus hypnosis
- Attention control, nondirective sessions with therapist
- All sessions were individual, four 1-hour sessions for 2 weeks

Outcomes

- Pre- and post-treatment and 1-month follow-up
- MPQ
- Activity log of time spent in sitting, standing/walking, and reclining

Notes

- Very weak design and unclear reporting of drop-outs and final number of subjects in each condition

Nicholas, Wilson, & Goyen, 1992

Method

- RCT
- Allocation concealment not described
- Subjects and providers not masked
- Assessor was independent in 14 of 18 evaluations
- Drop-outs were reported

Participants

- N = 20 adults
- Age range was 26 to 61 years, mean = 43.7 years
- 11 male and 9 female
- Chronic low back pain, mean = 5.5 years duration
- Equivalency of groups established on all measures and demographics at baseline

Interventions

- Attention-control condition was physiotherapy, education, and exercises plus psychology sessions
- CB treatment group received the same physiotherapy and psychology input plus education, goal setting, pacing, coping, and relaxation training
- Group format was used
- Five week duration with weekly sessions for both groups

Outcomes

- Pre- and post-treatment and 6-month follow-up
- Pain intensity measured by a Pain Rating chart
- Pain perception measured by Pain Beliefs Questionnaire
- Depression measured by the Beck Depression Inventory
- Activity level measured by the Sickness Impact Profile
- Coping measured by the Coping Strategy Questionnaire
- Self-efficacy measured by the Pain Self-Efficacy Questionnaire

Notes

- 18 of 20 subjects at post-treatment (drop-out in each group); 17 of 20 at follow-up (drop-out in control condition)

Philips, 1987

Method

- Randomization—treatment and control groups
- Allocation concealment was unclear
- Masking of subjects and assessor was unclear
- Drop-outs were not clearly reported
- Numbers given in data tables for each group

Participants

- N = 40 subjects at the start of the study
- Age range was 18 to 61 years
- Male:female ratio was not reported
- Multiple pain sites including back, head, and face
- Pain duration of more than 6 months

Interventions

- CB group treatment (N = 25), outpatient basis, 1.5 hours per week for 9 weeks. Included relaxation, graded fitness, pain control, anxiety management, and activity pacing
- Control condition (N = 15)—wait listed between 2 to 6 months

Outcomes

- Pre- and post-treatment and 1-year follow-up
- Pain behavior checklist
- Pain intensity diary
- Life Impact checklist
- Beck Depression Inventory
- MPQ

Notes

- Number of drop-outs indicated in data tables: treatment group dropped from 25 to 22 at post-treatment and 19 at follow-up

Turner & Jensen, 1993

Method

- RCT comparing cognitive-behavioural and relaxation treatment
- Masking is unclear
- Drop-outs reported

Participants

- N = 102; outpatients with chronic back pain
- 47 were male
- Mean age = 42 years

Interventions

- CB treatment outpatient group for 6 weeks, including adaptive thinking to decrease negative cognitions compared to standard relaxation treatment

Outcomes

- Pre- and post-treatment and 12-month follow-up
- Pain intensity
- Activity level
- Control
- Depression

Notes

- This study is a three-group comparison of cognitive, relaxation, and CB plus relaxation. This review compares the CB plus relaxation and relaxation treatment groups

Turner, 1982

Method

RCT

- Allocation concealment unclear
- Subjects not masked; assessor masking unclear
- Drop-outs reported

Participants

- N = 36 participants with chronic back pain
- Average 8.7 years duration

- 3 male and 33 female
- Average age 42 years, range 20 to 63 years
- 12 working full-time, 11 part-time

Interventions

- Cognitive-behavioural group treatment, including relaxation plus cognitive-behavioural goal setting, imagery, and coping strategies
- Progressive muscle relaxation only
- Wait list control group treatments in group format for 5 weeks, 90 minutes per week on an outpatient basis

Outcomes

- Pre- and post-treatment and 1-month follow-up
- Visual analog scale of pain severity
- Sickness Impact profile—self and other
- Diary of hours worked
- Beck Depression Inventory

Notes

- Two drop-outs reported
- For comparison of three conditions: 14 in CB group, 13 in relaxation group, and 9 in control group
- When two treatments compared pre and post: 18 in CB group and 16 in relaxation group

Turner & Clancy, 1988

Method

- RCT
- Allocation concealment unclear
- Subjects not masked; masking of assessor unclear
- Drop-outs reported

Participants

- N = 81 subjects with chronic low back pain
- Average 6.2 years duration of pain
- 51 male and 30 female; mean age = 46 years

Interventions

- Two treatments and one control (wait list) group
- Cognitive-behavioural treatment included relaxation, imagery, adaptive thinking, and home practice
- Operant behavioral treatment included social reinforcement, behavioral goals, and spousal education

- Both treatment groups held 2 hours per week for 8 weeks

Outcomes

- Pre- and post-treatment and 6- and 12-month follow-up assessments
- MPQ pain rating checklist
- Pain behavior checklist
- Videotapes of pain behavior
- Sickness Impact Profile—self and other
- Cognitive Errors Questionnaire

Notes

- Drop-outs reported for post-treatment assessment: Two in CB group, one in operant behavioral group, and four in wait list group—not included in analyses

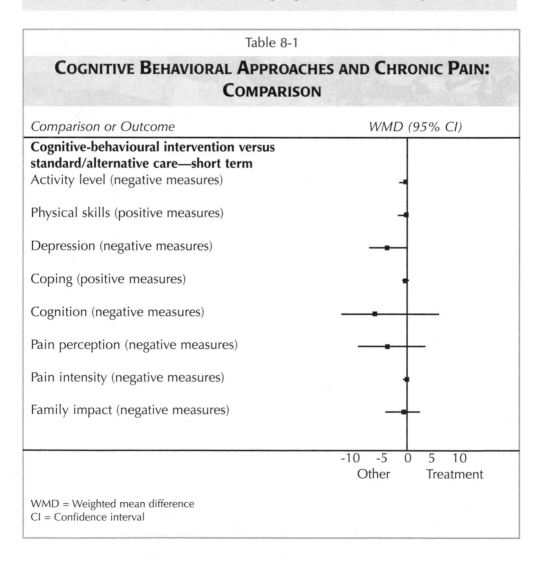

Table 8-1

COGNITIVE BEHAVIORAL APPROACHES AND CHRONIC PAIN: COMPARISON

Comparison or Outcome	WMD (95% CI)
Cognitive-behavioural intervention versus standard/alternative care—short term	
Activity level (negative measures)	
Physical skills (positive measures)	
Depression (negative measures)	
Coping (positive measures)	
Cognition (negative measures)	
Pain perception (negative measures)	
Pain intensity (negative measures)	
Family impact (negative measures)	

-10 -5   0   5   10
Other   Treatment

WMD = Weighted mean difference
CI = Confidence interval

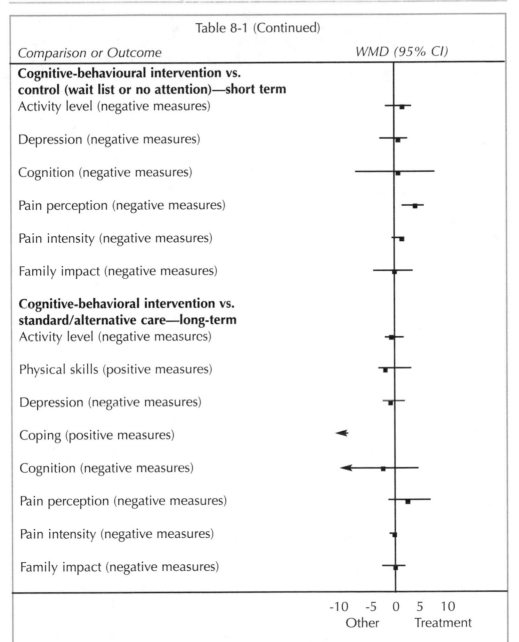

Table 8-1 (Continued)

Comparison or Outcome	WMD (95% CI)

Cognitive-behavioural intervention vs. control (wait list or no attention)—short term
Activity level (negative measures)

Depression (negative measures)

Cognition (negative measures)

Pain perception (negative measures)

Pain intensity (negative measures)

Family impact (negative measures)

Cognitive-behavioral intervention vs. standard/alternative care—long-term
Activity level (negative measures)

Physical skills (positive measures)

Depression (negative measures)

Coping (positive measures)

Cognition (negative measures)

Pain perception (negative measures)

Pain intensity (negative measures)

Family impact (negative measures)

-10 -5 0 5 10
Other   Treatment

Analysis and Interpretation of Table 8-1

This table indicates the summary statistic for the 10 studies that were systematically reviewed using RevMan software. The summary statistic for each of the outcomes listed is the "weighted mean difference," as all of the data was continuous. The WMD is a statistical calculation of the scores for all of the studies that measured the outcome listed. The confidence interval is set at 95%. The scale for the WMD statistic is from -10 to +10.

Table 8-1 (Continued)

In this table, the vertical line indicates "no difference" between the treatment and control groups. The summary statistic (i.e., the squares and lines) to the left of the vertical line indicates that the overall effect score for the outcome favours the control condition. The summary statistic to the right of the vertical line indicates that the overall effect score for that outcome favours the treatment condition (i.e, cognitive-behavioral intervention).

The outcomes that are compared in this table are listed on the far left of the page. They are organized into three main comparison groups:

1. Cognitive-behavioural intervention vs. standard/alternative care—short-term outcomes
2. Cognitive-behavioural intervention vs. control condition (wait list or no attention)—short-term outcomes
3. Cognitive-behavioural intervention vs. standard/alternative care—long-term outcomes

Please note that there are no comparisons for cognitive-behavioural intervention vs. control condition over the long-term, as there were insufficient data. Under each of these comparisons, there are six to eight different outcomes that were measured in the 10 studies. These outcomes were measured in two or more studies to be included in this analysis. The term *negative measures* means that the lower the score, the better the outcome, whereas *positive measures* means that the higher the score, the better the outcome.

Interpretation

The summary statistic (WMD), which is the overall effect size, is graphically displayed as lines and squares in Table 8-1. The squares represent the mean and the lines indicate the confidence interval for the summary statistic. The results would not be considered as strong if the lines and/or squares were touching the vertical (no difference) line. The majority of the summary statistics in Table 8-1 are touching the vertical "no difference" line, which indicates a weak overall effect for most of the outcomes. The outcomes that are clearly in one direction are pain perception and pain intensity, which both favour the treatment condition (cognitive-behavioural intervention) over a control (wait list or no attention) condition in the short-term.

An arrow to the far right or left of the scale indicates that the summary statistic (WMD) is off the scale. This means that the outcome scores, when calculated together as a summary statistic, strongly favour one condition. This only occurred with one outcome—coping under the comparison of cognitive-behavioural intervention vs. standard/alternative care. For this outcome, the standard/alternative care condition was favoured.

exclusion criteria narrowed this to 147 articles. Key words related to outcome studies, effectiveness, etc., resulted in selection of 51 articles for the initial, descriptive review. Hand searching and citation reviews found 20 more articles that met inclusion criteria. During the review process, many articles were excluded from the final list when they were read fully. The final number of accepted articles for this review was 29.

Data Extraction and Analysis

1. Descriptive review: Summary of Descriptive Review (p. 131) summarizes the important components of the accepted studies and provides an assessment of the main methodological issues and implications for occupational therapists.
2. Systematic review: Of the 29 studies included in the descriptive review, 13 were experimental or quasi-experimental in design. Three of these selected studies were subsequently excluded, as they compared different forms of cognitive-behavioural treatment programmes. The final number of selected studies for systematic review was 10.

Characteristics of Included Studies (p. 154) outlines the key methodological characteristics of the 10 studies selected for systematic review following the Cochrane Collaboration guidelines and the quality scale scores for each study. Table 8-1 provides a summary of the key outcomes that were measured in two or more of the selected studies.

DISCUSSION

The results of the descriptive review of 29 studies (see Summary of Descriptive Review on p. 131) appears to be positive for cognitive-behavioural approaches for people with chronic pain when compared with no treatment. However, the results are not as positive when cognitive-behavioural approaches are compared with alternative, or other forms, of treatment. Group treatment approaches appeared to be favoured over individual forms of treatment. Generally, it is difficult to make any strong conclusion about the effectiveness of cognitive-behavioural approaches from the descriptive review, as many of the studies used weak methodological designs.

The systematic review of 10 studies that used experimental or quasi-experimental designs found mixed results. Most of these studies used a randomized control design to examine the effects of a specific treatment programme as compared with no treatment and/or compared with another form of treatment (several studies did multiple comparisons at once). Multiple outcomes were studied, which was problematic for the analysis and interpretation of this systematic review.

The results of the systematic review indicate favourable results for cognitive-behavioural intervention compared with control (wait list or no attention) conditions in the short-term (i.e., immediately after intervention). The strongest effects were found in the short-term outcomes of pain perception and pain intensity. Weaker effects that favoured cognitive-behavioural intervention over control conditions include activity level, depression, and cognition.

When cognitive-behavioural interventions were compared with other/alternative forms of treatment, including standard medical care, physiotherapy, social support, and hypnosis, the results were less supportive of the cognitive-behavioural approach alone. No short-term outcomes were found to be clearly in favour of cognitive-behavioural interventions. Over the long-term, however (ranging from 6 to 18 months after intervention), some outcomes (e.g., depression, pain perception, and family impact) did move in the direction of favouring cognitive-behavioural intervention, but the overall effects of these outcomes were not strong.

In summary, it appears that cognitive-behavioural intervention may be beneficial for people with chronic pain. This critical review of the literature demonstrates some positive outcomes of cognitive-behavioural intervention, particularly when compared with no intervention. However, the evidence from this review is not conclusive. It is difficult to draw conclusions when the studies are "muddied" with different types of cognitive-behavioural interventions and multiple outcomes. This appears to mirror the clinical world, as cognitive-behavioural interventions are seldom used on their own. They are usually part of a multidisciplinary approach to the treatment of chronic pain.

Future research on the effectiveness of cognitive-behavioural interventions for people with chronic pain could focus on functional outcomes related to quality of life and participation in activities, which are important aspects of the role of an occupational therapist. It would be advantageous to use the same functional outcomes across different studies to allow for comparison across studies and to increase the strength of the findings.

Take-Home Messages

Background
- OTs are part of the interdisciplinary team and are interested in evaluating outcomes of their interventions.
- It is essential to base practice on best evidence.
- Cognitive-behavioural strategies teach skills that change the way people cope on a daily basis.
- Interested in reported effectiveness of cognitive-behavioural interventions in improving outcomes.

Materials and Methods
- Criteria:
  - types of studies (e.g., level of randomization)
  - types of participants (e.g., age)
  - types of intervention (e.g., three of cognitive-behavioural modalities)
  - types of outcome measures (clinically relevant)
- Search strategy for the identification of studies.
- Methods of review.
- Description of studies.
- Methodological quality of included studies.

Results
- Literature search (number of hits on electronic databases), hand searching, citation review.
- Data extraction and analysis (descriptive review).
- Systematic review (review based on design, decisions as to whether to include studies).

Discussion
- Often difficult to draw any real conclusions, as studies could use weak methodological designs.

- Conclusion that cognitive behavioural intervention may be beneficial for people with chronic pain, but the evidence is in no way conclusive.
- Direction for further research indicated —functional outcomes related to quality of life and participation in activities; advantageous to use same functional outcomes across different studies to allow for comparisons across studies as to increase the strength of findings.

LEARNING AND EXPLORATION ACTIVITIES

The purpose of this chapter is to provide students with an example of the process for undertaking a systematic review of the literature on a clinical topic and to provide them with the associated information concerning the effectiveness of cognitive-behavioural interventions.

1. Consider the results of this review. What has been learned? What knowledge is still required?
2. Create a one-page summary suitable for practicing therapists of the results of this review. Focus your summary on the clinical implications of the review findings.

REFERENCES

Altmaier, E. M., Lehmann, T. R., Russell, D. W., Weinstein, J. N., & Kao, C. F. (1992). The effectiveness of psychological interventions for the rehabilitation of low back pain: A randomized controlled trial. *Pain, 49*, 329-335.

Applebaum, K. A., Blanchard, E. B., Hickling, E. M., & Alfonso, M. (1988). Cognitive-behavioral treatment of a veteran population with moderate to severe RA. *Behavior Therapy, 19*, 489-502.

Basler, H. (1993). Group treatment for pain and discomfort. *Patient Education and Counseling, 20*, 167-175.

Basler, H., Jakle, C., & Kroner-Herwig, B. (1997). Incorporation of cognitive-behavioral treatment into the medical care of chronic low back patients: A controlled randomized study in German pain treatment centers. *Patient Education and Counselling, 31*, 113-124.

Bradley, L. A., Young, L. D., Anderson, K. O., Turner, R. A., Agudelo, C. A., McDaniel, L. K., et al. (1987). Effects of psychological therapy on pain behavior of rheumatoid arthritis patients. Treatment outcome and six-month follow-up. *Arthritis Rheum, 30*, 1105-1114.

Cinciripini, P. M., & Floreen, A. (1982). An evaluation of a behavioral program for chronic pain. *J Behav Med, 5*, 375-389.

Cochrane Collaboration. (1998). Review Manager, Version 3.1 for Windows. Updated March 1998.

Cohen, M. J., Heinrich, R. L., Naliboff, B. D., Collins, G. A., & Bonebakker, A. D. (1983). Group outpatient physical and behavioral therapy for chronic low back pain. *J Clin Psychol, 39*, 326-333.

Corey, D. T., Etlin, D., & Miller, P. C. (1987). A home-based pain management and rehabilitation programme: An evaluation. *Pain, 29*, 219-229.

Edelson, J., & Fitzpatrick, J. (1989). A comparison of cognitive-behavioral and hypnotic treatments of chronic pain. *J Clin Psychol, 45*, 316-323.

Flor, H., & Birbaumer, N. (1993). Comparison of the efficacy of electromyographic biofeedback, cognitive-behavioral therapy, and conservative medical interventions in the treatment of chronic musculoskeletal pain. *J Consul Clin Psychol, 61*, 653-658.

Heinrich, R. L., Cohen, M. J., Naliboff, B. D., Collins, G. A., & Bonebakker, A. D. (1985). Comparing physical and behavior therapy for chronic low back pain on physical abilities, psychological distress, and patients' perceptions. *J Behav Med, 8*, 61-78.

Jadad, A. R., Moore, R. A., Carroll, D., Jenkinson, C., Reynolds, D. J., Gavaghan, D. J., et al. (1996). Assessing the quality of report of randomized clinical trials: Is blinding necessary? *Control Clin Trials, 17*(1), 1-12.

Jensen, I., Dahlquist, C., Nygren, A., Royen, E., & Stenberg, M. (1997). Treatment for "helpless" women suffering from chronic spinal pain: A randomized controlled 18-month follow-up study. *Journal of Occupational Rehabilitation, 7*, 225-238.

Keefe, F. J., Dunsmore, J., & Burnett, R. (1992). Behavioral and cognitive-behavioural approaches to chronic pain: Recent advances and future direction. *J Consult Clin Psychol, 60*(4), 528-536.

Kerns, R. D. (1986). Comparison of cognitive-behavioral and behavioral approaches to the outpatient treatment of chronic pain. *Clin J Pain, 1*, 195-203.

Kerns, R. D., Turk, D. C., & Holzman, A. D. (1983). Psychological treatment for chronic pain: A selective review. *Clin Psychol Rev, 3*, 15-26.

Law, M., Stewart, D., Pollock, N., Letts, L., Bosch, J., Westmorland, M., et al. (1998). *Guidelines for critical review of the literature: Quantitative studies.* Retrieved March 14, 2002, from http://www.fhs.mcmaster.ca/rehab/ebp.

Linssen, A. C., & Spinhoven, P. (1992). Multimodal treatment programmes for chronic pain: A quantitative analysis of existing research data. *J Psychosom Res, 36*, 275-286.

Mulrow, C. D., & Oxman, A. D. (Eds.). (1997). *The Cochrane Handbook* (updated September 1997). In The Cochrane Library [database on disk and CD-ROM]. Issue 4. The Cochrane Collaboration, Oxford: Update Software.

Newton-John, T. R. O., Spence, S. H., & Schotte, D. (1995). Cognitive-behavioural therapy versus EMG biofeedback in the treatment of chronic low back pain. *Behav Res Ther, 33*, 691-697.

Nicholas, M. K., Wilson, P. H., & Goyen, J. (1991). Operant-behavioral and cognitive-behavioral treatment for chronic low back pain. *Behav Res Ther, 29*, 225-238.

Nicholas, M. K., Wilson, P. H., & Goyen, J. (1992). Comparison of cognitive-behavioral group treatment and an alternative non-psychological treatment for low back pain. *Pain, 48*(3), 339-347.

Nielson, W. R., Walker, C., & McCain, G. A. (1992). Cognitive behavioral treatment of fibromyalgia syndrome: Preliminary findings. *J Rheumatol, 19*(1), 98-103.

O'Leary, A., Shoor, S., Lorig, K., & Holman, H. R. (1988). A cognitive-behavioral treatment for rheumatoid arthritis. *Health Psychol, 7*(6), 527-544.

Parker, J. C., Frank, R. G., Beck, N. G., Smarr, K. L., Buescher, K. L., Phillips, L. R., et al. (1988). Pain management in RA patients. A cognitive-behavioral approach. *Arthritis Rheum, 31*, 593-601.

Philips, H. C. (1987). The effects of behavioral treatment on chronic pain. *Behav Res Ther, 25*, 365-377.

Richardson, I. H., Richardson, P. H., Williams, A. C., Featherstone, J., & Harding, V. R. (1994). The effects of a cognitive-behavioral pain management programme on the quality of work and employment status of severely impaired chronic pain patients. *Disabil Rehabil, 16*, 26-34.

Scheer, S. J., Watanabe, T. K., & Radack, K. L. (1997). Randomized controlled trials in industrial low back pain. Part 3: Subacute/chronic pain interventions. *Arch Phys Med Rehabil, 78*, 414-423.

Skinner, J. B., Erskine, A., Pearce, S., Rubenstein, I., Taylor, M., & Foster, C. (1990). The evaluation of a cognitive-behavioral treatment programme in outpatients with chronic pain. *J Psychosom Res, 34*(1), 13-19.

Spence, S. H. (1989). The differential effectiveness of group versus individual applications of cognitive-behaviour therapy in the management of chronic occupational pain of the upper limb. *Behav Res Ther, 27*, 435-446.

Spence, S. H. (1991). The differential effectiveness of group versus individual applications of cognitive-behaviour therapy in the management of chronic occupational pain of the upper limb: A 2-year follow-up. *Behav Res Ther, 29*, 503-509.

Turner, J. A. (1982). Comparison of group progressive-relaxation training and cognitive-behavioral group therapy for chronic low back pain. *J Consult Clin Psychol, 50*, 757-765.

Turner, J. A., & Chapman, C. R. (1982). Psychological interventions for chronic pain: A critical review. II. Operant conditioning, hypnosis, and cognitive-behavioral therapy. *Pain, 12*, 23-46.

Turner, J. A., & Clancy, S. (1988). Comparison of operant behavioral and cognitive-behavioral group treatment for chronic low back pain. *J Consult Clin Psychol, 56*, 261-266.

Turner, J. A., & Jensen, M. P. (1993). Efficacy of cognitive therapy for chronic low back pain. *Pain, 52*, 169-177.

White, K. P., & Nielson, W. R. (1995). Cognitive-behavioral treatment of fibromyalgia syndrome: A follow-up assessment. *J Rheumatol, 22*, 717-721.

Williams, A. C., Nicholas, M. K., Richardson, P. H., Pither, C. E., Justins, P. M., Chamberlain, J. H., et al. (1993). Evaluation of a cognitive-behavioural programme for rehabilitating patients with chronic pain. *Br J Gen Pract, 43*(377), 513-518.

Young, L. D., Bradley, L. A., & Turner, R. A. (1995). Decreases in health care resource utilization in patients with rheumatoid arthritis following a cognitive-behavioural intervention. *Biofeedback and Self-Regulation, 20*, 259-268.

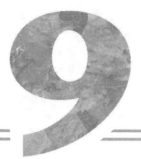

Evaluating the Evidence

Economic Analysis

Diane Watson, PhD, MBA, BScOT

LEARNING OBJECTIVES

After reading this chapter, the student/practitioner will be able to:
- Recognize the importance of assessing the value of intervention to ensure that it offers the most efficient treatment.
- Identify the different types of economic evaluations and when they are appropriate for use.
- Initiate research on a question related to economic analysis, including the development of a question and the use of various electronic databases.
- Critically appraise and communicate this research to his or her clients.

Over the past few years, evidence has increased regarding the effectiveness of certain types of occupational therapy services in enabling clients to attain specific, desirable outcomes. It would appear that clinical practitioners appropriately employ these interventions (Office of Inspector General, 1999) and are striving to shape their practice to become more evidence-based. The next challenge is clear—rehabilitation professionals must assess the value of effective interventions to ensure that they offer the most efficient means of attaining these outcomes. Only then will clients and consumers be able to evaluate the costs and outcomes associated with the choices they face when determining whether to participate in or offer rehabilitation services (Watson, 2000).

Clients participate in health programs and receive these services to attain desirable outcomes at minimal cost and risk. We often assume that health services are beneficial, but some interventions can be harmful to one's physical and financial health. For example, it has been estimated that approximately 20% of patients receive contraindicated chronic care and 30% receive contraindicated acute care (Schuster, McGlynn, & Brook, 1998). In addition, between 45,000 to 98,000 individuals die each year as a result of medical errors (Kohn, Corrigan, & Donaldson, 1999), and medical bills accounted for 40% of bankruptcies in the United States in 1999 (Gottlieb, 2000). These recent statistics draw attention toward the importance of balancing our understanding of potential benefits with insights regarding costs and risks.

Research evidence demonstrating the inappropriateness of some health services is mounting, and these findings are not unique to medicine. A recent review found that most Medicare patients in skilled nursing facilities who received occupational and physical therapy were appropriate candidates and benefited from intervention, but 10% of billed therapy was for services that were "not medically necessary" (Office of the Inspector General, 1999, p. 13). It was determined that patients who had similar diagnoses, goals, plans, and outcomes varied in the frequency and duration of the therapy services they received from different facilities. Evaluations such as this draw attention toward the importance of understanding the cost-effectiveness of rehabilitation services and excessive intervention.

The purpose of this chapter is to provide practitioners, administrators, and researchers with a basic understanding of, and appreciation for, research methods that have been used to appraise the costs and outcomes of health services. It is expected that this knowledge will enable these individuals to critically appraise and communicate evidence derived from the literature and stimulate enthusiasm among those who wish to conduct this type of evaluation. Other sections in this book highlight the process of seeking evidence regarding the effectiveness of specific services and incorporating this evidence into practice. By comparison, this chapter summarizes how research is conducted in order to evaluate the value of health services and describes how practitioners can obtain and appraise this evidence.

ASSESSING THE VALUE OF REHABILITATION SERVICES TO CLIENTS: ECONOMIC EVALUATION

Research methods have been developed to appraise, describe, and compare the relative value of health services. These methods have been called *cost-effectiveness analyses* (Russell, Gold, Siegel, Daniels, & Weinstein, 1996) and/or economic evaluations (Drummond, O'Brien, Stoddart, & Torrance, 1997). They are distinct from clinical evaluations in that they focus on costs and outcomes rather than the efficacy or effectiveness of a specific intervention. The effectiveness and appropriateness of a clinical intervention, however, should be established before being combined with an assessment of costs, as it would be wasteful to calculate the cost of providing ineffective services (Drummond, O'Brien, et al., 1997).

While effective research focuses on the impact of interventions on health, economic evaluations focus on the relative value of health services. Value refers to "a fair return or equivalent in goods, services, or money for something exchanged" (Merriam-Webster, 1984, p. 1303). Within the health care context, the term *value* refers to the relative worth, utility, or importance of a service in meeting the health needs of a defined clientele. For a service to be "valuable," clients should receive a fair return (i.e., service and outcome) for something exchanged (i.e., finances and time invested). In order to inform consumers and clients about the relative value of specific health and rehabilitation services for defined clientele, we must (a) conduct evaluations to determine whether specific interventions are effective at attaining desirable outcomes; (b) evaluate effective interventions to ensure that they offer the most efficient means of attaining specific outcomes; and (c) effectively communicate these results. Unfortunately, the number of evaluations that have been conducted to assess the relative value of rehabilitation services is small in comparison to the number of effectiveness studies (Watson & Mathews, 1998).

The intent and purpose of economic evaluations are to provide clients and consumers with information regarding value in order to inform their decisions. Therefore, these evaluations require that two or more services must be compared to assess "relative value." One of the comparisons, however, could be the "no service" alternative, which is equivalent to a control group in experimental research. In this context, a comparison would be made between the cost and benefit of receiving versus not receiving a rehabilitation service. For example, Rizzo, Baker, McAvay, and Tinetti (1996) conducted an economic evaluation when they compared the cost and outcomes of receiving versus not receiving a service to prevent falls among the elderly.

Types of Economic Evaluations

There are five different types of economic evaluation that have been defined in the literature: cost-consequences, cost-minimization, cost-effectiveness, cost-utility, and cost-benefit analyses (Canadian Coordinating Office for Health Technology Assessment, 1997; Drummond, O'Brien, et al., 1997). Table 9-1 illustrates how these different research methods might be applied to evaluate the relative worth of a rehabilitation service. Table 9-2 provides examples of economic evaluations that have been published in the literature and highlights the fact that investigators may conduct different types of economic evaluations when assessing the relative value of a health or rehabilitation service.

A cost-consequence analysis can be used to describe a health service or compare two or more health interventions. This type of analysis requires that investigators provide a descriptive profile of the costs (e.g., hospital costs, out-of-pocket expenses) and outcomes (e.g., impact on health and economic circumstances) of one or more interventions. For example, Hughes, Manheim, Edelman, and Conrad (1987) described the costs and outcomes of providing long-term home care.

A cost-minimization analysis is conducted to identify the least costly alternative when two or more services produce equivalent outcomes. Evidence that each service produces comparable outcomes must be demonstrated using evidence from the literature or tested as part of the analysis. When researchers determined that there was no significant difference in outcomes for patients who received hospital at home versus hospital inpatient care, a cost-minimization analysis was conducted to identify the least costly alternative (Jones et al., 1999).

Table 9-1

APPLYING ECONOMIC EVALUATION METHODS TO REHABILITATION SERVICES

Consider the following clinical scenario and the contribution of economic evaluation methods to the decision-making process.

Assume that an individual who had a stroke 10 days ago was given the choice to receive rehabilitation services using a number of different care approaches. Suppose that you have been given the responsibility to be a decision maker regarding the health care services received by this person. You have decided that his decision will primarily be based on the relative value (i.e., the relative costs and outcomes) of each alternative.

You have determined that the hospital offers poststroke rehabilitation services on a general unit or a specialized unit and that home-based rehabilitation services are available. Therefore, the following options are available: (1) hospital-based services on a general unit; (2) hospital-based services on a specialized unit; (3) early discharge from the hospital and home-based rehabilitation; or (4) early discharge and no rehabilitation services.

You have reviewed the literature to determine the relative value of institution-based versus home-based poststroke rehabilitation versus no intervention. A *cost-consequences analysis* would provide a descriptive profile of the costs and outcomes of each alternative and any evidence regarding significant differences between these alternatives. Assuming that the goals and objectives of the inpatient poststroke rehabilitation services were identical and, therefore, the types of outcomes expected of participants were similar, a *cost-effectiveness analysis* would provide insight regarding the relative value of the alternatives. Relative value would be measured by determining the cost per unit of health effect (e.g., cost per unit of change in functional status) derived from participation in each service delivery model in comparison to the no-service alternative.

Assume that the goals and objectives of the hospital-based programs were to increase independence in activities of daily living (ADL), while the goals of the home-based programs were to enhance participation of individuals who have experienced a stroke in community-based activities and support programs. In this context, it would be appropriate to conduct a cost-utility and/or cost-benefit analysis to compare the relative value of service alternatives that are directed toward different outcomes (i.e., independence in ADL versus enhance community participation). Both outcomes, however, impact health-related quality of life (HRQL). Therefore, a *cost-utility analysis* would require a comparison of the costs and HRQL of these two service alternatives. Alternatively, a *cost-benefit analysis* could be conducted to compare the costs, monetary outcomes, and net financial impact of participating in either of these two service alternatives.

Table 9-2

EXAMPLES OF ECONOMIC EVALUATIONS IN THE REHABILITATION LITERATURE

Type of Evaluation	*Health Service Area*	*Example Evaluation*
Cost-consequence	• Models of delivering home-based services • Providing versus not offering long-term home care	• Feldman, Latimer, & Davidson, 1996 • Hughes et al., 1987
Cost-minimization	• Stroke rehabilitation: Home or hospital • Group versus individualized services • Intensity of inpatient rehabilitation services • Economic consequences of early inpatient discharge to community-based rehabilitation for stroke in an inner-London teaching hospital	• Anderson et al., 2000 Jones et al., 1999 • Trahey, 1991 • Johnston & Miller, 1986 • Beech, Rudd, Tilling, & Wolfe, 1999
Cost-effectiveness	• Needle exchange program to prevent HIV transmission • Behavioural rehabilitation in chronic low back pain • Hip fracture and stroke • Hip and knee replacement surgery • Providing versus not offering a fall prevention program • Providing physical or occupational therapy versus not offering rehabilitation to individuals who have reflex sympathetic dystrophy • Intensity of rehabilitation services in nursing home	• Gold, Gafni, Nelligan, & Millson, 1997 • Goossens et al., 1998 • Kramer et al., 1997 • Rissanen et al., 1997 • Rizzo et al., 1996 • Severens et al., 1999 • Przybylski et al., 1996

Table 9-2 (Continued0

Type of Evaluation	Health Service Area	Example Evaluation
Cost-utility	• Intensive versus nonintensive care to very low-birth-weight infants	• Boyle, Torrance, Sinclair, & Horwood, 1983
	• Hip and knee replacement surgery	• Rissanen et al., 1997
	• Cardiac rehabilitation	• Oldridge et al., 1993
Cost-benefit	• Intensive versus nonintensive care to very low-birth-weight infants	• Boyle et al., 1983
	• Needle exchange program to prevent HIV transmission	• Gold et al., 1997
	• Providing versus not offering a fall prevention program	• Rizzo et al., 1996
	• Maintaining seniors in the community: emergency alarms	• Ruchlin & Morris, 1981
	• Home versus institutional-based psychiatric services	• Margolis & Petti, 1994

A cost-effectiveness analysis is conducted when an investigator is interested in describing and comparing the relative costs and outcomes of two or more services. These evaluations require that the services being compared produce the same type of outcome. For example, Severens et al. (1999) compared the costs and outcomes of individuals who have reflex sympathetic dystrophy receiving physical therapy, occupational therapy, or no rehabilitation service. A cost-effectiveness analysis was used to study the value of each service option because the goal of each service was to achieve the same type of outcome (i.e., reduce upper extremity impairment and improve health status).

In contrast, cost-utility and cost-benefit analyses are conducted to compare the relative costs and outcomes of two or more services that produce different types of outcomes. Cost-utility analyses consider both health status and the value of that status to the client when evaluating outcomes, while cost-benefit analyses require that investigators measure the monetary value of outcomes. Consider the challenge of trying to determine which clients should receive occupational therapy, given that demand for your services exceeds your ability to offer care. Should you offer occupational therapy services to individuals who have had a physical injury or to those who have a psychiatric condition? Consider making this decision on the basis of which alternative would maximize outcomes for the amount of cost (e.g., monetary and time) invested. One way to compare outcomes for services that produce different types of outcomes is to measure change in health status (i.e., cost-utility analysis). In other words, measure whether changes in the health status of patients with physical injuries are more, less, or the same as those with psychiatric conditions. Another way to compare outcomes is to measure outcomes in financial terms (i.e., cost-benefit analysis). See Tables 9-1 and 9-2 for more examples of economic evaluations.

Conducting Economic Evaluations

Economic evaluations are conducted using a multistep process (Mathews & Watson, 2000). A research question is initially posed to define the purpose and scope of the assessment. The question should describe a service or identify interventions being described or compared, outline the perspective and time horizon of the analysis, specify the scope of the intervention, and detail the costs and outcomes considered. Economic evaluations can be descriptive, comparative, or both. Descriptive evaluations simply describe the goals and objectives of the service, the population for whom the program was provided, the type of intervention offered, the costs of providing and/or consuming the intervention service, and the outcomes or effects of the service. Comparative assessments require that two or more services be compared with appropriate alternative interventions or no intervention. The perspective of the analysis is important to consider and identify prospectively, as evaluations that are conducted from the same viewpoint as the "user" of the assessment tend to be more relevant and useful (Stoddart, 1982). Evaluations can be conducted from the perspective of society, payers, providers, and/or consumers. The important and relevant costs and outcomes should be specified and included in an evaluation. These elements can be identified through a process that considers the goals, objectives, and activities of the health service; the needs of the target population and service recipients; and the preference of the audience for whom the evaluation report is intended. The most relevant and important costs and outcomes to include are those that are valued by all stakeholders. The majority of economic evaluations published in the literature appear to be authored by a team of investigators who have diverse backgrounds. It appears, therefore, that the successful generation of evidence regarding the cost and outcomes of medical and rehabilitative services may require a team of individuals who have clinical, research, methodological, and health economic backgrounds.

A literature review is important to conduct during the initial planning stages of an evaluation to enhance understanding of the particular issue and to capitalize on what others have previously done. Evidence regarding the costs and/or the effectiveness of the services being described and/or compared is compiled and evaluated. The process by which evidence can be located in the literature and critically appraised is profiled in Chapters 5 and 6. Economic evaluations should employ rigorous methodologies to determine the efficacy and effectiveness of an intervention and estimate as realistically as possible the true costs of intervention.

Good evaluations should include an assessment regarding the robustness of the findings. These assessments—termed *sensitivity analyses*—are required, as investigators must make a number of judgments or assumptions throughout the course of the analysis. A sensitivity analysis presents the range of possible values resulting from variations of a critical judgment (Drummond, O'Brien, et al., 1997). Evaluators should also make judgments regarding the internal and external validity of their assessments. Sources of bias, contamination, and noncompliance should be described and documented. All studies are hampered by limitations, but a final report that includes a description of these shortcomings will ultimately help decision-makers to weigh the merits of the evaluation and, thereby, make judgments based on evidence and reason.

Critically Reviewing Economic Evaluations

The characteristics that describe rigorous economic evaluation projects are those that can be used to critically appraise those articles summarizing the findings of one of these evaluative efforts. Table 9-3 provides a listing of questions that can be used when evaluating evidence in the literature regarding the relative value of health service interventions. This list

---

Table 9-3

CRITICALLY APPRAISING THE INTERNAL AND EXTERNAL VALIDITY OF ECONOMIC EVALUATIONS

Internal Validity

1. Did the research question clearly and accurately define the options compared?
2. Was the perspective of the analysis defined?
3. Were the important and relevant costs and outcomes identified?
4. Were the costs and outcomes properly measured and valued?
5. How rigorous was the methodology that was used to establish costs?
6. How rigorous was the methodology that was used to establish the effectiveness of the service alternatives?
7. Were the differences in costs and outcomes between the options analyzed and compared?
8. Was appropriate allowance made for uncertainties in the evaluation by including a sensitivity analysis incorporating clinically sensitive variations in important variables?

External Validity

1. Are the outcomes worth the costs?
2. Could my patients expect similar health outcomes?
3. Could I expect similar costs?

---

was developed after reviewing formats that have been used by others to appraise the quality of economic evaluation evidence (Drummond, O'Brien, et al., 1997; Drummond, Richardson, O'Brien, Levine, & Heyland, 1997).

The National Health Service Research and Development Centre for Evidence Based Medicine (CEBM) in Oxford, England was established in 1995 to promote the teaching and practice of evidence-based health care. The CEBM has published guidelines for ranking the level of evidence of effectiveness studies and economic evaluations, and this document is available on the World Wide Web at http://cebm.jr2.ox.ac.uk/docs/levels.html.

Locating Economic Evaluations in the Literature

Economic evaluations that have been published in the literature can be found using traditional databases. The National Library of Medicine provides free Internet access to enable people to search on-line databases such as MEDLINE and HealthSTAR. The World Wide Web address for these resources is www.nlm.nih.gov. MEDLINE is considered to be a premier bibliographic database that contains references and abstracts for journal articles in life sciences with a concentration on biomedicine and the clinical sciences. HealthSTAR is the bibliographic database that provides access to the published literature of health services technology, administration, and research. The National Information Centre on Health Services Research and Health Care Technology provides free Internet access to enable people to search their on-line databases. The World Wide Web address for this resource is http://text.nlm.nih.gov/hsrsearch/hsr.html.

There are two databases that provide abstracts and critical appraisals of economic evaluations. The National Health Service Centre for Reviews and Dissemination at the University of York in the United Kingdom offers free Internet access to their Economic Evaluation Database (NHS EED). The World Wide Web address for this valuable resource is http://agatha.york.ac.uk/welcome.htm. This database contains structured abstracts and critical appraisals of economic evaluations from 1994 onward. The Office of Health Economics and the International Federation of Pharmaceutical Manufacturers Association offers access to their Health Economic Evaluations Database (HEED) on a subscription basis. This database contains abstracts and structured reviews of economic evaluations, cost analyses and cost of illness studies from 1967 onwards. HEED is available in CD format or via the Internet and can be accessed at most university libraries.

CONCLUSION

The number of evaluations that have been conducted to evaluate the effectiveness of rehabilitation interventions and programs has grown rapidly in the last few years. By comparison, the number of evaluations that have been conducted to assess the relative value of these services is small. This is not unexpected, as it is important to establish clinical effectiveness before calculating costs. It would be wasteful to determine the relative cost of providing ineffective services.

Research methods have been established to appraise the costs and outcomes of health services to provide clients and consumers with information regarding relative value. It is hoped that these insights will inform their decisions. There are five types of economic evaluations, but these methodological approaches simply differ in how they measure and/or quantify outcomes. A number of good evaluations have been published in the literature, and Table 9-2 (p. 175) provides examples of studies that may be of interest to rehabilitation professionals. Information has been provided to enable the reader to locate and appraise this literature, in hopes that this exercise will inform clinical practice and stimulate enthusiasm among those who wish to conduct this type of research. The next challenge for the rehabilitation profession is clear. We must assess the value of effective interventions to ensure that they offer the most efficient means of attaining specific outcomes and effectively communicate these findings to our clients.

Take-Home Messages

- Rehabilitation professionals must assess the value of effective interventions so that clients and consumers can evaluate costs and outcomes when deciding to participate, and so that they can offer the most efficient types of interventions.
- We cannot always assume that the potential benefits from receiving a service outweigh the costs and risks.
- When making a decision about which service to offer or which intervention to receive, clinicians and clients must consider the costs, risks, and outcomes of each alternative.

Economic Evaluation
- Focus on appraising, describing, and comparing the relative value of specific interventions in order to inform decision making.
- *Value* is the relative worth, utility, or importance of a service in meeting the health needs of a defined clientele.
- There are three aspects to an economic evaluation:
    1. Evaluate whether specific interventions are effective at attaining outcomes.
    2. Evaluate effective interventions to ensure they offer the most efficient means.
    3. Effectively communicate these results.

Types of Economic Evaluations
- Cost-consequence—descriptive profile of the costs and outcomes of one or more interventions.
- Cost-minimization—identifies the least costly alternative for services that result in equivalent outcomes.
- Cost-effectiveness—describes and compares the relative costs and outcomes of two or more interventions that result in the same type of outcome.
- Cost-utility—describes and compares the relative costs and outcomes of two or more interventions in which the outcomes of interest include health status and the value of the status to the individual.
- Cost-benefit—describes and compares the relative costs and outcomes of two or more interventions in which both the costs and outcome can be measured in monetary values.

Conducting Economic Evaluations
- Research question defines the purpose and scope of assessment.
- Descriptive analysis or comparative assessment.
- Important to consider the perspective of the analysis (i.e., from society, payers, providers, and/or consumers).
- Evaluators of economic analyses should make judgments regarding the internal and external validity of their assessments, including source of bias, contamination, and noncompliance.
- When critically analyzing economic analyses, it is important to look at both internal and external factors.

Locating Economic Evaluations in the Literature
- Research can be found with traditional databases like MEDLINE and HealthSTAR.
- National Health Service Centre for Reviews and Dissemination (University of York, UK) contains structured abstracts and critical appraisals of economic evaluations from 1994 onward (web-based).
- Health Economic Evaluations Database contains abstracts and structured reviews from 1967 onward (subscription).

LEARNING AND EXPLORATION ACTIVITIES

The purpose of this chapter is to provide a basic understanding and appreciation of the research methods that have been used to appraise the costs and outcomes of health services.

Upon completion of this chapter, students should be aware of the role that economic evaluations play in evidence-based practice.

1. You are the manager for a program providing home-based rehabilitation services for older adults discharged home after total hip replacement surgery. It is important to conduct economic evaluations of this program. For each type of economic analysis, describe the purpose of the evaluation and what specific information would be collected to complete such an evaluative study.

   a. Cost-consequences

   b. Cost-minimization

   c. Cost-effectiveness

   d. Cost-utility

   e. Cost-benefit analyses

2. Select one of the economic evaluation studies listed in Table 9-2. Using the questions in Table 9-3, complete a critical appraisal of this article. What are the implications of the findings for rehabilitation practice?

REFERENCES

Anderson, C., Mhurchu, C. N., Rubenach, S., Clark, M., Spencer, C., & Winsor, A. (2000). Home or hospital for stroke rehabilitation? Results of a randomized controlled trial. II: Cost minimization analysis at 6 months. *Stroke, 31*, 1032.

Beech, R., Rudd, A. G., Tilling, K., & Wolfe, C. D. (1999). Economic consequences of early inpatient discharge to community-based rehabilitation for stroke in an inner-London teaching hospital. *Stroke, 30*, 729-735.

Boyle, M. H., Torrance, G. W., Sinclair, J. C., & Horwood, S. P. (1983). Economic evaluation of neonatal intensive care of very-low-birth-weight infants. *N Engl J Med, 308*, 1330-1337.

Canadian Coordinating Office for Health Technology Assessment. (1997). *Guidelines for economic evaluation of pharmaceuticals: Canada* (2nd ed.). Ottawa, Ontario: Author.

Drummond, M. F., O'Brien, B. J., Stoddart, G. L., & Torrance, G. (1997). *Methods for the economic evaluation of health care programmes* (2nd ed.). Oxford, UK: Oxford University Press.

Drummond, M. F., Richardson, W. S., O'Brien, B. J., Levine, M., & Heyland, D. (1997). Users' guide to the medical literature. How to use an article on economic analysis of clinical practice: Are the results of the study valid? *JAMA, 277*, 1552-1557.

Feldman, P. H., Latimer, E., & Davidson, H. (1996). Medicaid-funded home care for the frail elderly and disabled: Evaluating the cost savings and outcomes of a service delivery reform. *Health Serv Res, 31*, 489-509.

Gold, M., Gafni, A., Nelligan, P., & Millson, P. (1997). Needle exchange programs: An economic evaluation of a local experience. *Canadian Medical Association Journal, 157*, 255-262.

Goossens, M. E., Rutten-Van Molken, M. P., Kole-Snijders, A. M., Vlaeyen, J. W., Van Breukelen, G., & Leidl, R. (1998). Health economic assessment of behavioral rehabilitation in chronic low back pain: A randomized clinical trial. *Health Econ, 7*, 39-51.

Gottlieb, S. (2000). Medical bills account for 40% of bankruptcies. *British Medical Journal, 320*(7245), 1295.

Hughes, S. L., Manheim, L. M., Edelman, P. L., & Conrad, K. J. (1987). Impact of long-term home care on hospital and nursing home use and cost. *Health Serv Res, 22*, 19-47.

Johnston, M. V., & Miller, L. S. (1986). Cost-effectiveness of the Medicare three-hour regulation: Physical plus occupational therapy. *Arch Phys Med Rehabil, 67*, 581-585.

Jones, J., Wilson, A., Parker, H., Wynn, A., Jagger, C., Spiers, N., et al. (1999). Economic evaluation of hospital at home versus hospital care: Cost minimization analysis of data from randomized controlled trial. *British Medical Journal, 319*, 1547-1550.

Kohn, L., Corrigan, J., & Donaldson, M. (1999). *To err is human: Building a safer health system.* Washington, D.C.: National Academy Press.

Kramer, A. M., Steiner, J. F., Schlenker, R. E., Eilertsen, T. B., Hrincevich, C. A., Tropea, D. A., et al. (1997). Outcomes and costs after hip fracture and stroke: A comparison of rehabilitation settings. *JAMA, 277*, 396-404.

Margolis, L. H., & Petti, R. D. (1994). An analysis of the costs and benefits of two strategies to decrease length in children's psychiatric hospitals. *Health Serv Res, 29*, 155-167.

Mathews, M., & Watson, D. (2000). Designing and managing an evaluation. In D. E. Watson (Ed.), *Evaluating costs and outcomes: Demonstrating the value of rehabilitation services* (pp. 25-42). Bethesda, MD: American Occupational Therapy Association.

Merriam-Webster. (1984). *Merriam-Webster's ninth new collegiate dictionary.* Springfield, MA: Author.

Office of Inspector General. (1999). *Physical and occupational therapy in nursing homes: Medical necessity and quality of care.* Washington, D.C.: Department of Health and Human Services.

Oldridge, N., Furlong, W., Fenny, D., Torrance, G., Guyatt, G., Crowe, J., et al. (1993). Economic evaluation of cardiac rehabilitation soon after acute myocardial infarction. *Am J Cardiol, 72*, 154-161.

Przybylski, B. R., Dumont, E. D., Watkins, M. E., Warren, S. A., Beaulne, A. P., & Lier, D. A. (1996). Outcomes of enhanced physical and occupational therapy service in a nursing home setting. *Arch Phys Med Rehabil, 77*, 554-561.

Rissanen, P., Aro, P., Sintonen, H., Asikainen, K., Slätis, P., & Paavolainen, P. (1997). Costs and cost-effectiveness in hip and knee replacements: A prospective study. *Int J Technol Assess Health Care, 13*, 575-588.

Rizzo, J. A., Baker, D. I., McAvay, G., & Tinetti, M. E. (1996). The cost-effectiveness of a multifactorial targeted prevention program for falls among community elderly persons. *Med Care, 34*, 954-969.

Ruchlin, H. S., & Morris, J. N. (1981). Cost-benefit analysis of an emergency alarm and response system: A case study of a long-term care program. *Health Serv Res, 16*, 65-80.

Russell, L. B., Gold, M., Siegel, J. E., Daniels, N., & Weinstein, M. C. (1996). The role of cost-effectiveness analysis in health and medicine. *JAMA, 276*, 1172-1177.

Schuster, M., McGlynn, E., & Brook, R. (1998). How good is the quality of health care in the United States? *Milbank Q, 76*, 517-563.

Severens, J. L., Oerlemans, H. M., Weegels, A. J., van Hof, M. A., Oostendorp, R. A., & Goris, R. J. (1999). Cost-effectiveness analysis of adjuvant physical and occupational therapy for patients with reflex sympathetic dystrophy. *Arch Phys Med Rehabil, 80*, 1038-1043.

Stoddart, G. L. (1982). Economic evaluation methods and health policy. *Evaluation and the Health Professions, 5*, 393-414.

Trahey, P. J. (1991). A comparison of the cost-effectiveness of two types of occupational therapy services. *Am J Occup Ther, 45*, 397-400.

Watson, D. E. (2000). *Evaluating costs and outcomes: Demonstrating the value of rehabilitation services.* Bethesda, MD: American Occupational Therapy Association.

Watson, D. E., & Mathews, M. (1998). Economic evaluation of occupational therapy: Where are we at? *Can J Occup Ther, 65*, 160-167.

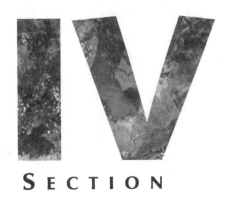

SECTION

Using the Evidence

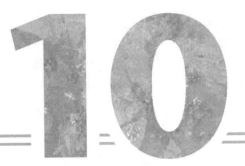

Building Evidence
in Practice

Mary Law, PhD, OT(C)

LEARNING OBJECTIVES

After reading this chapter, the student/practitioner will be able to:

- Develop an understanding of building evidence for practice.
- Identify the essential components and different types of critically appraised topics (CATs).
- Understand and explain the use of CATs in evidence-based practice.

Using evidence-based practice as an occupational therapist or a physical therapist means processing and organizing a lot of information from the research literature. Each time you use your evidence evaluation skills (i.e., identifying new clinical questions, searching for relevant studies in the literature, and integrating your findings into practice) you will be exposed to vast amounts of information. The critically appraised topic, or CAT, is one method for organizing your thoughts and keeping your evidence straight.

CATs

CATs are the preferred categorization format for quick studies in evidence-based practice. The CAT was originally developed at McMaster University (Sauve et al., 1995), but several CAT formats have evolved since then. Simply put, a CAT is a one- or two-page "summary of a search and critical appraisal of the literature related to a focused clinical question, which should be kept in an easily accessible place so that it can be used to help make clinical decisions" (Center for Evidence-Based Emergency Medicine, n.d.a). The most essential characteristics of CATs are that they be simultaneously brief, informative, and useful.

To give a more general understanding of the basis for CATs, it is important to be able to place them in the complete EBP process. The University of Oxford's Centre for Evidence-Based Medicine breaks up the evidence-based information search process into five parts (n.d.). They suggest that once you have realized that you have an information need, you should:

1. Translate these needs into answerable questions.
2. Track down the best evidence to answer them.
3. Appraise that evidence for its validity and applicability.
4. Integrate that evidence with clinical expertise and apply it in practice.
5. Evaluate the performance of the intervention.

This definition meshes with that of the Centre for Evidence-Based Emergency Medicine's (n.d.b) definition of a CAT, which states, "A CAT is a one- or two-page summary of all of the preceding steps involved in your evidence-based approach to the literature. It provides immediate access to your method and results."

CATs have a hand in all of the steps of the evidence-based process. They require that one have a focused question, categorize the evidence found, allow for the evaluation of that evidence, and produce a clinical bottom line which will be developed into practice. Finally, CATs can be reviewed on a regular basis and their successes passed on for further analysis.

Different Types of CATs

There are five major types of CATs: those for diagnosis; prognosis; evaluating risk and harm in a case-control study; evaluating risk and harm in a cohort study; and treatment, prevention, and screening.

Diagnosis/Screening

CATs for diagnosis are the easiest to understand. They involve simply finding relevant studies that identify disease symptoms and assessing the diagnostic accuracy of those symptoms. If the symptom in question is present, how likely is it that the patient has the disease or condition? Diagnostic CATs compare new diagnoses with the medical "gold standard," or the most highly accurate diagnostic test that currently exists. The CAT for diagnosis has a

Figure 10-1. Two-by-two table used for diagnostic calculations.

	Disease Present	Disease Absent
Test Positive	a	b
Test Negative	c	d

two-by-two table for entering the evidence numbers (Figure 10-1) and a formula for calculating the likelihood ratios for the new diagnosis, or how likely it is that a person has the disease if he or she shows the symptom.

A likelihood ratio is a simple calculation of the probability that a client has a certain condition given the results of a test. There are two equal and opposite types of results to consider when examining the results of clinical tests—sensitivity and specificity. These two factors interplay with each other to produce results. The *sensitivity* of a diagnostic test is the proportion of people who actually have the disease or problem in question who come up with a positive test. The *specificity* of a test is the equal and opposite result—the proportion of people who do not have the disease who come up (rightfully) with a negative test. From the above graphic:

$$\text{Sensitivity} = \frac{a}{(a + c)}$$

$$\text{Specificity} = \frac{b}{(b + d)}$$

Thus, the likelihood ratio is the sensitivity of the test (the chance that it will rightly include clients with the condition) divided by the opposite of the specificity (1 - specificity, or the chance that it will wrongly exclude clients with the condition). A likelihood ratio (LR) is thus:

$$LR = \frac{sensitivity}{(1 - specificity)}$$

$$LR = \frac{\dfrac{a}{(a + c)}}{\dfrac{b}{(b + d)}}$$

If this is still unclear, we suggest that you consult a medical statistics textbook or online resources such as the Centre for Evidence-Based Medicine's Glossary, which is located at http://cebm.jr2.ox.ac.uk/docs/glossary.html. LRs are most often used by physicians for medical diagnostic questions, but they are also used in rehabilitation for screening issues (e.g., the identification of a developmental delay).

Prognosis

A CAT for prognosis will assess the ability of a symptom to forecast probable outcomes. The difference between a diagnosis CAT and a prognosis CAT is that diagnosis CATs attempt to establish whether or not persons have a condition, while prognosis CATs try to predict the future of a condition for one person. An example in rehabilitation is the predictive validity of screening tests, such as the Motor Assessment of Infants.

Risk and Harm in Case-Controlled Studies

Risk is very simply defined as the probability that an event will occur, and the next two types of CATs discussed attempt to find the risk for patients with a certain condition in two different ways. A case-controlled study is a study "which starts with the identification of persons with a condition of interest and a control group without the condition" (Gray Cancer Institute, n.d.).

The case-controlled CAT, therefore, analyzes information on the presence of risk factors using a statistical technique called an *odds ratio* (OR). An OR is simply the odds of a patient in the experimental group suffering an adverse event relative to the odds of a patient in the control group suffering the same event. There are two numbers to consider when calculating an OR: the experimental event odds (EEO) and the control event odds (CEO). The OR is:

$$OR = \frac{\dfrac{EEO}{1 - EEO}}{\dfrac{CEO}{1 - CEO}}$$

Once again, if this is not clear, consult a text or the CEBM (NHS Research and Development, n.d.a).

Risk and Harm in Cohort Studies

Cohort studies differ from case-controlled studies in that the two types of studies approach populations differently. Cohort studies are studies in which subsets of a defined population are identified. These groups may or may not be exposed to factors hypothesized to influence the probability of the occurrence of a particular outcome. The cohorts are then followed forward in time to determine differential outcomes based on exposure or no exposure.

In cohort studies, it is necessary to calculate the relative risk of the experimental and control groups. A relative risk is simply the number of people exposed to a risk factor who developed the unwanted outcome taken as a percentage of the whole. The relative risk will differ for groups that are categorized differently, as the population considered is different. An easy analogy that illustrates this concept is the example of taxation. Each year, a percentage of citizens in a country who file tax returns are randomly chosen and are subjected to an in-depth audit. The number of citizens audited taken as a percentage of the total number of citizens who file tax returns is the relative risk of an audit. For those who are not legally required to file tax returns (e.g., children), the relative risk of an audit is different; for those who decide to illegally refrain from filing a tax return, the relative risk of an audit is different again. It is crucial to understand that while each subgroup has its own relative risk, the complete sample (the entire population of the country) has its own relative risk as well (which would be a weighted average of the relative risks of its subgroups).

Intervention Studies (Treatment, Prevention, and Screening)

CATs in this category deal with the strongest type of available evidence—randomized controlled trials. This type of CAT distills information from an article on a treatment into a final conclusion on the Number Needed to Treat (NNT). The NNT, as defined by the NHS Research and Development Centre (n.d.b), is as follows:

> *The Number Needed to Treat (NNT) is the number of persons you need to treat to prevent one additional bad outcome (stroke, poor function, etc.). ...An NNT of 5... means you have to treat 5 people with the intervention to prevent one additional bad outcome.*

Elements Present in Reliable CATs

No matter what type of CAT you use, whether you use a general form or tailor it specifically to each individual situation, there are elements of the CAT that will always be present. Those elements, and a discussion of their purpose in the CAT, are provided below.

The Date of Completion

Although this seems straightforward, all CATs require a date of completion be prominently displayed. As will be discussed, CATs are inherently transitory creations, with a "shelf life" hovering between a few months and a few years (depending on the advance of knowledge in the field). When you are reviewing your CATs, or if others are examining them for use with their clients, it is imperative that they know when you completed your evidence-based analysis of the literature, and whether or not they should do their own search to find out if any advances in knowledge have been made in the interim.

The Question

At the heart of the CAT is your clinical question. Care should be taken in preparing and wording this question, as its structure will dictate the course of your research. It has been suggested (Richardson, Wilson, Nishikawa, & Hayward, 1995) that a question's "anatomy" should consist of these four parts:

1. The person or problem being addressed.
2. The intervention or exposure being considered.
3. The comparison intervention or exposure, when relevant.
4. The outcomes of interest.

If a question encompasses all four aspects, it will be usable in a literature search and will yield results that will be helpful. A sample question could be phrased as follows: For persons with condition A, will treatment X be more effective than treatment Y in leading to outcome P, or increasing function in outcome P? If a question cannot be made to fit these criteria, more work needs to be done in defining it.

The Clinical Bottom Line

The clinical bottom line is where you summarize your findings for all to see. After your examination of the evidence (discussed next), your final evaluation and the actions you will take based on that evidence are briefly summarized here. The clinical bottom line is more than the results of the article you read. Rather, you should report your critical evaluation of the evidence you've reviewed and your clinical judgment on how those results could be generalized to apply to your client.

The Evidence

As this is evidence-based practice, there is room on the CAT to list the evidence you've found that pertains to the question. It is a good idea to summarize the evidence you are using to make your case. The CAT is your clinical lifeline—it is the backup you have for your decision on a person's treatment. If required, you can refer back to the CATs and explain them as the basis for your clinical judgment. It is important to cite the article's source on the CAT and, if your institution uses paper CATs, advisable to attach the article and proof you found to the final document. The information (or critical review) written up in the CATs also includes the numerical and statistical bases of the evidence.

The Gold Standard

On CATs that specifically have to do with diagnosis or screening (e.g., asking if test A can accurately diagnose condition B), there is room to describe the current "gold standard" test. The gold standard will be a known, valid diagnostic or screening tool. Your diagnostic tool (based on the evidence you've found) should be offered up for comparison to the gold standard in its likelihood ratios. You can also input information gleaned from journal articles to calculate LRs (discussed previously). Other types of CATs, such as those for evaluating Risk and Harm, don't have a "gold standard" treatment with which to be compared, but they should be measured against other existing treatments for the specific condition in question.

Notes

This section, sometimes titled "comments" or "additional information," is where information goes that does not fit into any of the other categories, but which you feel should be added to the CAT. It is a good idea to note any important issues that came up in the critical appraisal or any other costs or consequences of a proposed "clinical bottom line" that were not mentioned before. This section could also be used to record your personal reflections on the evidence you've found and its application. This section will be especially helpful if your CAT is used by others in the field, as it provides a human dimension to the making of the CAT.

SAMPLE CAT FORMAT

The sample CAT format (Table 10-1) is from the Centre for Evidence-Based Emergency Medicine and is posted on-line at www.ebem.org/cats/formulate.html.

Table 10-1

SAMPLE CAT

Title

- This is the same as the clinical question. Identify the type of question that has been asked (therapy, diagnosis, prognosis, harm).

Reviewer

- Name of CAT author.

Search

- The resource selected (MEDLINE, EMA, etc.) and the specific search strategy used are summarized, including MeSH terms, specification of publication type(s), and years searched. The number of citations found and the number selected are given.

Date

- Date of the search and the proposed date for re-evaluation of the topic. Base the latter upon your estimate of how fast knowledge in this area is changing.

Citation(s)

- Use a standardized format such as MEDLINE or *Annals of Emergency Medicine*, and use standard abbreviation for journal identification.

Summary of Study

Summarize the study using the following format:

1. Population—what patients were included and excluded.
2. Interventions—therapeutic interventions, diagnostic interventions, exposures, time.
3. Outcomes—what was measured and/or counted.
4. What happened—track flow through study; how many patients presented, were excluded, or dropped out; completed protocol, etc.

Appraisal

1. Validity checklist—A one- or two-line summary of the results of the validity tests for your question type.
2. Results—Summarize results of appraisal. Calculate important parameters such as number needed to treat, likelihood ratio, include confidence intervals or P values whenever possible.
3. Applicability—Review clinical significance, applicability to your patient population, and potential tradeoffs between harm and benefit.

Conclusions

- Two- or three-line summary and conclusions. Do not make recommendations stronger than justified by the literature. Make value judgments explicit (e.g., "this is not a good test for X because of this clinical reason").

There are other excellent examples of CAT forms available on the web. Students should look at the following sample CATs:

→ Centre for Evidence-Based Medicine, Oxford University
   http://cebm.jr2.ox.ac.uk/docs/catbank.html

→ University of Rochester Medical Center
   www.urmc.rochester.edu/MEDICINE/RES/CATS/index.html

Finally, the Centre for Evidence-Based Medicine has developed a software program called the *CATmaker*, which assists in the creation of computerized CATs. A demonstration version of the software is available for download at www.jr2.ox.ac.uk/cebm/docs/catmaker.html.

USING CATs

As was stated at the beginning of this chapter, CATs are used to summarize and organize evidence for specific clinical situations in practice. However, they are even more useful if they are available to a network of health care professionals. Some health care centres have set up collections of CATs called *CATbanks*, which contain all of the CATs their staff have put together. This way, each practitioner's evidence-based work is made available to the entire unit. Several good examples of CATbanks are

→ The Centre for Evidence Based Medicine's CATbank:
   http://cebm.jr2.ox.ac.uk/cats/catsearch.html

→ The Southwestern Ontario Regional Academic Health Science Network CATs:
   http://ahsn.lhsc.on.ca/cat/

→ The University of Washington Pediatric EBM Page:
   http://students.washington.edu/garrison/topic/index.htm

→ The University of Rochester:
   www.urmc.rochester.edu/medicine/res/cats/indexmaster.html

→ University of North Carolina CATs:
   www.med.unc.edu/medicine/edursrc/!catlist.htm

→ University of Michigan CATs:
   www.med.umich.edu/pediatrics/ebm/cat.htm

DRAWBACKS OF CATs

Despite their usefulness as a tool in evidence-based practice, CATs have their drawbacks. It must be remembered that each CAT is the product of either one individual or a small group of individuals and, as such, is subject to error, bias, and other limitations that are inherent to non-peer-reviewed material. CATs are designed to be dated as well and are only used as short-term or interim guides until more conclusive evidence in the form of RCTs or systematic reviews can provide more conclusive evidence on the topic in question. Sauve et al. (1995) suggest that "when others research and reappraise the same clinical problem the next time a client presents it, the old CAT may be used as the starting point rather than the last word."

SUMMARY OF CATs

CATs are quick, easy, and intuitive organizational tools for using evidence-based practice. They can be created around a variety of topics and methods of looking at evidence. Despite some differences in format, they consist of several basic categories that must be completed. CATs are useful in that they can be collected and can serve as a pool of the evidence-based practice knowledge created by a specific unit; however, CATs can be flawed because of the inherent speed of their creation. CATs represent an advance in the organization and dissemination of research-transfer knowledge and should be integrated into the repertoire of the evidence-based practitioner.

Take-Home Messages

CATs (Critically Appraised Topics)
- A CAT is a one- or two-page summary of a search and critical appraisal of the literature related to a focused clinical question.
- CATs are brief, informative, and useful.
- Five types of CATs: diagnosis/screening; prognosis; evaluating risk/harm in a case controlled study; evaluating risk/harm in a cohort study; treatment, prevention, and screening.
- Necessary elements of CATs: date of completion, question, clinical bottom line, evidence, gold standard, and notes.
- CATs are a quick, easy, and intuitive tool, but they are also subject to error or bias.
- They should be seen as a starting point in a decision-making process rather than a final word.

LEARNING AND EXPLORATION ACTIVITIES

The purpose of this chapter is to introduce the definition and uses of CATs to students. The following exercises allow students to practice developing and using CATs so that they become an effective tool of evidence-based practice.

1. Compare the different CAT templates suggested in this chapter. Which one makes the most sense to you? Which information do you think is the most crucial in a CAT? Which the least important? Why? Using the CAT templates given as examples, create your own CAT template which incorporates the information you feel is essential.

2. Choose a topic in rehabilitation and make a CAT about it. This can be something you have been studying in class or a topic of personal interest. Do this exercise along with a number of your classmates, and when you have finished, exchange CATs and discuss their strengths and weaknesses. If you are really energetic, the class may want to create a paper or electronic CATbank of your collected CATs, which can be expanded as you collectively continue your studies in evidence-based practice.

REFERENCES

Center for Evidence-Based Emergency Medicine. (n.d.a). *Critically appraised topics bank*. Retrieved January 11, 2002, from http://www.ebem.org/cats/catbank.html.

Center for Evidence-Based Emergency Medicine. (n.d.b). *Formulating a critically appraised topic*. Retrieved January 11, 2002, from http://www.ebem.org/cats/formulate.html.

Gray Cancer Institute. (n.d.). *The on-line medical dictionary*. Retrieved January 14, 2002, from http://www.graylab.ac.uk/cgi-bin/omd?case-control+studies.

NHS Research and Development Centre for Evidence-Based Medicine. (n.d.a). *Odds ratios*. Retrieved January 14, 2002, from http://cebm.jr2.ox.ac.uk/docs/oddsrats.html.

NHS Research and Development Centre for Evidence-Based Medicine. (n.d.b). *NNT*. Retrieved January 14, 2002, from http://cebm.jr2.ox.ac.uk/docs/nnt.html.

Richardson, W., Wilson, M., Nishikawa, J., & Hayward, R. (1995). The well-built clinical question: A key to evidence-based decisions. *ACP J Club, 123*, A12-13.

Sauve, S., Lee, H. N., Meade, M. O., Lang, J. B., Faroukh, M., Cook, D. J., et al. (1995). The critically appraised topic: A practical approach to learning critical appraisal. *Annals of the Royal College of Physicians and Surgeons of Canada, 28*(7), 396-8.

University of Oxford Center for Evidence-Based Medicine. (n.d.). *What is a CAT?* Retrieved January 11, 2002, from http://www.jr2.ox.ac.uk/cebm/docs/cats/catabout.html.

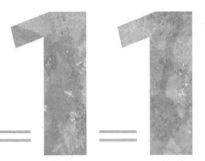

Practice Guidelines, Algorithms, and Clinical Pathways

Donna Nicholson, PTReg(C), OTReg(C)

LEARNING OBJECTIVES

After reading this chapter, the student/practitioner will be able to:

- Critically evaluate the need for clinical practice guidelines and care pathways in the more challenging health care environment.
- Identify the key characteristics of clinical practice guidelines, algorithms, and clinical pathways.
- Recognize some of the barriers to developing these guidelines and identifying ways to circumvent these obstacles.
- Use the appropriate terminology associated with care pathways.
- Recognize and understand the various factors involved in the implementation of this practice, including technology, legality, and documentation.

RECENT TRENDS IN HEALTH CARE

The increasing incidence of earlier hospital discharges and emergency visits without admissions means that patient/clients with a higher level of risk and severity are now returning to or remaining in the community. Those who are admitted now experience shortened lengths of stay with a focus on efficiency and effectiveness in order to maintain access for those who need an acute care bed. Caregivers are experiencing increased burden as communities lack adequate levels of support services due to insufficient funding and lack of available skilled workers. With the move to managed care in community health care, and a vision for patient/client choice and family involvement in planning services in all settings, the goal is to achieve a more appropriate and responsive mix of services and support by adopting new models of service planning and delivery that blend quality with responsiveness and equity. Newly emerging directions are now pointing us toward a focus on accountability, quality, and efficient utilization of health care services at all points of the continuum of care. There is recognition for the need to coordinate and organize care within agencies/institutions and beyond. Stakeholders expect and are beginning to demand that key clinical and cost outcomes be identified. Enhanced consumer participation in developing and implementing plans of care means the focus is on increased collaboration and improved communication between care receivers and care providers and also between the multidisciplinary providers themselves.

STRATEGIES TO ADDRESS TRENDS AND NEW DIRECTIONS

The emerging trends in health care demand approaches that embrace increased efficiency and improved quality with enhanced responsiveness. Some effective mechanisms for achieving quality standards include care pathways, continuous quality improvement, resource management, outcome measurement, clinical protocols, information systems management, and *clinical practice guidelines* (CPGs). Outcome measures are effective tools that indicate the value and impact of the intervention but do not guide practice other than point to the need to change interventions to achieve the desired results. On the other hand, care pathways based on clinical practice guidelines or protocols and incorporating outcome measures can standardize practice that is both responsive and accountable to funders as well as consumers. The focus of this chapter will be to provide the reader with introductory information regarding two of these strategies, clinical practice guidelines and care pathways.

Clinical Practice Guidelines

The Institute of Medicine defines CPGs as "systematically developed statements that assist practitioner and patient decisions about appropriate health care for specific clinical circumstances" (Field & Lohr, 1992; Canadian Medical Association, 1994). In 1994, the Canadian Medical Association (CMA) adopted this definition (Verhulst, 1994). To date, few CPGs have been developed for disciplines other than physician interventions, and although many professional colleges are currently debating the feasibility of developing discipline-specific guidelines, it may be some time, if ever, before these become available for and are embraced by all professions.

Guidelines may be based on expert opinion/consensus and/or evidence-based practice as identified by research and may be regional, facility-wide, program based, unit specific, or based on case types. CPGs offer recommendations for care and are prescriptive in nature, helping the practitioner determine the appropriateness of selected interventions. They are often official statements or policies on the proper indications for performing a clinical procedure or treatment or the proper management for specific clinical problems. They can be either evidence-based or nonevidence-based, but generally, those CPGs developed more recently have been based on well-researched evidence supported by internationally recognized collaborative bodies such as the Cochrane Collaboration and CANARIE (Canadian Network for the Advancement of Research, Industry, and Education). CPGs may also be referred to as practice parameters, practice policies, appropriateness criteria, or consensus statements and may be endorsed or supported by a group of experts. They can help the practitioner determine the most effective and appropriate interventions, inform or educate practitioners, and provide a strategic method for describing what should be done. There are more CPGs available in the United States than in Canada, possibly due to the lack of funding and dedicated resources for development, testing, and implementation of CPGs. There appears to be a wide variation across the country in setting priorities and guidelines for development of CPGs, while at the same time there are few available and validated measurement and feedback tools. The best approach to development of CPGs is one that capitalizes on the strengths of various models, using a combined approach of both evidence-based and expert consensus. This ensures that the best available evidence is used in an unbiased way to inform recommendations while building on the experience of experts who assist with interpretation of evidence, judge applicability of evidence in specific clinical situations, and address trade-offs between alternative interventions according to the balance between benefit, harm, and affordability (Canadian Medical Association, 1996).

Currently, there are approximately 1,500 CPGs recognized by the CMA. Definitions, examples, explanations, and a list of CPGs are available on the CMA web site (www.cma.ca) or the National Guidelines Clearinghouse (www.guidelines.gov). Since standards on development of guidelines have only recently been released and use of the standards is voluntary, many CPGs lack indications on how the guideline was developed (research basis) and those developing the guideline may have lacked the expertise to critically appraise the literature. This makes it difficult to discern what methods underlie the CPG, since there are varying approaches and capabilities to carry out reviews and, thus, different conclusions can be drawn from the same evidence. Organizations such as the Agency for Health Care Research & Quality (formerly the Agency for Health Care Policy and Research [AHCPR]) initially developed CPGs but now restrict its activity to dissemination only of guidelines that are available in formats suitable for health care practitioners, the scientific community, educators, and consumers. The CMA also disseminates guidelines as they are developed but does not participate in their development. Agencies such as the Cochrane Collaboration aim to help people make informed decisions about health by preparing, maintaining, and ensuring the accessibility of rigorous, systematic, and up-to-date reviews (and where possible, meta-analyses) of the benefits and risks of health care interventions. This international research organization makes available manuals, tools, and training materials that facilitate the design and conduct of the reviews as well as allowing easy access to the reviews and continuous open peer review (Jadad, Haynes, Hunt, & Browman, 2000).

Table 11-1 lists the names of some typical Canadian (CMA) and American (AHCPR) CPGs. Table 11-2 shows an example of a published and internationally recognized CPG, the Ottawa Ankle Rule.

Table 11-1

TYPICAL CPGs

CMA	*AHCPR*
Ottawa Ankle Rules	Management of Postoperative Pain
Cataract Management	Prediction and Prevention of Pressure Ulcers in Adults
Management of Cardiovascular Risks	Management of Urinary Incontinence in the Elderly
Lab Testing for Thyroid Dysfunction	Detection, Diagnosis, and Treatment of Depression in Primary Care
Management of Prostate Cancer	Managing Early HIV Infection

Table 11-2

GUIDELINE FOR RADIOGRAPHY OF THE ANKLE AND FOOT (OTTAWA ANKLE RULE)

An ankle x-ray series is required only if there is pain in the malleolar zone and any one of the following:
- Bone tenderness along the distal 6 cm of the posterior edge of the fibula or tip of the lateral malleolus
- Bone tenderness along the distal 6 cm along the posterior edge of the tibia or tip of the medial malleolus
- Inability to bear weight for four steps, both immediately and in the emergency department

A foot X-ray series is required only if there is pain in the midfoot zone and any one of the following:
- Bone tenderness at the base of the fifth metatarsal
- Bone tenderness at the navicular bone
- Inability to bear weight for four steps, both immediately and in the emergency department

Exclusions:
- Less than 18 years
- Intoxication
- Multiple painful injuries
- Pregnant
- Head injury
- Diminished sensation due to neurological deficit

Adapted by the Alberta Clinical Practice Guidelines Program Working Group (Alberta Medical Association) from Stiell, I. G., Wells, G., Laupacis, A., et al. (1995). Multicentre trial to introduce the Ottawa Ankle Rules for use of radiography in acute ankle injuries. *British Medical Journal, 311,* 594-597. Reprinted with permission of the Alberta Clinical Practice Guidelines Program Working Group.

Barriers to Implementation and Uptake of CPGs

Although the benefits of implementing CPGs appear obvious (evidence-based practice, standardized approach/reduced variation, increased practitioner and patient knowledge, enhanced quality, efficiency, accountability, and effectiveness), practitioners continue to be reluctant to embrace them for many reasons:

→ Development of the guidelines is a time-consuming and labour-intensive effort (guidelines do not implement themselves and can take up to 3 years for completion of one guideline).

→ Current information and reporting systems are inadequate.

→ To succeed in implementing, there must be intense dissemination efforts followed by dedicated resources for evaluating and generating feedback (follow-up and reporting of variances from established practice). This level of intensity is generally unsupported in most settings. (Education alone fails to produce sustained changes in clinical practice.)

→ Practitioners often remain suspicious because they are also beginning to see conflicting CPGs on the same topic and are plagued by fears about the purpose and ultimate use of CPGs, as well as concerns about legal issues.

→ Many of the guidelines developed are not executable at the point of care (too complicated, time-consuming, or inconvenient).

→ There is often no system for monitoring the impact of the guideline on current practice, no feedback mechanism, and no process for iterative refinement.

→ There is a fear that guidelines may decrease individualized care.

Factors for Ensuring Successful Implementation of CPGs

Those who have been more successful in implementing CPGs have identified certain key factors. They recommend that the type of clinical problem or task chosen for CPG development should be a single, well-defined task versus a complex or complicated task. There must be practitioner participation during development of the guideline, and the resulting document should be in a simple, clear language and format. Financial incentives for development and uptake were seen to facilitate the success of CPGs as did reducing administrative barriers. Peer review processes more often resulted in behaviour change. The CPG must prove itself cost-effective while improving care. Critical to the entire process was the strength of the evidence upon which the guideline was to be based.

Evaluation of CPGs

If CPGs are to become integral components of health care practice, they are best viewed as integral components, not stand-alone strategies. They must be developed with a focus on adequate funding for the entire process, including evaluation, and should ultimately affect practice and/or policy. There must be a shift of focus from development to changing behaviour and measuring performance (outcomes). The climate is right for a move to alternative approaches that may be more cost effective. Funders are not interested in financing practice that is not evidence-based. CPGs must be "part of the fabric of the organization and evaluation must be a built-in component" (Bell & Wilson, 1998). Graham, Calder, Hebert, Carter, & Tetroe (2000) reviewed 12 guideline appraisal instruments according to their context, developer information, methods, recommendations, dissemination, implementation, and evaluation. There were limitations of the review, since the appraisal instruments included had poor or unknown reliability and validity and incomplete or unknown methodology. Several

Table 11-3

PRACTICE GUIDELINE EVALUATION AND ADAPTATION CYCLE

Step 1   Conduct systematic search for practice guidelines
Step 2   Select a validated guideline appraisal instrument
Step 3   Assess quality of how guidelines were developed and quality of recommendations
Step 4   Assess clinical content
Step 5   Develop local protocol based on adaptation and adoption of existing guideline recommendations
Step 6   Return to step 1 for continual review and revision of guideline

Reprinted from Graham, I., Lorimer, K., Harrison, M., & Piercianowski, T. (2000). Evaluating the quality and content of international clinical practice guidelines for leg ulcers: Preparing for Canadian adaptation. *Canadian Association for Enterostomal Therapy Journal, 19*(3), 15-31.

guideline appraisal instruments now gaining international recognition include the AGREE Instrument, a valid and reliable tool developed by an international consortium of researchers that uses a four-point lichart scale to evaluate CPGs according to their scope/purpose, stakeholder involvement, clarity, editorial independence, formulation of recommendations, application, monitoring, and identification of evidence (AGREE Collaboration, n.d.). A recently developed conceptual framework, the Practice Guideline Evaluation and Adaptation Cycle (Graham, Lorimer, Harrison, & Piercianowski, 2000) (Table 11-3), involves a systematic search for practice guidelines, appraisal of the quality of the guidelines by an interdisciplinary committee using a guideline appraisal instrument, content analysis of guideline recommendations, and coming to a consensus about which recommendations should be adopted locally. Based on review of existing guideline appraisal instruments, these researchers chose the Appraisal Instrument for Clinical Guidelines, Version 1 (Cluzeau, Littlejohns, Grimshaw, & Feder, 1997). This instrument has been shown to have easy applicability with acceptable reliability and evidence of validity. It is also the instrument of choice for the Independent Appraisal Service of the National Health Service (NHS) in the UK to assess all guidelines funded by the NHS through the National Clinical Guidelines Group. This guideline appraisal instrument consists of 37 items inquiring whether information is present and the quality of the information in three dimensions—rigour with which the guideline was developed, context and content, and dissemination and monitoring. The developers found that using this appraisal instrument and the Practice Guideline Evaluation and Adaptation Cycle was a feasible process and facilitated local adaptation of international guidelines. Only by applying rigorous appraisal tools and methods such as these will guidelines be recognized as valid by practitioners. The result may then be an actual difference in practice.

Using the Practice Guideline Evaluation and Adaptation Cycle, the developers formed recommendations that are the basis for the clinical practice guideline for Leg Ulcer Care in Ottawa-Carleton. The guideline was adapted from four existing guidelines and local consensus with the grades of recommendation and types of evidence clearly referenced right within the guideline, clearly speaking to the evidence basis for the guideline (Tables 11-4 and 11-5).

Table 11-4

OTTAWA-CARLETON COMMUNITY CARE ACCESS CENTRE
LEG ULCER CARE PROTOCOL

Grades of Recommendation	Type of Evidence
A	Evidence obtained from at least one randomized clinical trial or meta-analysis of randomized clinical trials
B	Evidence from well-designed clinical studies but no randomized clinical trials
C	Evidence from expert committee reports or opinion and/or clinical experience or respected authorities. Indicates absence of directly applicable studies of good quality

Reprinted with permission of Ottawa-Carleton Community Care Access Centre.

Algorithms

To facilitate the move to evidence-based practice and the development of CPGs and care pathways, practitioners who are unfamiliar with these strategies may find it useful to begin the process by developing algorithms or decision trees. *Algorithms* are "written guidelines to stepwise evaluation and management strategies that require observations to be made, decisions to be considered, and actions to be taken" (Hadorn, McCormick, & Diokno, 1992). Algorithms are simply CPGs arranged in a decision-tree format. Rehabilitation practitioners may be familiar with the algorithm concept found in the well-known outcome measure, the Functional Independence Measure (Guide for the Uniform Data Set, 1997) (Appendix G). Developers of CPGs have found that algorithms facilitate decision making for practitioners and make it easier for them to list essential clinical steps that can then be used during the development of a guideline and then a subsequent care pathway, if desired. The algorithm itself does not become part of the guideline or pathway but is used in conjunction with it. For example, in the case of overall management of persons with stroke, the results of the history and physical examination could lead to the use of a guideline for management of poststroke. The recommendations concerning routine tests and other diagnostic procedures could be incorporated into the "Tests/Diagnostics" section of a care pathway (see section on Care Pathways for more detailed information regarding pathways). The development of an algorithm can be a straightforward, nonthreatening way to introduce the process of development for CPGs and pathways to practitioners who may not be familiar with these concepts. They can help to clarify the key decision points requiring action while maintaining a simplistic approach. The decision tree example in Table 11-6 (p. 204) shows the process that was used in assisting case managers in a community intake setting to determine the essential information required at the point of referral. The decision tree was applied to every intake question and the decision to keep (collect) or discard (don't collect) the assessment question was made based on the outcome.

Table 11-5

Ottawa-Carleton CCAC
Leg Ulcer Care Protocol Reference Guide[A]

Assessment

Clinical history, physical exam, and lab testing to assess etiology and factors contributing too the leg ulcer[b,d] C

Ankle brachial pressure index (ABPI) to screen for arterial disease[b-e] . . . . A

| Venous . . . C ABPI *at least* 0.8[b-d] | Nonvenous or mixed[b-d] . . . . C ABPI *between* 0.5 *and* 0.8 OR Unusual ulcer presentation[b-d] OR Presence of other disease[b-d] Refer to the appropriate specialist[b] | Arterial . . . C ABPI *less than* 0.5. Refer to a vascular surgeon[f] |

| Treatment | Graduated multilayer compression bandaging for the uncomplicated ulcer. High compression (35 to 40 Hg) is more effective than low compression.[b-d] Applied by trained practitioner[b,d] . . . . A, B |

| Wound management | Measure surface area serially over time[b,c] . . . . C Wash ulcer with tap water or saline[b-d] . . . . A Simple, nonadherent dressing[b,c] . . . . A Acceptable to client[b] . . . . C Dressing appropriate to stage of healing and amount of exudate[e] . . . . C Moist wound environment[e] . . . . A |

| If ulcer is painful | Hydrocolloid or foam dressing[c] . . . . A Pain management plan:[b,c,e] Compression, exercise, elevation, and analgesia[b] . . . . B |

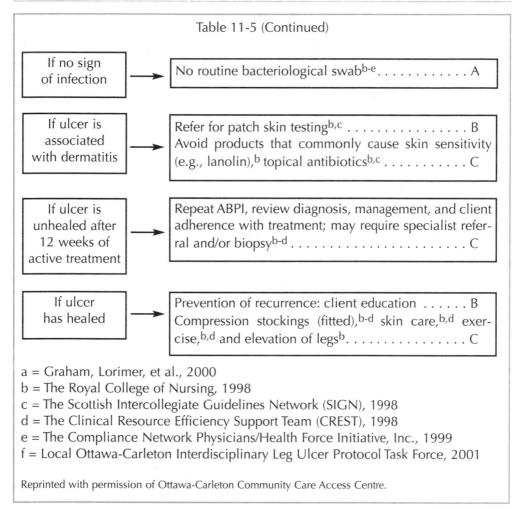

Table 11-5 (Continued)

| If no sign of infection | → | No routine bacteriological swab[b-e] . . . . A |

| If ulcer is associated with dermatitis | → | Refer for patch skin testing[b,c] . . . . B
Avoid products that commonly cause skin sensitivity (e.g., lanolin),[b] topical antibiotics[b,c] . . . . C |

| If ulcer is unhealed after 12 weeks of active treatment | → | Repeat ABPI, review diagnosis, management, and client adherence with treatment; may require specialist referral and/or biopsy[b-d] . . . . C |

| If ulcer has healed | → | Prevention of recurrence: client education . . . . . . B
Compression stockings (fitted),[b-d] skin care,[b,d] exercise,[b,d] and elevation of legs[b]. . . . . C |

a = Graham, Lorimer, et al., 2000
b = The Royal College of Nursing, 1998
c = The Scottish Intercollegiate Guidelines Network (SIGN), 1998
d = The Clinical Resource Efficiency Support Team (CREST), 1998
e = The Compliance Network Physicians/Health Force Initiative, Inc., 1999
f = Local Ottawa-Carleton Interdisciplinary Leg Ulcer Protocol Task Force, 2001

Reprinted with permission of Ottawa-Carleton Community Care Access Centre.

Clinical Pathways

With over 1,500 CPGs developed and available for uptake in Canada but few incorporated into routine practice, it is clear that guidelines by themselves do not change practice. CPGs, however, can form the foundation of evidence upon which clinical pathways are built and together these tools can assist in the provision of optimal quality of care in an environment of fiscal restraint and public accountability. They enable us to systematically measure, analyze, and improve health care delivery.

A *clinical pathway* is defined as "a cause and effect grid or framework, which identifies expected measurable patient/client outcomes (or behaviours) against a timeline for a specific case-type or group" (Zander & Hill, 1995). Because the model's initial conception was primarily focused on nursing and physician activities, it has become "a multidisciplinary tool, which makes explicit the usual problem and activities that must occur to facilitate the achievement of expected outcomes in a defined length of time" (Cancer Care Ontario, 1999). The clinical pathway is a tool that sets locally agreed clinical standards based on the best available evidence for managing specific groups of clients. It can form part or all of the clinical record and enables the care given by members of the multidisciplinary team, together

Table 11-6

EXAMPLE OF A SIMPLE DECISION TREE

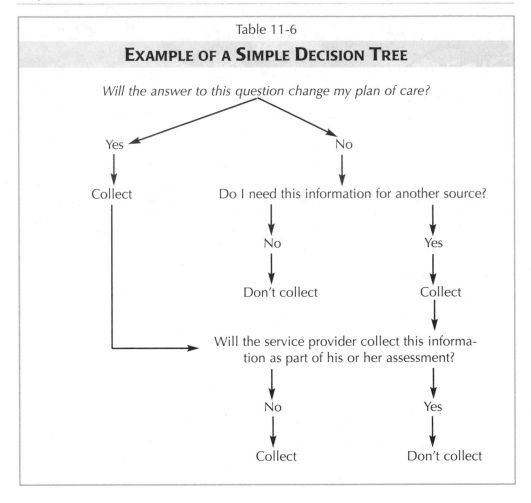

Will the answer to this question change my plan of care?

Yes → Collect

No → Do I need this information for another source?

   No → Don't collect

   Yes → Collect

Will the service provider collect this information as part of his or her assessment?

   No → Collect

   Yes → Don't collect

with the progress and outcome, to be documented. Variations from the pathway are record-ed, and analysis allows a continuous evaluation of the effectiveness of clinical practice. Obtained information is used to revise the pathway to improve the quality of client care (Kitchiner & Bundred, 1996, 1999). Clinical pathways have been developed in an attempt to improve quality of care and patient satisfaction, and to reduce variations in practice, compli-cations, errors, resource utilization, and costs. They identify anticipated outcomes, health care provider interventions, and anticipated intervention times. Pathways have been utilized in the American health care system since the late 1980s when Karen Zander of the Centre for Case Management developed a patented model named CareMap (Center for Case Management, South Natick, MA). The model applied the engineering project management principles of those effective critical paths utilized since the late 50s and early 60s in the auto-motive industry and manufacturing, first gaining international recognition in the American Aerospace Industry at NASA. The concept, which began as a nursing and case management initiative in Boston's New England Medical Center in 1985, was quickly adopted by the hos-pital sector in both the United States and larger centres in Canada, as well as internationally. Soon after this, we began to see the trend to focus care planning in American health care organizations for clusters of patient/clients with similar conditions called *case mixed groups*

(CMGs) or *diagnostic related groups* (DRGs). Subsequent to this, the American health care system was quick to move to capping service by dictating maximum costs based on the projected episode of care in a model known as managed care.

We are now experiencing an explosion of coordinated care models both in the United States and Canada similar to Zander's original CareMap model, using names synonymous with the original but unique to each particular setting and application both for the purpose of avoiding copyright and to achieve user participation by ensuring provider involvement during development and commitment to the use of the pathway, once implemented (Appendix H).

Framework for Clinical Pathways

Developers have coined a multitude of names for their particular coordinated care model (e.g., case path, care path/plan/pathway/compass/track/guide, multidisciplinary action plan, target track, critical path, anticipated recovery path, clinical pathway, care management/case management, collaborative care path, care process), but the framework and components of all are similar and recognizable as having roots in the CareMap concept. Recently, we have also seen the emergence of other copyrighted systems sold for profit and providing education and support for development and implementation within a unique setting. These systems bear names such as Interqual, PtCare System, Interpath, VNAFirst, and CareWare (see Purchased Care Pathway Systems at the end of the chapter). The obvious advantages of using such purchased systems include reaping time and cost savings by avoiding the prolonged and expensive development process. They facilitate the ability to compare results across other settings and institutions using the same tool and provide the availability of expert support for implementation and evaluation and, in some cases, the confidence that the tool is based on solid research evidence. Drawbacks to commercial systems include the potential for lack of buy-in from staff who may refuse to support what is perceived as "cookie-cutter" medicine, the possible poor fit of a model that is generic with a service that is unique, and little to no opportunity for consumers to be involved in development of the care plan. Although home built pathways are generally viewed by staff with less suspicion than purchased systems, some concerns may still be expressed by staff who are newly introduced to the concept. Pathways may be seen as cookbook medicine or cost-cutting mechanisms for administrators. Difficulty may be experienced when attempting to address comorbidity. The pathway may be perceived as being too simplistic, too inflexible, and just one more piece of paper to complete. There may also be the fear that information collected will be used to penalize.

Critical pathway models have a matrix listing interventions along one axis and time along another. Interventions typically included are consultations and referral; assessments and observations; tests, treatments, measurements and diagnostics; nutrition, medication, activity, and mobility; safety, patient/client, and family education/teaching; and discharge planning. Within the timeline, we may see identified typical problems, desired clinical outcomes, intermediate goals or *key indicators*, as well as physician orders. Some "next generation" pathways now include not only variance tracking records but also admission and discharge indicators/status, as well as key indicator and outcome records (clinical and client/patient).

Choosing Case Types for Pathway Development

Experts with experience in developing pathways recommend that a systematic review of the particular population served, such as cost of care, volume, level of risk, etc., be undertaken. When choosing a particular area for development of a pathway, the greatest impact will be achieved if the initial focus is directed toward groups with demonstrated:

→ High volume

- → High cost
- → High risk
- → High practice variability
- → Potential for improvement
- → Predictable course
- → Provider interest
- → Potential to cross multiple settings and disciplines in continuum
- → Physician interest, initiative, and acceptance.

Development Strategies

Many of the first pathways developed were based on current practice not only due to the paucity of available research, particularly in the area of rehabilitation, but also because of the lack of support from their organization for the time and effort involved in doing the literature searches. Now, most developers recognize the importance of basing their pathways on best practice supported by solid research evidence. They begin the work of building pathways by reviewing whatever background information is available, including completing a critical review of similar pathways currently in use within other sites. This is (or should be) complemented by an extensive literature review, both of pathways as well as information regarding practice for the clinicians involved in providing care for the particular case type for which the pathway is being developed. Many developers begin the process by bringing together the key partners involved in care for the case type to be addressed, provide key research articles, samples of pathways, a description of the development task, and then send the development committee off with the homework of researching information on their individual practice for the specific client group. If multiple agencies are involved in the development, each agency should be asked to review and provide current available data regarding practice for comparative purposes. In this way, if it is discovered that evidence in the literature is lacking in a particular area, the preimplementation data can provide the foundation for further investigation and evaluation following implementation of the pathway. Since all members of the development team must have a thorough understanding of the concept and philosophy of the clinical pathway model, it is also necessary to provide staff with education and teaching materials regarding the pathway model prior to embarking on the development task.

Important factors to remember when developing both CPGs and pathways include using a suite of tools, rather than rigidly attempting to apply one model or format to every situation. Build on variability to target your tool to your audience. Think about who you are, where you are going, and where you wish to end. Most importantly, make sure the tool that is developed meets the needs of the clients and the clinicians who will use the tool.

First generation pathways were usually diagnosis-based (as in the management of stroke, diabetes, acute myocardial infarction) or symptom-based (as for the investigation and treatment of clients presenting with chest pain). They could also focus on a specific procedure (total joint replacement, coronary artery bypass graft, transurethral resection of prostate) or encourage the use of therapeutic guidelines such as postoperative analgesia. Second generation pathways that highlight activity or function are now emerging (continence, enteral feeding, memory loss, self-injection) with a resulting focus on education, teaching, and client outcomes rather than specific medical interventions.

Continuum Pathways

The first pathways to emerge usually reflected only the activity within a single institution or service but developers are now realizing the importance of linking pathways along the continuum of care (e.g., hospital to home, home to long-term care). This enables the person receiving care to have knowledge of the entire episode of care, while the providers can ensure gaps between settings and services are minimized. Chronic conditions such as asthma, obstructive pulmonary disease, diabetes, and palliative care have been managed through the development of pathways that coordinate care across the primary-secondary care interface (Dowsey, Kilgour, Santamaria, & Choong, 1999). The effort involved in developing such transorganizational, multidisciplinary pathways is enormous, but the benefits far outweigh the risks. Studies are now emerging that show that when pathways are introduced, better client outcomes are achieved (Ellershaw, Foster, Murphy, Shea, & Overill, 1997). Results indicate that pathways contribute to client-focused care, as they constantly monitor quality and any deviation from the pathway identifies complications early. The plan of care is clearly defined and shared with the client and, in some instances, clients are involved in the actual development of the plan. Discharge or transition planning is facilitated because the median length of stay is defined and length of stay can often be reduced without an increase in complications or unscheduled re-admissions.

When developing such continuum pathways, it is important for developers to do the following:

1. Choose the target group for which the pathway will be developed together.
2. Concentrate on the interface between the pathways and clearly define the transition status (functional level or point at which the client/patient moves from one setting to another).
3. Reach a consensus regarding common definitions (e.g., develop a multisite terminology guide).
4. Use international diagnostic codes.
5. If computerized, use a common electronic interface.

Often, the resulting benefits of developing and implementing continuum pathways for the care providers are the emergence of new partnerships and increased collaboration between agencies, decreased duplication of effort, increased knowledge of available services, and recognition for expertise.

Pathway Development Teams

It is important that the development team select the specific client group for the pathway to ensure interest and enthusiasm for the task at the front line rather than solely at an administrative level. Many excellent pathways have failed because those affected by the tool were not involved with its formulation and implementation, were thus disinterested, and did not see the importance of the work. Interested participants who are involved in the actual care delivery must be identified and selected to form working groups. In situations in which providers have never before had the opportunity of debating practice or reviewing literature, it may be necessary to form single discipline working groups prior to moving to multidisciplinary groups. In this way, scope of practice for each discipline can be determined and agreed upon prior to determining the scope of the pathway (beginning and end). If the literature search identifies any related CPGs that direct practice for the patient/client group for which a pathway is being developed, the CPG can become the foundation for the pathway with the addition of a timeline plus admission and discharge indicators or criteria. Table 11-7 provides a comprehensive process checklist for CPG and clinical pathway development.

Table 11-7

CHECKLIST FOR DEVELOPMENT OF CPGs AND CLINICAL PATHWAYS

Assemble multidisciplinary teams
↓
Define clinical problems and current practice
↓
Conduct literature search

Locate and appraise systematic reviews   Locate and appraise primary studies
↓   ↓
Update systematic reviews   Generate systematic reviews
↓   ↓
Describe and classify research according to levels of evidence
↓
Formulate or reformulate guideline recommendations
↓
Link guidelines to form clinical pathways
↓
Select process and outcome measures
↓
Identify documentation requirements and preferences
↓
Adapt effective strategies from systematic reviews to local culture
↓
Disseminate and pilot test guidelines and pathways
using effective strategies from systematic reviews
↓
Collect and analyze process and outcome measures
↓
Combine with updated literature review and appraisals
↓
Correct problems and make revisions

Adapted from Dook, D. J., Greengold, N. I., Elrodt, A. G., & Weingarten, S. R. (1997). The relation between systematic reviews and practice guidelines. *Ann Intern Med, 127*(3), 210-216.

Documentation System

Clinical pathways and their documentation systems have often been implemented without follow-up such as chart audits and milestone tracking. In the past, there has been a lack of congruence between clinical pathway tools and nonpathway tools, such as flow charts and outcome measures. When they were first developed, clinical pathways initially were tools that were used only as a guide, being housed in policy and procedure manuals. With some pathways, staff were asked to "sign-off" at the end of a shift. Others were used in conjunction with flow sheets to facilitate being able to trend information over the episode of care. There is the danger that staff may see the clinical pathway as an "add-on" or "one more form to sign" if documentation is not integrated. With the introduction of clinical pathways comes the need to introduce staff to an entirely new approach to recording and charting, requiring the development of a documentation system to complement the model and ensure that organizational, legal, and professional standards are met. Clinical pathways force the move to a *charting by exception* model, resulting in many immediate advantages being realized. Any trends in a client's or a group of clients' status can be seen without having to wait an extended period of time for a trending report to be generated. Abnormal data recorded on a client's record is immediately highlighted and easily retrieved. Transcription and duplication of charting is eliminated, resulting in documentation time being cut significantly. Information that has already been recorded isn't repeated. Clients are evaluated against well-defined goals because assessments are standardized so providers evaluate and document findings consistently. All providers now can use the same approach for the same case type and begin to compare outcomes without being dependent on formalized research. This is due to the fact that an accurate representation of the course of treatment, changes in condition, and care rendered for the particular case type are readily available—an ideal format for conducting applied research.

Clinical Pathway Evaluation

Preimplementation Review of Design: An Appraisal Instrument for Clinical Pathways

A collaborative effort between Cancer Care Ontario and McMaster University has recently produced an appraisal instrument for clinical pathways called *The Markers of Quality in Paths* (Weinstein & Hockley, 1999). The instrument includes recommendations for development standards, purpose, process of approval, format for paper and electronic versions, and makes recommendations for ongoing review. A companion tool, the Checklist for Path Appraisal, includes questions related to process, outcomes, and content and defines various levels of achievement with respect to each dimension. Use of the Markers of Quality in Paths in conjunction with the Checklist for Path Appraisal will assist developers of pathways to describe their system and tools, helping them to look at the phase or generation their organization is in with respect to pathways. It will also assist in looking for areas to be redeveloped within the system and tools so that they properly support the organization's needs.

Postimplementation Review of Process and Experience

Evaluation following initial implementation or pilot of a clinical pathway should collect data from multiple sources, including surveys or focus groups for users (staff surveys), consumers, families, and physicians. Chart audits should be carried out to validate information collected from surveys and also give important information regarding documentation practices. It is helpful to develop a data collection template with details that have been chosen for review such as length of stay and visit frequencies, client's discharge status, clinical (functional status), and client outcomes (negotiated goals achieved), as well as any positive or negative variances along the pathway.

Identifying Outcomes: Variances

By tracking information on clinical pathways, it will be possible to identify the critical success factors for case types that will define optimal steps in clinical processes, reduce unnecessary variation in these processes, and provide data for continuous improvement (Zander, 1992). When making a decision regarding the process by which to define patient/client progress and outcome, it is necessary to carefully consider the plan for analysis and the available supports (clerical, technical, systems, etc.). Many large institutions embarking on the clinical pathway model have made the error of implementing complex tracking systems for determining outcomes, only to be quickly overwhelmed by data without having the ability to effect change based on the reports generated. A *variance* is defined as the difference between what is expected and what actually happens. Variances can be the result of patient/client, practitioner, or system issues and can be either positive or negative. Factors usually resulting in a variance include the patient/client's condition such as an unexpected complication, an issue of the support network such as availability or burden of care, a provider or agency issue such as presence of a wait list, or availability of test results; there may also be variances regarding provision of equipment and supplies (e.g., delivery, availability) as well as environmental issues (e.g., unsanitary conditions, lack of water, heat, electricity, food, telephone). If the recording and reporting system is computerized, it may be possible to track variances concurrently (at the same time the variance is identified) and thus affect change immediately to address the variance. However, because most agencies lack this degree of technical support, variances are usually tracked retrospectively (after the patient/client has been discharged from the pathway). Variances that focus on the program level rather than patient/client level include factors such as length of stay, number and frequency of visits, readmission rates, infection rates, and length of time waiting for service. This concept of refining variance data down to the vital few leads to the identification of key indicators (Appendix I).

Identifying Outcomes: Key Indicators

More recently there has been a move away from variance tracking toward identification of performance capability that indicates the patient/client's recovery status—a type of health report card. These key indicators or outcomes form milestones that coincide with a change in level of care or resource utilization, such as weight-bearing status for an orthopaedic intervention, ability to self-inject insulin for diabetes care, or first day of ambulation following stroke. With this move has also come a new focus away from "micromanaging" an episode of care (e.g., extubation, catheter removal, tolerance of fluids) to a broader focus on the continuum of care, identifying key admission and discharge indicators to facilitate a smooth transition throughout levels of care (Appendix J). Key indicators such as length of stay, readmission rates, or incidence of complications have statistical value that can provide a direction over time of a specific process. Standard tools used for quality improvement such as control charts are useful methods for interpreting and presenting the data collected (Appendix K).

A template for developing a key indicator record is included in Appendix L for student practice in identifying decision points in a plan of care.

Pathway Computerization and Impact of Technology

A systematic review of the effects of computer-based clinical decision support systems on physician performance and patient outcomes revealed the trends for physicians answering questions regarding their practice. The study showed that 76% asked colleagues, 14% used

CPGs, and 10% accessed Medline (Hunt, Haynes, Hanna, & Smith, 1998). The implementation of an electronic system that includes links to supporting evidence has been shown to facilitate access for the users to the evidence supporting the guidelines and pathways at the point of care. This can often result in more effective uptake of new protocols.

Point of care tools that allow timely data access/capture plus order entry/result reporting help to facilitate concurrent interdisciplinary documentation. They allow multiple user access to information and have the potential for comparison of data on many levels (provider, agency, provincial, national, international). As well as the benefit of reduced documentation time and the potential for concurrent variance analysis (impossible with a paper-based system), there is also the potential for complete integration of information across the full continuum of care so that data can be easily shared and is only entered once. This allows all providers to easily retrieve complete and current information from a common health database. It is then possible to build in decision support and education tools (staff and client/patient) consistent with the protocol. Several Internet-based novel design concepts, which have recently emerged into what is being called *clinical* or *disease guidance systems*, enhance the management of clients/patients through the use of "just-in-time, evidence-based medical literature and practice guidelines" (Penn, Lau, & Wilson, 1996). Not only do these systems generate a set of client/patient care activities or orders individualized to each person, but it is done in such a way that the individual activities are linked to available evidence, providing practitioners the ability to enroll clients/patients into active research trials via the Internet. All components of the system, literature, and guidelines are maintained and distributed by a robust publishing system through an expanded Web technology, which allows commercial control of copyright and royalties. Several international (USA, UK, Netherlands, Germany) evaluation studies are underway to determine the effectiveness of such clinical guidance systems. Other computer-based projects underway include the Alberta WellNet, an initiative that links pharmacy information, providing distance health services and development of a common financial system; StrokeNet, a collaborative effort researching best practice for stroke care; and CQIN, the Clinical Quality Improvement Network (another Alberta initiative), linking randomized controlled trial evidence and its application in clinical practice.

LEGAL IMPLICATIONS OF CLINICAL PATHWAYS AND CPGS

Integration of clinical pathways and CPGs into a documentation system that moves to charting by exception often raises legal questions from practitioners regarding the security of the electronic chart, rigour of the record in a court of law, and professional documentation responsibility (notion that if it isn't documented, it wasn't done). In response to such concerns, lawyers indicate that the use of practice standards does not create significant new risks and actually may reduce the risk and cost of litigation when the tool is approved as a permanent part of the care record (Stradiotto, 1997). Signatures must follow completion of interventions, outcomes must be entered, and variances identified and documented as lack of progress with identification of plans to deal with them. The feeling in the legal community is that exception charting is likely stronger documentation than the documentation consistently recorded in the previous system since casebooks are filled with examples showing poor record keeping and conflicting professional notes as sources of liability. Clinical pathways aid in defence because they are a complete plan of care, they encourage clear communication, and enhance uniform record keeping (Burke & Murphy, 1995). Exception charting provides consistent documentation of *standards of care* and meets federal, provincial, and

Table 11-8

SIMILARITIES AND DIFFERENCES BETWEEN CPGs, ALGORITHMS, AND CLINICAL PATHWAYS

CPGs and Algorithms	Clinical Pathways
Focus on identifying best clinical option	Focus on operationalizing options
Useful across clinical settings; apply generally	Setting/institution specific; tailored to fit local conditions
May or may not be provider specific	Require multi- or transdisciplinary approach
Based on evidence, expert opinion, or consensus	Based on evidence
Developed and supported by a group of experts	Produced by a multidisciplinary team
Guide practice in an explicit manner	Define optimum sequence and timing of interventions

municipal, as well as professional, standards. It is a legally and financially defensible documentation system if followed consistently by those who use it. If documentation policy is consistently applied and staff can testify to consistent application of policy while understanding the importance of switching to detailed charting as soon as there is any reason to believe the client/patient has fallen outside the norm, defence should not be difficult (Hill, 1995).

CPGs, ALGORITHMS, AND CLINICAL PATHWAYS: COMPARISON

Table 11-8 is provided to highlight the similarities and differences between CPGs, algorithms, and clinical pathways. Although it is not essential to develop a CPG or algorithm before developing a pathway, it can be an excellent foundation upon which to build a clinical pathway.

Benefits and Limitations

Successful strategies to improve the quality and utilization of health care services must take into account relevant scientific information and clinical experience; identify optimal ways to manage individual episodes of care; and achieve acceptance by physicians, other health care professionals, and patient/clients/families. Properly developed practice parameters (guidelines) and clinical paths, modified as necessary to meet institution-specific and patient/client-specific needs, are important mechanisms to facilitate these goals (American Medical Association, 1990a; Spath, 1993).

Practice guidelines provide the valuable scientific foundation for the development of clinical pathways, while clinical pathways provide an effective mechanism to facilitate dissemination and implementation of the recommendations in practice guidelines. Numerous challenges remain in the development of CPGs and clinical pathways, such as the adaptation of guidelines and pathways to individualized patient/client management and the maintenance of appropriate clinical flexibility. Nevertheless, CPGs and pathways are promising approaches in the design of effective methods to improve the quality and utilization of health care services (American Medical Association, 1990b).

Pathways are not an end unto themselves, but a means of achieving a better understanding of the systems and processes used to help achieve the desired outcomes. Well built CPGs and pathways based on solid research can facilitate conforming to the guidelines (standards of care, practice) of regulatory bodies. As a result, accountability models and outcome-based practice are established. Patient/client and family understanding of the process and the desired outcome is improved and collaboration between disciplines is enhanced. Documentation becomes more streamlined and focused, facilitating preparation for future electronic recording. Equity in services from community to community is improved and a more appropriate mix of services and supports is achieved.

With the move in some provincial health care systems to managed competition, it will become increasingly important for those agencies competing for limited resources to demonstrate evidence of quality care, resource management, and controlled costs. The development and implementation of CPGs and clinical pathways will put many community health care agencies in a competitive mode to obtain contracts and will surely become important marketing tools, giving agencies a competitive edge while negotiating contracts (Freeman & Chambers, 1997). Recently, the National Health Service in the UK introduced the concept of clinical governance. This involves a process of continuous quality improvement for which senior clinicians and managers are directly responsible. It has moved the emphasis from cost containment, as demonstrated in the US model of managed care, to a process of managing clinical care to improve quality within the resources available (Scally & Donaldson, 1998). Pathways have been recognized as one option for facilitating this process, allowing changes to be driven by clinicians rather than managers. An evidence-based approach that incorporates the explicit, conscientious, and judicious use of the best available evidence from health care research in the management of individual clients and in program planning will help to identify the best approach—one that capitalizes on the strengths of various models to achieve a balance between benefit, harm, and affordability (Brouwers, 2000).

LEARNING AND EXPLORATION ACTIVITIES

Material is provided in Appendices L, M, and N to assist the practitioner who is beginning to develop clinical pathways.

1. Appendices L and M: use the template (Appendix M) for developing a specific pathway. Begin by choosing a particular diagnostic group or condition and record the expected admission status, critical interventions, timeline, and discharge status. Use Appendix L to develop a key indicator record.

2. Appendix N: Complete the outcome statements for each of the conditions listed.

DEFINITIONS

Algorithm: Written guidelines to stepwise evaluation and management strategies that require observations to be made, decisions to be considered, and actions to be taken.

Ankle brachial index pressure index (ABPI): A measurement that uses a portable Doppler ultrasound to screen for arterial disease.

Charting by exception: A method of documenting normal findings about a patient/client (sometimes using symbols) and based on clearly defined guidelines for practice (i.e., plan of care, predicted outcomes).

Clinical pathway: A multidisciplinary tool that makes explicit the usual client/patient problem and activities that must occur to facilitate the achievement of expected patient/client outcomes in a defined length of time.

CPGs: Clinical practice guidelines, which are systematically developed statements to assist practitioner and patient decisions about appropriate health care for specific clinical circumstances

Case mixed group: A grouping of clients/patients based upon the different types (mix) of diagnoses (cases) for which they are being treated.

Diagnostic related group: A code of classifying illnesses according to principal diagnosis and treatment requirements.

Key indicator: An event or intervention deemed to be critical for achieving the anticipated outcome. May also be called *milestones* or *benchmarks*.

Outcomes: Factors that identify the results of the interventions (e.g., functional health status, morbidity, mortality, quality of life, satisfaction, cost).

Performance indicator: A measurement tool, screen, or flag that is used as a guide to monitor, assess, and improve the quality of client/patient care, support services, and organizational functions that affect outcomes.

Protocol: A written statement or plan that defines the management of broad patient/client problems or issues and may include decision trees, algorithms, flowcharts, and research plans.

Standards of care: A level of performance or a set of conditions considered acceptable by some authority or by the individual(s) engaged in performing or maintaining the set of conditions in question.

Variance: A deviation in the implementation or occurrence of a stated critical indicator (i.e., the difference between what is expected to happen and what actually happens).

Positive variance: A deviation that occurs when the patient/client progresses at a rate faster than anticipated usually, resulting in a shorter length of stay or fewer visits per episode of care.

Negative variance: A deviation that occurs when the patient/client progresses at a rate slower than anticipated, usually resulting in a longer length of stay or a greater number of visits per episode of care.

Variance analysis: The process of collecting, managing, reviewing, analyzing, and reporting variance occurrences.

Concurrent variance analysis: The immediate review of current variance data for a particular population or individual patient/client to identify the need to alter interventions.

Retrospective variance analysis: The analysis of aggregated variance data for a particular population after discharge to identify patterns and trends.

WEB LINKS

Cancer Care Ontario Practice Guidelines Initiative
http://hiru.mcmaster.ca/ccopgi
Care Paths in Oncology: Information from the Program in Evidence-Based Care (PEBC) is a collaborative effort between Cancer Care Ontario and McMaster University. Site includes an extensive literature search on care maps, critical paths, etc., 1986-1999 from MEDLINE, Embase, CINAHL, and HealthStar.

Cochrane Collaboration
www.cochrane.org
An international research effort that prepares, maintains, and promotes the accessibility of meta-analysis of randomized controlled trials and systematic reviews of the effects of health care interventions. Available on CD or Internet by subscription. Some parts available free on Internet. Includes five major databases that are searched simultaneously.

Canadian Medical Association InfoBase
http://mdm.ca/cpgsnew/cpgs/index.asp
Database of guidelines produced or endorsed in Canada by a national, provincial/territorial, or regional medical or health organization; professional society; government agency; or expert panel.

CMA ePractice Tools
www.cma.ca/cma/common/linkNavigate.do?skin=129
 Site includes PSD applications and clinical practice guidelines produced or endorsed in Canada by a national, provincial, or territorial medical or health organisation; professional society; government agency; or expert panel.

GERGIS—German Guideline Information Service (English sitemap)
www.leitlinien.de/sitemapenglish.htm
Content in English is marked with "English version." Information on guideline appraisal, dissemination, implementation, German guideline clearinghouse (English version).

The National Guideline Clearinghouse (NGC)
www.guideline.gov/index.asp
This is a public resource for evidence-based clinical practice guidelines sponsored by the Agency for Health Care Research and Quality (formerly the Agency for Health Care Policy and Research) in partnership with the American Medical Association and the American Association of Health Plans. Structured abstracts of guidelines only.

Scottish Intercollegiate Guidelines Network (SIGN)
www.show.scot.nhs.uk/sign/guidelines/index.html
Sixty evidence-based clinical guidelines—published, in development, or under review—cover a wide range of topics that relate to the NHS priority areas of cancer, cardiovascular disease, and mental health.

VNA First—Home Care Steps
www.vnaf.org/hsp/index.htm
Home Care Steps is a patented pathway system that is used by more than 600 home health agencies across the United States, Canada, and Brazil.

Center for Case Management
www.cfcm.com
This site offers CareMap pathways for purchase, educational resources, and an on-line copy of *The New Definition* newsletter.

National Pathway Association (U.K.)
www.the-npa.org.uk
Web site provides members with a network of professionals interested in developing, sharing, and promoting the use of care pathways. Includes a membership list and register of care pathways being developed by members.

Journal of Integrated Care Pathways
www.rsm.ac.uk/pub/jicp.htm
Access to the journal on the Internet. A membership fee is required.

Medic8
www.medic8.com
Medic8 is a leading medical portal for healthcare professionals, providing quick, easy access to the best medical resources on the Internet. Includes comprehensive listing of UK and overseas guidelines, links to all major international guidelines groups plus free search engine.

Royal College of Nursing Professional Clinical Guidelines
www.rcn.org.uk/professional/professional_clinical_guidlines.html
Royal College of Nurses web site explaining what are guidelines, where to find them, plus RCN developed CPGs for pressure ulcer risk, assessment and prevention; management of venous leg ulcers; pain management in children; and vaccine administration. Also included are CPGs that the RCN has been involved in developing asthma in adults, stable angina, management of diabetes, and management of imminent violence.

Alberta Wellnet
www.albertawellnet.org
Alberta Wellnet was formed in mid-1997 as the umbrella for a series of province-wide and regional initiatives to build an integrated health information network in Alberta that facilitates improvements to the delivery of health services by improving access to health information.

Australian National Health and Medical Research Council Clinical Practice Guidelines
www.health.gov.au/nhmrc/publications/synopses/cp30syn.htm
1999 update of the 1995 guidelines—a guide to the development, implementation, and evaluation of clinical practice guidelines. It includes a new section on evaluation and can be downloaded as a PDF file.

Evidence-Based Medicine Resource Center
www.ebmny.org/cpg.html

The page contains references, bibliographies, tutorials, glossaries, and on-line databases to guide those embarking on teaching and practicing evidence-based medicine. It offers practice tools to support critical analysis of the literature and MEDLINE searching, as well as links to other sites that help enable evidence-based medical care.

Guideline Appraisal Project (GAP)
www.cche.net/usersguides/main.asp

GAP brings health service researchers, policy makers, and practitioners together in appraising, summarising, and disseminating information about clinical practice guidelines. The project studies what clinicians want from clinical practice guidelines and how to equip them with practical strategies for meeting their needs. GAP investigators have surveyed clinicians about guidelines, conducted guideline appraisal workshops, developed users guides for guidelines, promoted a standardised approach to summarising guidelines, and initiated guideline summary inventories.

eGuidelines
www.eguidelines.co.uk

National and European clinical guidelines developed by clinicians and sponsored by the relevant independent professional bodies are summarized and included free of charge. Primary care guideline summaries, news of new guidelines and related issues, and links to over 200 clinical governance and medical sites. Registration is required.

Alberta Clinical Practice Guidelines Program
www.albertadoctors.org/resources/guidelines.html

The Alberta Clinical Practice Guidelines Program administered by the Alberta Medical Association under the direction of a multi-stakeholder advisory committee. The CPG Catalogue includes a vast array of CPGs developed in Canada and also by other North American agencies such as US Preventive Services Task Force, the AHCPR, etc. The guidelines are indexed and categorized as one of the following: consensus statement, guideline, laboratory index, patient guideline, policy paper, quick reference guide.

PURCHASED CARE PATHWAY SYSTEMS

CareMap
Interqual
PtCare System
Interpath
VNAFirst
CareWare

RESOURCES

1. Shunk, C., & Reed, K. (2000). Clinical practice guidelines: Examination and intervention for rehabilitation. Gaithersburg, MD: Aspen Publishers, Inc.

2. Database of Physical Therapy Related Consensus Statements (CS), Systematic Reviews (SR), Meta-analyses (MA), and Clinical Practice Guidelines (CPGs)
Ontario Physiotherapy Association/Ontario Physiotherapy Association
October 2000
3. Practice Guidelines Series
The American Occupational Therapy Association, Inc.
4720 Montgomery Lane, PO Box 31220
Bethesda, MD 20824-1220

REFERENCES

AGREE Collaboration. (n.d.). *Introduction to the AGREE collaboration.* Retrieved March 26, 2002, from http://www.agreecollaboration.org.

American Medical Association. (1990a). *Attributes to guide the development of practice parameters.* Chicago, IL: Author.

American Medical Association. (1990b). *The interface of clinical paths and practice parameters.* Chicago, IL: Author.

Bell, N., & Wilson, D. (1998, April). *Alberta Clinical Practice Guidelines Program.* Presentation to "Putting Evidence into Practice." Alberta Medical Association, Edmonton, Alberta.

Brouwers, M. (2000, June). *Program in Evidence-Based Care, Cancer Care Ontario.* Presentation to "Pathways 2000," Institute for International Research, Toronto, ON.

Burke, L. J., & Murphy, J. (1995). *Charting by exception applications: Making it work in clinical settings.* Albany, NY: Delmar Publishers.

Canadian Medical Association. (1994). *Guidelines for Canadian clinical practice guidelines.* Ottowa, Ontario: Author.

Canadian Medical Association. (1996). *Implementing clinical practice guidelines: A handbook for practitioners.* Ottowa, Ontario: Author.

Cancer Care Ontario. (1999). *Neuro-oncology clinical practice guidelines.* Retrieved March 26, 2002, from http://hiru.mcmaster.ca/ccopgi/neucpg.html.

Clinical Resource Efficiency Support Team (CREST). (1998). *Guidelines for the assessment and management of leg ulceration: Recommendation for practice.* Belfast: CREST.

Cluzeau, F., Littlejohns, P., Grimshaw, J., & Feder, G. (1997). *Appraisal instrument for clinical guidelines.* London: St. George's Hospital Medical School.

Compliance Network Physicians/Health Force Initiative, Inc. (1999). *Guideline for the outpatient treatment of venous and venous-arterial mixed leg ulcers.* Retrieved March 26, 2002, from http://www.cnhfi.org/GL/LU-C.htm.

Dowsey, M., Kilgour, M., Santamaria, N., & Choong, P. F. M. (1999). Clinical pathways in hip and knee arthroplasty: A prospective randomised controlled study. *Med J Aust, 170,* 59-62.

Ellershaw, J., Foster, A., Murphy, D., Shea, T., & Overill, S. (1997). Developing an integrated care pathway for the dying patient. *Eur J Palliat Care, 4,* 203-207.

Field, M. J., & Lohr, K. L. (Eds.). (1992). *Guidelines for clinical practice: From development to use.* Washington, D.C.: National Academy Press.

Freeman, S. R., & Chambers, K. A. (1997). *Nursing Management, 28*(6), 45-48.

Graham, I., Calder, L., Hebert, P., Carter, A., & Tetroe, J. (2000). Review of Guideline Assessment Instruments. *International Journal of Technology Assessment in Health Care, 16*(4), 1024-1038.

Graham, I., Lorimer, K., Harrison, M., & Piercianowski, T. (2000). Evaluating the quality and content of international clinical practice guidelines for leg ulcers: Preparing for Canadian adaptation. *Canadian Association for Enterostomal Therapy Journal, 19*(3), 15-31.

Guide for the Uniform Data Set for Medical Rehabilitation (including the FIMTM Instrument), Version 5.1. (1997). Buffalo, NY: State University of New York at Buffalo.

Hadorn, D. C., McCormick, K., & Diokno, A. (1992). An annotated algorithm approach to clinical guideline development. *JAMA, 267,* 3311.

Hill, M. (1995). Integration of CareMap tools into the documentation system. In K. Zander (Ed.), *Managing outcomes through collaborative practice* (pp. 149-163). South Natick, MA: American Hospital Publishing Inc.

Hunt, D. L., Haynes, R. B., Hanna, S. E., & Smith, K. (1998). Effects of computer-based clinical decision support systems on physician performance and patient outcomes: A systematic review. *JAMA, 280*(15), 1339-1346.

Jadad, A. R., Haynes, R. B., Hunt, D., & Browman, G. P. (2000). The Internet and evidence-based decision-making: A needed synergy for efficient knowledge management in health care. *Canadian Medical Association Journal, 162*(3), 362-365.

Kitchiner, D. J., & Bundred, P. (1996). Integrated care pathways. *Arch Dis Child, 75,* 16-168.

Kitchiner, D. J., & Bundred, P. (1999). Clinical pathways [Editorial]. *Medical Journal of Australia, 170,* 54-55.

Local Ottawa-Carleton Interdisciplinary Leg Ulcer Protocol Task Force. (2001). *Recommendations.* Ottawa, Ontario: Author.

Penn, A., Lau, F., & Wilson, D. (1996). *An internet-based clinical guidance system for managing stroke.* Alberta: University of Alberta and Capital Health Authority, Synapse Publishing Inc.

Royal College of Nursing. (1998). *Clinical practical guidelines: The management of patients with venous ulcers.* Retrieved March 26, 2002, from http://www.rcn.org.uk/professional/professional_clinical_guidlinesrcn_guidelines.html.

Scally, G., & Donaldson, L. J. (1998). Clinical governance and the drive for quality improvement in the new NHS in England. *BMJ, 317,* 61-65.

Scottish Intercollegiate Guidelines Network (SIGN). (1998). *The care of patients with a chronic leg ulcer: A national clinical guideline.* Edinburgh, UK: SIGN.

Spath, P. (1993). *Succeeding with critical paths.* Forest Grove, OR: Brown-Spath & Associates.

Stradiotto, R. A. (1997, November). *Clinical pathways in the continuum of care: Are they a defence to medical malpractice claims?* Presentation to Clinical Pathways, Toronto, Ontario.

Verhulst, L. (1994, August). Implementing clinical practice guidelines. Paper presented at the meeting of the Advisory Committee on Health Services, Ottawa, Canada.

Weinstein, J., & Hockley, J. (1999). *Appraisal instruments for clinical pathways.* Hamilton, Ontario: Hamilton Health Sciences Corporation, Lakeridge Health Corporation and Cancer Care Ontario.

Zander, K. (1992). Quantifying, managing, and improving quality. Part III: Using variance concurrently. *The New Definition, 7*(4), 1-4.

Zander, K., & Hill, M. (1995). *Managing outcomes through collaborative practice: Integration of CareMap tools into the documentation system* (pp. 149-163). South Natick, MA: American Hospital Publishing Inc.

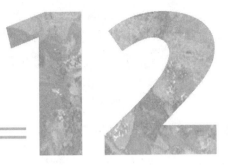

Communicating Evidence to Clients, Managers, and Funders

Linda Tickle-Degnen, PhD, OTR/L

LEARNING OBJECTIVES

After reading this chapter, the student/practitioner will be able to:

- Recognize the role that effective communication about evidence plays in being an evidence-based practitioner.
- Understand the various clinical roles of potential decision makers.
- Critically evaluate the body of evidence on a clinical situation, including distinguishing between different types of evidence.
- Use appropriate communication techniques to discuss the evidence and make treatment decisions based on the persons involved.

> *Imagine that next Monday you have your first appointment with Mr. Davis, a man with Parkinson's disease. As an evidence-based practitioner, you would seek recent research evidence on the daily lives of persons with this disease to supplement the knowledge you have accrued through your clinical experience and training. One important clinical outcome of gathering this evidence is that you would become a more knowledgeable practitioner. The evidence hopefully would inform your own practice actions. For example, during the appointed meeting time, you might have a list of issues to discuss with Mr. Davis and his family that is expanded beyond what you normally would have addressed. More importantly, beyond informing your own practice actions, you would possibly be able to expand Mr. Davis' knowledge in a manner that would enable him to become a collaborative partner in the clinical process. The more Mr. Davis knows about how his own life relates to others with similar circumstances, the more he can make reasoned choices that work for him.*

The point of the above scenario is to demonstrate that the purpose of evidence-gathering does not stop with the personal edification of the practitioner. The evidence is put to use to achieve many purposes, some of which require direct communication with others about the content of the evidence. A collaborative relationship requires this direct communication so that the client and family members become informed clinical partners. They are active rather than passive (i.e., they act with as much autonomy as possible and the least amount of dependency); clients and those acting upon their behalf must be informed rather than uninformed or misinformed.

As an expert consultant, the therapist must directly communicate about evidence with other decision makers besides clients and their family members. The therapist talks about evidence with managers and funders of services so that management and funding decisions are informed. The focus of this chapter is on communicating about research evidence so that decision makers can make informed decisions that relate to clients' lives and the provision of rehabilitation services.

EFFECTIVELY COMMUNICATING EVIDENCE

Talking about evidence alone will not guarantee that decision makers will become more informed. The therapist must take steps to effectively communicate about the evidence. An effective communication regarding clinical evidence is one in which a message has not only been sent, but also received, understood, and acted upon. A therapist may talk about evidence, but if the message is irrelevant, not framed in a manner that enables decision making and action, or incomprehensible, it will not be listened to, comprehended, and acted upon. Messages that are relevant, framed to enable decision making and action, and comprehensible are most effective for making a communication bridge between sender and receiver. Although the terms *sender* and *receiver* are used here, this is not to suggest that the information travels in a unidirectional path from therapist to the decision maker. Rather, as stated by the National Center for the Dissemination of Disability Research (NCDDR) (1996), "...knowledge is not an inert object to be 'sent' and 'received,' but a fluid set of understandings shaped both by those who originate it and by those who use it" (p. 4). With this bidirectionality of knowledge construction as the underlying premise, this chapter describes four steps on the path to effective evidence-based communication:

1. Identify the clinical role of the decision maker with respect to the therapist.
2. Identify the decisions that the decision maker will be involved in making with the therapist.

3. Gather and interpret research evidence that is guided by the information needs of the decision maker and the clinical population of interest.

4. Translate the evidence into a comprehensible communication that enables an informed discussion with the decision maker so that decisions can be made and actions taken.

Identify the Clinical Role of the Decision Maker With Respect to the Therapist

This chapter addresses three types of decision makers with whom therapists are likely to communicate—client or family member, manager, and funder. Effective communication begins with identifying the distinctions between the communication recipients' clinical roles and the contexts surrounding the performance of those roles. Different clinical roles generate different perspectives and needs. People are more likely to understand and respond to communication messages that are consistent with their own experiences and perspectives and based on their own needs and objectives (Falvo, 1985; NCDDR, 1996).

The clinical role of clients and family members is to receive therapy services to improve their lives. Communication with clients and family members often occurs face-to-face in periodic and repeated appointments. The clinical role of managers is to develop therapy programs; allocate resources, such as space, budget, materials, and staff support; and guide the therapist's provision of services. Managers must work within a set of multiple and complex organizational objectives (e.g., provide effective and efficient services to a particular population), initiatives (e.g., increase client satisfaction while increasing therapists' caseload), and constraints (e.g., limited building space). Communication with managers may occur frequently and informally, or infrequently and formally, and is often face-to-face. The clinical role of funders is to decide whether to fund the development of future clinical programs and the provision of current clinical services from an array of possible services and programs. Communication with funders is often formal and in written form.

Identify the Decisions That the Decision Maker Will be Involved in Making With the Therapist

Communication is a two-way street. The therapist also has a clinical role that determines what types of decisions will be important to communicate about. In rehabilitation, the therapist and client are concerned with helping the client to participate more competently and with more satisfaction in daily living and valued activities that occur in the home, community, and society at large. Throughout the chapter, the term *participation* is used to mean this activity and societal participation. A simple model of the clinical role with respect to participation issues involves the following three tasks:

1. Determine and describe participation issues that are relevant to a particular client population.

2. Select assessment procedures to measure client attributes related to participation.

3. Plan and implement intervention to maintain or improve client participation.

There are other tasks as well; however, these central ones are useful as a basis for demonstrating what types of information, or evidence, therapists will be most likely to communicate. Decision making is required around all of these tasks, whether the decision making occurs in the context of direct service provision to clients, in the context of program development or resource allocation discussions with managers, or in the context of written communication with funders around program funding and service compensation.

When the clinical tasks of the therapist are intersected with the clinical roles of the decision makers who interact with therapists, it becomes clear that different decision makers need to make different decisions. Specifically, clients and their family members need *descriptive* information from the therapist about the importance of participation in their lives. With this information they can begin to understand and give voice to their life experiences and begin to plan an adaptive course of action in response to their own rehabilitation needs. They need *assessment* and *intervention* information to make informed decisions related to choosing in assessment and intervention procedures.

Managers need *descriptive* information about participation from the therapist in order to develop and support clinical programs that are likely to be responsive to client rehabilitation needs. They need *assessment* and *intervention* information to decide which assessment and intervention procedures should be supported and provided by the organization.

Funders need *descriptive* information about participation from the therapist in order to determine whether or not a clinical program addresses or will address, if in the planning phase, important client rehabilitation needs. They need to determine if there is a reasonable rationale for funding. They need *assessment* information to determine whether or not assessment procedures currently or will effectively document important attributes of clients and their responses to rehabilitation intervention. Finally, they need *intervention* information to decide whether or not the current or predicted level of effectiveness and feasibility of a clinical intervention program is worth funding.

Gather and Interpret Research Evidence that Is Guided by the Needs of the Decision Maker and the Clinical Population of Interest

Steps 1 and 2 provide a general conceptual territory for the kind of evidence that the therapist will have to gather to meet the needs of decision makers. At step 3, the therapist begins to narrow this territory to address the specific and unique needs of decision makers and the client population that is involved in the decisions. The therapist creates a clinical question to guide the retrieval of information (Sackett, Richardson, Rosenberg, & Haynes, 1997). As the therapist gathers and interprets information, the therapist formulates possible answers to the question. The therapist then presents these possible answers to the decision maker for discussion.

Tables 12-1 through 12-3 show sample questions for organizing the gathering and interpretation of descriptive, assessment, and intervention evidence, separately for different types of decision makers. Each question is composed of at least three elements: the type of evidence that is being sought, an attribute related to participation, and a description of a clinical population. Keeping in mind this chapter's opening clinical scenario involving Mr. Davis, all of the questions in the tables are about the clinical population with Parkinson's disease. The questions that guide the search for evidence for communicating with clients and their family members are written with the specific attributes of the client in mind (e.g., age and gender are specified). The questions that guide the search for evidence for communicating with managers and funders are written with a more general clinical population in mind. Based upon the particular context and timing of decision-making activities, the therapist can develop the wording of the questions independently or in collaboration with the decision maker. The questions can be written with as much specificity or generality as is needed for decision-making, as long as two conditions are met. The questions cannot be written so specifically that the evidence will be extremely restricted and hard to find (e.g., a question about quality of life for 75-year-old men with Parkinson's disease who live in Minnesota and are retired busi-

	Table 12-1	
	ORGANIZING THE SEARCH FOR DESCRIPTIVE EVIDENCE TO DISCUSS WITH DIFFERENT DECISION MAKERS	
Decision Maker	*Decision Maker's Use of Evidence*	*Question that Guides the Search for Evidence*
Client and family members	To understand and give voice to one's own life experience and to begin to plan an adaptive course of action	What factors are associated with high quality of life and life satisfaction among 75-year-old men with Parkinson's disease?
Manager	To develop and support clinical programs that are likely to be responsive to client rehabilitation needs	What factors are associated with high quality of life and life satisfaction among persons with Parkinson's disease?
Funder	To determine whether a clinical program will address important client rehabilitation needs	Same question as for manager

	Table 12-2	
	ORGANIZING THE SEARCH FOR ASSESSMENT EVIDENCE TO DISCUSS WITH DIFFERENT DECISION MAKERS	
Decision Maker	*Decision Maker's Use of Evidence*	*Question that Guides the Search for Evidence*
Client and family members	To make informed decisions related to choosing assessment procedures	Is goal attainment scaling a reliable and valid method for assessing personally meaningful goal achievement among 75-year-old men with Parkinson's disease?
Manager	To decide which assessment procedures should be supported and provided by the organization	What are the most reliable and valid methods for assessing personally meaningful goal achievement among persons with Parkinson's disease?

Table 12-2 (Continued)

Decision Maker	Decision Maker's Use of Evidence	Question that Guides the Search for Evidence
Funder	To determine whether or not assessment procedures will effectively document important attributes of clients and their responses to rehabilitation intervention	Same question as for manager

Table 12-3

ORGANIZING THE SEARCH FOR INTERVENTION EVIDENCE TO DISCUSS WITH DIFFERENT DECISION MAKERS

Decision Maker	Decision Maker's Use of Evidence	Question that Guides the Search for Evidence
Client and family members	To make informed decisions related to choosing intervention procedures	What are the most effective and feasible interventions for achieving participation in successful and safe meal preparation among 75-year-old men with Parkinson's disease?
Manager	To decide which intervention procedures should be supported and provided by the organization	What are the most effective and feasible interventions for achieving personally meaningful goals among persons with Parkinson's disease?
Funder	To decide whether or not the predicted level of effectiveness and feasibility of a clinical intervention program is worth funding	Same question as for manager

ness executives). Nor can they be written so generally that they would require years of evidence-searching and be of no particular consequence to the decision makers (e.g., a question about concerns of patients in hospitals).

The questions vary across the three tables in terms of the type of evidence and the attribute of interests that are involved. The descriptive questions in Table 12-1 involve evidence about associations and attributes related to quality of life and life satisfaction. The assessment questions in Table 12-2 involve evidence about reliability, validity, and attributes related to personally meaningful goal achievement. The intervention questions in Table 12-3 involve evidence about effectiveness and feasibility and attributes related to meal preparation and, more globally, goal achievement. The attributes in all of these questions are the measured or outcome variables of interest in the research studies that the therapist retrieves in the literature search.

The emphasis in this chapter is on communicating about information from published research articles. This source of information is particularly important when the therapist does not have readily available data that have been systematically collected in his or her own setting. It should be noted, however, that in actuality, therapists will most likely draw upon a variety of information sources for meeting the decision-making needs of clients, managers, and funders. They can gather information by talking to clinical experts and clients, recalling their own clinical experience and training, and systematically collecting data in their clinical setting.

Using key words or related words and synonyms in the questions to search the literature, the therapist retrieves research articles. Table 12-4 shows some possible terms that could be used to search for evidence relevant to the sample questions in Tables 12-1 through 12-3. The most effective and efficient use of the therapist's time is to first search for research syntheses and meta-analyses (with "synthesis" or "meta-analysis" as key words). These types of research articles describe a whole body of research that might be relevant to answering a clinical question. Their strength is that they amass evidence in one location; however, this strength is the limitation of the research synthesis in that it may provide evidence that is highly summarized and general. Therefore, it is often useful to supplement synthesis and meta-analytic articles with research articles that report the findings from single studies to find detailed evidence about situations and issues related to the clinical population of interest. Once retrieved, the therapist must interpret the findings before communicating about them. The later section in this chapter, "Examples of Interpreting and Communicating Evidence," (p. 229) gives details about how to interpret findings from sample research articles found in response to the questions in Tables 12-1 through 12-3.

Translate the Evidence into a Comprehensible Communication to Facilitate an Informed Discussion With the Decision Maker

Once the therapist has gathered and interpreted the evidence, it is time to have the direct face-to-face or written communication. By following steps 1 through 3, the therapist has assured that the evidence collected is important and relevant to the decision maker. Now the therapist must help make the evidence comprehensible. Individuals understand and retain information better when the content and presentation of the communication has the following attributes:

1. Nontechnical, simple, and concrete language with simple grammatical structure.
2. Terms that cross cultures and perspectives. The words and images have the same meaning for the sender and receiver of the communication.

Table 12-4

SEARCH TERMS FOR THE SAMPLE QUESTIONS IN TABLES 12-1, 12-2, AND 12-3

Table	Type of Evidence		Attribute of Interest		Client Population	
	Key Words	*Related Words*	*Key Words*	*Related Words*	*Key Words*	*Related Words*
12-1	Association	Correlation Regression Descriptive Qualitative Cross-sectional Longitudinal	Quality of life Life satisfaction	Well-being Coping Happiness Use of time Daily activities Depression	Parkinson's disease	Neurological Older adult Gerontology Geriatric Rehabilitation
12-2	Reliability Validity	Consistency Trustworthiness Assessment Outcome measure Instrument development	Goal assessment scaling Personally meaningful Goal achievement	Self-report Value Attainment Quality of life Personal projects	Same as above	Same as above
12-3	Effectiveness Feasibility Intervention	Efficacy Outcome Rehabilitation Treatment Experiment Randomized trial Quasi-experiment	Same as above Meal preparation	Same as above, Cooking aids Food Activities of daily living	Same as above	Same as above

3. Brevity, with just enough detail for decision making.

4. Checks for confusion or lack of comprehension.

5. Suggestions for concrete actions related to the information.

These attributes are discussed in the patient education literature (Bradshaw, Ley, Kincey, & Bradshaw, 1975; Davis et al., 1996; Doak, Doak, & Root, 1996; Falvo, 1985; Redman, 1997) and literature on the dissemination of research findings (NCDDR, 1996), and they apply to persons regardless of their level of education or comprehension.[1] Although it is always best to use common, everyday language and simple phrasing, the therapist should be prepared to give a detailed report of synthesized evidence should the listener ask for this information.

For clients who have comprehension disabilities, limited education, or a primary language other than the therapist's, the therapist adjusts the language and concepts appropriately. In these cases, pictures and visual images are helpful supplements. It is important to keep distractions at a minimum and create a comfortable communication environment. Despite the listener's level of comprehension and scientific background, the therapist should allow enough time for the listener to absorb and discuss the communicated information before engaging in any decision making.

The most important attribute of the communication to keep in mind is that the therapist is providing possible answers, not the one correct answer, to a clinical question. Research with human beings is based upon a model of tendencies and variations in living organisms and complex events, not upon determined facts. As a result, the therapist offers information to work with, not to dictate. Examples for how to communicate about a body of evidence are given in the sections below.

Examples of
Interpreting and Communicating Evidence

Using a clinical case of a person with Parkinson's disease is useful for talking about communicating about evidence because evidence relevant to this disease is not found easily in the rehabilitation literature. Such is the case with many of the clinical populations with whom therapists work. Even more challenging is the fact that most of the research literature on Parkinson's disease is about medical symptoms, pathology, and pharmaceutical treatment. Despite these challenges, there is hope for the evidence-based therapist who works with populations about which there is seemingly little research evidence. There is a small but growing body of research on quality of life and life satisfaction descriptions, assessments, and interventions for persons with chronic illness and disability. The terms *quality of life* and *life satisfaction* tap into aspects of persons' lives related to their everyday participation in activities and satisfaction with their activities. Knowledge that these terms are highly relevant to therapists is one of the first steps in bridging the communication gaps that face the evidence-based therapist. In the next few sections, the case of Mr. Davis as an individual client and Parkinson's disease as a clinical population is used to demonstrate how the research literature is interpreted and communicated to clients and their family members, managers, and funders. Three types of evidence are discussed: descriptive, assessment, and intervention. There are two illustrations for each of these areas of evidence: one from an article that is a synthesis of more than one study and one from an article on a single study.

To begin to interpret the evidence given in each article, the therapist—let's call him or her Therapist Foster—must first determine if the research participants are relevant to Mr. Davis or the general population of clients with Parkinson's disease with whom he or she works at the clinic. For the findings to be highly relevant for discussion with Mr. Davis and his family, some of the research participants should be similar to him with respect to important attributes that could affect the answers to the clinical questions. These attributes of interest may be disease severity, gender, age, cultural background, marital status, and socioeconomic status. For the findings to be relevant for discussions with managers and funders, the participants should be similar to the Parkinson's disease population seen in Therapist Foster's own clinic. Table 12-5 summarizes the fictional characteristics of the case of Mr. Davis, as well as the therapist's Parkinson's disease caseload and the actual characteristics of research participants in six research articles that are reviewed in the sections below. Second, the therapist should determine what possible answers this study gives to the clinical questions that guided the search for the evidence. Therapist Foster will be concerned with answering those questions listed in Tables 12-1 through 12-3. Table 12-6 shows the types of data analytic findings that would most likely provide answers to the questions. Third, and finally, the therapist should determine the strength of the evidence in answering the questions. The therapist conducts this final step by evaluating the quality of the study design, procedures, and measures. This chapter addresses the first two steps but gives only cursory attention to the third step.

Evidence That Describes the Lives and Needs of Clients With Parkinson's Disease

Interpretation of a Synthesis of Studies

Using the clinical questions in Table 12-1 to organize a literature search, Therapist Foster found a research synthesis article on factors associated with quality of life and life satisfaction among older adults. No synthesis was found specifically for the Parkinson's disease population. Pinquart and Sörensen (2000) conducted a meta-analysis on a set of factors associated with subjective well-being in later life. *Subjective well-being* is a construct that encompasses quality of life and life satisfaction concepts. The meta-analysis combined the findings of 286 relevant research studies, examining specifically the factors of socioeconomic status; quantitative and qualitative aspects of older persons' social networks; and competence, defined as skills to manage basic, instrumental, and leisure daily life activities.

Therapist Foster begins the interpretation of this meta-analytic study by determining how relevant it is to Mr. Davis' case and to Therapist Foster's larger Parkinson's disease caseload. Table 12-5 shows that the meta-analysis included studies that had research participants similar to Mr. Davis in many respects. Although the meta-analysis included studies with participants who were chronically ill, it did not report information about specific diseases. However, some findings were reported separately for males and females and separately for participants of different age groups. Therefore, Therapist Foster could pay attention to the findings for males and the oldest adults for communicating with Mr. Davis.

Therapist Foster, having determined that the meta-analytic report is relevant, turns to locating the findings that will help to answer the clinical questions. Table 12-6 shows the types of findings that are often important to descriptive evidence. In the case of Pinquart and Sörensen's report (2000), correlations are the primary findings of interest. It was found that the higher the participants' socioeconomic status, the higher their life satisfaction ($r = .17$), but this association was smaller for adults who were 75 years and older ($r = .10$). The quality of social contacts had a higher association with life satisfaction ($r = .22$) than quantity of contacts ($r = .12$). The quality of contacts association was highest for participants over the

Table 12-5

CHARACTERISTICS OF THE THERAPIST'S CLINICAL POPULATION AND THE REVIEWED STUDIES' RESEARCH PARTICIPANTS

Client Identity	Disease	Degree of Disability	Age	Gender	Race and Ethnicity	Family and Living Context	Work Status	Socio-economic Status
Mr. Davis	Parkinson's	Moderate	75	Male	Black, US	Lives with disabled wife (post-stroke) in community with adult children near	Retired banker	Upper middle
Therapist Foster's Parkinson's caseload	Parkinson's	Mild to severe, inpatient and outpatient rehabilitation	≥ 50	60% male and 40% female	Diverse races, US	Diverse	Retired	Diverse
Research participants in Pinquart & Sörensen (2000)	Well and ill	None to severe	≥ 55	Male and	NR, North female European	Diverse American,	Diverse	Diverse
Research participants in Koplas et al. 1999)	Parkinson's	Mild to severe	51 to 87	59 males and 27 females	79 white, 5 black, and 2 other	68 married, 14 widowed, and 4 divorced	Diverse	Diverse

Table 12-5 (Continued)

Client Identity	Disease	Degree of Disability	Age	Gender	Race and Ethnicity	Family and Living Context	Work Status	Socio-economic Status
Research participants in Stolee, Stadnyk, Myers, & Rockwood (1999)[a]	Diverse	Diverse, inpatients of geriatric rehabilitation unit	61 to 96	40 males and 133 females	NR, Canadian	Diverse, discharged to institutions and community	NR	NR
Research participants in Yip et al. (1998)	Diverse	Diverse, inpatients of geriatric rehabilitation unit	77 (average)	55 males and 88 females	NR, Canadian	50 married and 93 other discharged to institutions and community	NR	NR
Research participants in Murphy & Tickle-Degnen (2001)	Parkinson's	Mild to severe	70 (average)	Male and female	NR, North American, European	NR	NR	NR
Research participants in Kondo, Mann, Tomita, & Ottenbacher (1997)	Diverse	Fine/gross motor or vision disability	62 to 92	4 females and 1 male	NR, US	1 married, 4 alone in the community	Retired	NR

NR = Not reported or unable to infer from article.
[a] This presents three studies, but the participant characteristics are from the third study. The authors did not report specific participant characteristics for the first two studies; however, those studies occurred in settings similar to the third study.

Table 12-6

STUDY RESULTS THAT PROVIDE PROBABLE ANSWERS
TO DIFFERENT TYPES OF QUESTIONS

Type of Question	*Data Analytic Results*
Descriptive	• General and unique qualitative themes, categories • Means, medians, modes • Frequency distributions, ranges, variances • Sign and magnitude of measures of association (e.g., *r*) and difference (e.g., *d*)
Assessment[a]	• Reliability coefficients • Validation coefficients and measures of difference (e.g., *d*, t, F)
Intervention	• Mean and variation of change scores • Magnitude of difference between intervention change and control change (e.g., *r* or *d*)[b] • Confidence intervals • Tests of significance (e.g., t, F)

[a] See Tables 12-7, 12-8, and 12-9 for more detail.
[b] See Table 12-10 for more details.

ages of 70 ($r = .29$). Finally, the higher the participants' competence in basic and instrumental daily living skills, the higher their life satisfaction ($r = .23$) regardless of age. In general, the differences between genders in the associations appeared to be less relevant to Mr. Davis' case than the differences between different ages, so they are not discussed here.

Two important pieces of evidence to note from the correlations described above are their signs and magnitude (i.e., how big they are). The signs are positive, indicating that on the average participants tended to have higher life satisfaction when they had higher socioeconomic status, stronger social networks, and more competence in performing daily living activities. As far as magnitude is concerned, Cohen (1988) suggests that correlations with absolute values of about .10 are of a small magnitude, of about .30 are of a moderate magnitude, and of about .50 or higher are of a large magnitude. Using these criteria, the magnitude of the correlations in the meta-analytic report of Pinquart & Sörenson (2000) were of a small to moderate magnitude. Another way of thinking about these magnitudes is that it was a small to moderate majority of people, not a large majority, that fell within the pattern of having high life satisfaction with high socioeconomic status, strong social networks, and competent performance, or of having low life satisfaction with low status, weak networks, and less competent performance. Another important piece of evidence is the statistical significance of the findings. The correlations and comparisons between correlations reported in the above paragraph were reported to be statistically significant below the traditional level of .05. This statistical significance indicates that the findings were strong enough, given the sample size, to feel confident in ruling out chance as the factor responsible for the strength. Studies that have large sample sizes, such as meta-analyses (this one having thousands of research participants represented), often have significant findings, thus effectively ruling out chance as an explanation for the findings.

Therapist Foster can take away from this examination of the Pinquart and Sörensen (2000) meta-analysis the following possible answer to the questions in Table 12-1: high quality of social contacts, continued competence in daily living activities, and socioeconomic status may be important aspects of life satisfaction for clients with Parkinson's disease. For Mr. Davis, in particular, socioeconomic status may not be an important factor unless he has financial concerns at this time. This possibility is based upon the meta-analytic findings that socioeconomic status was not an important quality of life factor for participants who were at least 75 years old, the age of Mr. Davis.

Descriptive evidence, unless it is derived from experimental or, sometimes, from longitudinal studies, does not usually give strong indication of causality. The associations found in the Pinquart and Sörensen (2000) meta-analysis are not causal patterns despite the authors' questionable use of the word "influence" in the title and throughout the text, a word that implies causality.[2] The quality of social contacts could affect a person's life satisfaction, but the reverse could be true as well. A person who feels satisfied may engender high quality social interactions. There may be a different, unmeasured factor that may explain why both life satisfaction and quality of contacts are high together or low together—perhaps, good physical and mental health. Descriptive evidence helps the therapist to understand possible patterns that exist in human behaviour and experience, but it does not provide definitive prescriptions for intervention. Intervention decisions require evidence of a causal nature, as when individuals are randomly assigned to intervention and control conditions, or when interventions are systematically provided and withdrawn. Descriptive evidence, on the other hand, helps a therapist to recognize important issues, and to have a language for discussing and exploring these issues with clients, managers, and funders.

Interpretation of a Single Study

There is a recent, small, growing body of research that describes quality of life issues for people with Parkinson's disease. Take for example a study by Koplas et al. (1999) that examined the association between quality of life and the following factors: physical disability, depression, self-perceived mastery, and health locus of control. Table 12-5 shows that the participants in this study were similar to Mr. Davis and Therapist Foster's broader Parkinson's disease caseload in many respects. The associations between quality of life and these factors were demonstrated with a multiple regression analysis and a multivariate analysis of variance. Many quantitative descriptive studies of quality of life issues use complex statistical association analyses, since quality of life itself is a complex construct and there are many factors associated with it. The therapist, however, need not be an expert in multivariate analysis to glean evidence from the article.

One of the primary findings of this study was that mastery, which was defined as the degree to which an individual believes that his or her behaviour can influence important personal outcomes, was found to have the largest association with quality of life, with all the other measured factors being statistically controlled in the regression analysis. The association was statistically significant. No other association with quality of life was found to be statistically significant in the regression model; however, this lack of significance may be an artifact of high correlations between mastery and the other factors, a possibility that the authors failed to discuss. Unfortunately, the authors did not present simple correlations, which would give a clearer picture of the findings. Nonetheless, Therapist Foster would still learn from the article, primarily through the text, the direction of the associations and the relatively high magnitude of the mastery association relative to the other factors' associations. The higher the participants' mastery beliefs were, the higher their self-reported quality of life. The statistical significance suggests that the findings were not attributable to chance.

The authors provide some basic means and standard deviations that are informative. For example, they show the distribution of mastery scores for individuals in the early, mild stage of the disease; in the middle, moderate stage of the disease; and in the late, severe stage of the disease. The middle stage group, who would be most similar to Mr. Davis in disease severity, had an average mastery score of 25.5 (on a possible scoring range of 10 through 40) with a standard deviation of 3.7. One property of a normal distribution of scores, described in any statistics textbook (e.g., Portney & Watkins, 2000), is that 68% of the sample's scores fall within one standard deviation, in either direction, of the average score. Another property is that 95% of the sample's scores fall within two standard deviations. Assuming that the scores are distributed normally, then 95% of the scores of individuals in the middle stage of the disease fall within the range of $25.5 - (2 \times 3.7) = 18.1$ to $25.5 + (2 \times 3.7) = 32.9$. This range of 18.1 to 32.9 indicates that there is variation from a relatively low mastery score to a relatively high mastery score among people with a moderate degree of disease severity.

Just as Pinquart and Sörensen (2000) suggest that the factors they describe "influence" subjective well-being, so do Koplas et al. (1999) draw incorrect causal implications from their correlational study. They infer from their findings that health care professionals may be able to improve their Parkinson's disease clients' quality of life by trying to optimize clients' perceptions of control. A more appropriate "take-to-the-clinic message" would be to think of quality of life as a multidimensional phenomenon that, for clients with Parkinson's disease, is likely to include feelings related to mastery.

Koplas et al. (1999) did not examine social networks as a possible factor associated with quality of life; however, they did note that when participants were asked to discuss aspects of Parkinson's disease that were most difficult for them, the participants "frequently" (no statistical evidence given) discussed the loss of the ability to effectively communicate in speech and writing, difficulty in the workplace, loss of emotional control, and concerns with the progression of the disease.

Therapist Foster can take away from this examination of the Koplas et al. (1999) findings the following possible answer to the questions in Table 12-1: high feelings of mastery may be an important component of quality of life among clients with Parkinson's disease. Mr. Davis and other clients currently may have low or high feelings of mastery. Other quality-of-life factors may be related to communication ability, workplace factors, emotional control, and thoughts about the progression of the disease.

Communication Examples

Therapist Foster would probably want to peruse other research articles about quality of life and Parkinson's disease, but the two reviewed in this section provide enough evidence to compose initial communications to Mr. Davis, managers, and funders. The following example might be a way to begin a discussion with Mr. Davis:

> *I would like to get to know you better by discussing what it is like for you to go about your daily life while living with Parkinson's disease. It may be helpful for us to discuss some recent research findings about older people and people with Parkinson's disease. It has been found that people are more satisfied with life when they can continue to be with their friends and family members, have*

loving and good times with them, and give one another useful support and help. [Discuss]. It has also been found that being able to keep doing activities inde- pendently and skillfully is important for feeling satisfied with life for many peo- ple. [Discuss.] One study of people with Parkinson's disease found that many people are more satisfied with their lives when they feel in control over things that happen in their lives. Have you thought about whether or not you feel in con- trol and whether or not this matters to you? [Discuss.] Communication can be a problem for people with Parkinson's disease. Is this a concern for you? [Discuss, and raise other remaining issues in a similar fashion]. We've talked a lot about what makes life satisfying and worth living for you today. Are there any changes in your day-to-day life that would make your life more satisfying to you, your wife, and others who are important to you?

A communication with a manager or funder could be stated more formally. It could be used to start a discussion about the development of an evidence-based rehabilitation program for a Parkinson's disease population. If the communication is in written form, it is appropri- ate to include research literature citations. Locations where citations would be appropriate are marked next:

A research synthesis [citation] found that older people, including those with chronic illnesses, had higher life satisfaction when they had active and high qual- ity relationships with friends and family members, were able to perform their daily living and leisure activities competently, and were of a higher socioeconomic sta- tus. A study [citation] of people with Parkinson's disease, in particular, found that people with high feelings of mastery were more likely to report having a high quality of life than people with low feelings of mastery, regardless of their level of disability or depression. Further quality-of-life concerns in this Parkinson's dis- ease sample were the ability to communicate in speech and writing, difficulties in the workplace, loss of emotional control, and concerns about disease progression. These quality-of-life factors should be taken into consideration when developing an rehabilitation program for people with Parkinson's disease.

Evidence That Guides the Choice and Use of Assessment Tools for Clients With Parkinson's Disease

Every score or conclusion drawn from an assessment procedure is a measure of several simultaneous elements; the client's performance is only one of those elements. Other ele- ments are called *error* and include the context of the assessment, the attributes of the thera- pist, and the testing tool itself. For example, a measure of a client's dressing performance could also be a measure of the client's familiarity with the room in which the dressing is per- formed and with the clothing used; a measure of the therapist's emotions, expectations, and behaviour with the client; and a measure of the scale used in scoring. Imagine a client put- ting on an unfamiliar blouse, in an unfamiliar environment, with a harried therapist who was using a two-point rating scale (0 = dependent, 1 = independent) to judge the performance. Now imagine this client putting on a familiar blouse, in a familiar environment, with a relaxed therapist who was using a five-point scale (graduated from 0, requires another to per- form every step to 4, able to perform every step with no assistance) to judge the performance. This client may receive two very different recommendations based upon these two different types of testing situations; perhaps a recommendation for further rehabilitation in the first sit- uation, and for immediate discharge home in the second situation. Standardized assessment procedures that are reliable and valid are, by definition, less likely to result in inconsistent and incorrect conclusions compared to unstandardized, low reliability or low validity procedures. Obviously, therapists, clients, funders, and managers, at the very least, do not want to waste the client's and therapist's time and resources in assessments that will result in incorrect conclusions and, at the most, have the client receive incorrect recommendations that could have major life consequences.

The challenge of the evidence-based practitioner is to use assessment procedures that have demonstrated reliability and validity, are feasible in the therapist's clinical context, and are the right fit for the client. The research literature on the measurement properties of assessment procedures uses a dizzying array of terminology to discuss and report reliability and validity findings. What is most crucial to the selection of an assessment tool is whether or not that tool has been tested for the particular forms of reliability and validity most pertinent to the purpose of the assessment. See Tables 12-7, 12-8, and 12-9 for common forms, methods, and standards derived from a quantitative paradigm that are used with many assessments relevant to rehabilitation.

Interpretation of a Synthesis of Studies

Using the clinical questions in Table 12-2 to organize a literature search, Therapist Foster found an article by Stolee et al. (1999) that reviewed two previous studies by their research group and a newly completed one. The researchers studied the measurement properties of Goal Attainment Scaling (GAS) with a geriatric rehabilitation population. Table 12-5 shows that there were participants in this study that were similar to Mr. Davis and Therapist Foster's broader Parkinson's disease caseload with respect to age and disability. Let's assume that Mr. Davis is coming to Therapist Foster as an outpatient, whereas the participants in the study were inpatients. Stolee et al.'s research participants were predominantly female, unlike Mr. Davis and Therapist Foster's caseload, but males were represented in the sample. Finally, the participants were in Canada rather than the United States, but Canada and the United States. are similar in that they are Western cultures that put strong values on individual goal achievement. The research participants were of unknown race and socioeconomic status, so they cannot be compared to the therapist's caseload in this respect.

With GAS, clients and therapists create individualized goals and then measure the achievement of the goals against a graded set of behavioural outcomes. Even though the goals can be different for every client, the score derived from the GAS can be compared and averaged across different clients in a meaningful way. The higher the score, the more successfully the client and therapist achieved the goals. For example, suppose Mr. Davis wanted to be able to cook more quickly and with less spilling. His meal preparation activities have declined in quality and efficiency as his tremors, bradykinesia, and fatigue have increased. A goal for Mr. Davis' meal preparation activities would be scaled from –2 , the worst plausible outcome, such as the home delivery of meals, to +2, the best plausible outcome, such as the efficient and safe preparation of nutritious and pleasant meals.

Stolee et al. (1999) found that interrater reliability of the GAS outcome score was high, ranging from intraclass correlations of .87 to .93 across the three studies. An earlier study had found beginning evidence of adequate interrater reliability for the development of the goals. In addition to reliability findings, Stolee et al. reported evidence related to several types of descriptive and evaluative validity. A descriptive form of content validity was supported through an analysis of the content of individualized goals. The goals were found to fall into 10 primary categories (including mood/motivation and cognition, but predominantly activities of daily living, future care, and mobility), all of which were appropriate for geri-

Table 12-7

A RELIABILITY PRIMER

Form of Reliability	Tested when the score or assessment conclusion is expected to be consistent across different...	Examples of assessments that should demonstrate an adequate degree of this form of reliability	The degree of reliability is commonly summarized with a coefficient that represents the consistency between different raters, times, or items, such as...	What is an "adequate" degree of reliability?
Inter-rater	Therapists or raters	• Therapist's judgment of ADL independence from observing client's performance	Correlation (e.g., intraclass) Cohen's kappa	≥ .70 ≥ .40
		• Therapist's summary of a client's feelings or experiences	Percentage agreement	≥ 80%
Test-retest	Testing times, as long as the client has not changed	• Client's ADL performance before receiving intervention	Correlation (e.g., intraclass)	≥ .70
		• An interest checklist	Difference in standard deviation units (e.g., d)	≤ .20
Internal consistency	Items of a measure	• A 20-item short-term memory test	Correlation	≥ .40
		• A 10-item self-esteem questionnaire	Cronbach's alpha	≥ .70

Note: Reliability testing methods and standards vary across different research areas. See a research methods textbook (e.g., Portney & Watkins, 2000) for general and common methods and interpretation standards.

Table 12-8

A VALIDITY PRIMER, I

General form of validity	Tested when the score or assessment conclusion is expected to be a valid (true) measure of...	Why tested?	Specific forms of validity testing (see Table 12-9)
Descriptive	Current client attributes at one point in time, such as current ADL performance or feelings about self	To see if the measure differentiates between clients who have different attributes	Content Criterion-related Construct
Predictive	Client attributes in the future, such as ability to successfully perform work activities or to adjust to disability	To see if the current measurement predicts future attributes	Content Criterion-related Construct
Evaluative	Change over time in client attributes, such as change in ADL performance, change in feelings of self-efficacy	To see if the measure is responsive to change in the client	Content Criterion-related Construct

Note: Validity testing terminology, methods, and standards vary across different research areas (see Portney & Watkins, 2000).

atric inpatient rehabilitation needs. Descriptive and evaluative forms of criterion-related validity were reported as well. In terms of descriptive validity, the GAS outcome scores were highly correlated with outcome scores on the Barthel Index (r's ranging from . 59 to .86) and with scores on the Older Americans Resources and Services (OARS) Index of Instrumental Activities of Daily Living ($r = .54$). These correlations suggest that the GAS can be used to measure goal achievement related to activities of daily living (ADL). Evaluative criterion-related validity was demonstrated on change scores, from before to after rehabilitation. Change on the GAS correlated with change on the Barthel ($r = .60$) and the OARS ($r = .48$). In addition, the standardized response mean, a measure of the magnitude of the change in the score in standard deviation units, was 1.73 for the GAS compared to .97 and .80 for the Barthel and the OARS. This finding means that participants' scores increased by more than 1 standard deviation on the GAS, whereas their scores increased by almost 1 standard deviation on the two ADL measures. All of these magnitudes are considered large (> .80 according to Cohen, 1988). Other validity tests consistently suggested the GAS to adequately

Table 12-9

A VALIDITY PRIMER, II

Specific Form of Validity	Addresses the question...	Example	How this form of validity is assessed	What is an "adequate" degree of validity?
Content	Does the content of the measure cover all aspects or elements of the attribute of interest being measured?	Does a basic ADL instrument measure all important self-care activities?	• Documented expert opinion • Comparison with relevant theory	• Relative congruence between content and expert opinion • There is a logical and direct relationship between the measure and the theory
Criterion-related	Does the score or conclusion drawn from the measure relate to a score or conclusion drawn from a valid criterion?	• Does the score from a new ADL instrument (the one that is yet to be validated) lead to the same conclusions as a score from an established ADL instrument? • Do clients with brain damage have a different score on a cognitive test than clients without brain damage?	• Administration of both new and established measure to clients and calculation of correlation between the two measures • Administration of the test to different populations of clients and comparison of the scores	• A level of association that should theoretically exist between the two (e.g., $r \geq .60$) • A difference that should theoretically exist between the two (e.g., $d \geq .30$)

Table 12-9 (Continued)

Specific Form of Validity	Addresses the question...	Example	How this form of validity is assessed	What is an "adequate" degree of validity?
Criterion-related (continued)		• Do clients who are known to have improved their ability to drive show this improvement in a new driving test?	• Administration of a test before and after an intervention and comparison of the two scores	• A difference that should theoretically exist between the two (e.g., $d \geq .80$)
Construct (convergent and discriminant)	Does the score or conclusion drawn from the measure relate more to validated measures of the same attribute than to validated measures of a different attribute?	• Does a dementia test relate more to another dementia test than it does to a test of depression?	• Administration of measures designed to measure similar and different attributes and comparisons of the relationships between the various measures	• Larger correlations between similar measures compared to smaller correlations between different measures

Note: Validity is not normally determined by comparison to one absolute standard. It is established through a variety of means that make scientific and theoretical sense and is best determined by comparison with standards in a specific field of research.

describe differences in goal achievement among the participants, and to adequately evaluate changes in goal-related behaviours from before to after rehabilitation.

Stolee et al. (1999) also began an investigation of the descriptive and evaluative construct validity of the GAS scores. They found that the GAS outcome and change scores correlated more highly with the ADL outcome and change scores than with scores on a quality of life measure. This finding was unexpected but several explanations are possible. Stolee et al. noted that ADL and mobility problems were the most prevalent presenting problems in the research participants, and possibly goals addressing these problems are not quality of life goals, or at least, not a comprehensive representation of quality of life goals. Alternatively, there may have been a validity problem with the quality of life measure, given that many of the participants reported that the questions on the measure were inappropriate for their situation (no details given).

Together these findings suggest a possible answer to the questions in Table 12-2: GAS is a reliable and valid method for assessing goal achievement among individuals in a geriatric rehabilitation program. It is one possible method to be compared against others for determining which is the most reliable and valid one for assessing goal achievement in a Parkinson's disease population.

Interpretation of a Single Study

The GAS may be an appropriate tool for measuring goal achievement; however, the traditional form of GAS takes extra work compared to simpler rating scales or checklists. The extra work and time needed to make meaningful, measurable, and consistently set goals for each client in a busy clinical setting may not be feasible. Therapist Foster might continue to search the literature to determine if there were other individualized goal achievement measures with acceptable measurement properties. The therapist might find a study by Yip et al. (1998) that tested a simpler, less time-consuming version of GAS. The research participants in this study were similar to that of Stolee et al.'s (1999), as shown in Table 12-5. Yip et al. reported the development of a standardized menu to use with GAS. This menu, which operates as a checklist, retains the primary elements of GAS. The authors reported the new form of the GAS to be feasible, with goal setting taking 10 to 15 minutes per client and subsequent attainment discussions taking 2 to 3 minutes. These steps were completed during team conferences with the client and family members' preferences in mind but not with these individuals present. Yip et al. did not report interrater reliability for the menu. They reported the standardized menu to have acceptable content validity, with content similar to that reported by Stolee et al. In addition, Yip et al. found that evaluative criterion-related validity coefficients were supportive of sufficient validity but were of a slightly lower magnitude than those found with the traditional GAS in Stolee et al.'s study. The correlation between the GAS menu form outcome score and the changes on standardized ADL measures (including the Barthel and OARS) ranged from .43 to .45, compared to the .48 to .60 found in Stolee et al.'s study. This is probably not a meaningful validity difference. The standardized response mean, a measure of the magnitude of the change in the score in standard deviation units, was 1.56 for the menu GAS compared to .82 and .72 for the Barthel and the OARS, respectively. This finding was similar to that for the more traditional GAS.

This study builds the repertoire of possible answers to the questions in Table 12-2: the measurement properties of the menu GAS suggest that it would be an equally adequate, yet more feasible, measure of goal attainment than the traditional GAS in a busy clinical setting.

Communication Examples

Therapist Foster would probably want to find syntheses and study reports about other goal attainment and client-centred assessments (McColl & Pollock, 2001), but the two reviewed in this section provide enough evidence to compose initial communications to Mr. Davis, managers, and funders. The following example might be a way to begin a discussion with Mr. Davis and his wife, who comes with Mr. Davis to every rehabilitation appointment. The terms *validly* and *reliably* have been replaced in this example with *accurately* and *precisely* because of people's more intuitive understanding of the latter terms:

> *One of the first steps of rehabilitation is to determine accurately and precisely the needs and goals of a client. Then the client and therapist can design a program to directly meet these needs and goals. One method that has been found to be accurate and precise involves you and me writing down very concrete goals. Then for each goal we write easier versions and harder versions. [Discuss examples based upon some needs already identified with Mr. Davis.] From these goals, we then design therapy to achieve the easiest version of the goals first, then try to reach the version that is most acceptable to you. Then we might even try to achieve one that is more difficult to achieve. We can start either by writing the goals ourselves or by using a checklist of goals. Would you like to be involved in writing the goals?*

A communication with a manager or funder could be stated more formally, as in the example below, to start a discussion about the development of assessment tools in rehabilitation with a Parkinson's disease population. If the communication is in written form, it is appropriate to include research literature citations. Locations where citations would be appropriate are marked below:

> *The geriatric rehabilitation literature has demonstrated that Goal Attainment Scaling is one reliable and valid procedure for writing rehabilitation goals with clients like those with Parkinson's disease [citation]. One form of the scaling is to identify goal areas, such as dressing, mobility, or visiting friends, that are important for an individual client, and then to write a series of concrete behavioural objectives related to each goal area. Usually five objectives are written and graded from the worst to best possible outcome for the client. Because the development of objectives can be somewhat time-consuming, another form of doing the scaling has been created [citation]. This form involves a behavioural outcome checklist that is completed for each client. This form, like the other one, has been found to demonstrate good interrater reliability as well as descriptive and evaluative validity. The scaling has been used effectively to both plan the intervention programs for individual clients as well as to evaluate their progress in response to intervention. Both forms yield scores that can be entered into a database for tracking outcomes of therapy. (Therapist Foster goes on to describe and compare other client-centred assessment tools.)*

Evidence That Guides the Choice of Interventions Used With Clients With Parkinson's Disease

Suppose that Mr. Davis decides to try GAS with the therapist to develop and track the achievement of his rehabilitation goals. Through discussion with him and his wife, Therapist Foster finds that successfully and safely preparing meals is a major concern for the couple.

Since Mrs. Davis' stroke some years back, Mr. Davis has assumed primary responsibility in preparing meals. He derives satisfaction from his ability to prepare nutritious and delicious meals. Over the years, as his symptoms of bradykinesia and tremors have increased, he has found it fatiguing and inefficient to prepare meals. He also worries that he will burn himself or spill cooked food as he pulls it out of the oven, which is at knee level. Both he and his wife are concerned that the meals are not as nutritious or satisfying as they once were because Mr. Davis has reduced the amount and type of food that he prepares. With the therapist, Mr. Davis and his wife write goal attainment levels aimed at improving the success and safety of Mr. Davis meal preparation activities. Next, based on the clinical question in Table 12-3, the therapist searches for the latest evidence on interventions for improving meal preparation performance among individuals like Mr. Davis. Table 12-3 also shows a broader question for communication with managers and funders that addresses client-centred intervention designed to achieve clients' personally meaningful goals.

Interpretation of a Synthesis of Studies

To start to develop possible answers to these questions, Therapist Foster retrieves a meta-analysis recently published in the rehabilitation literature that examined the effectiveness of rehabilitation-related interventions for persons with Parkinson's disease (Murphy & Tickle-Degnen, 2001). Table 12-5 demonstrates that the participants in the studies included in the meta-analysis are similar to the therapist's Parkinson's disease population in many respects. After determining that the meta-analysis is relevant to this population, the therapist looks for the major meta-analytic result, the average effect size estimate. Meta-analysts convert every relevant statistical finding to an effect size that can be averaged across all studies. Tests of significance (such as t or F and their *p* values) cannot be compared across studies because their magnitudes are a function of both the size of the effect and the sample size (Rosenthal & Rosnow, 1991). The most common estimates of effect size used in the rehabilitation and psychological literature are the effect size *r* and the effect size *d*. Table 12-10 shows interpretations and calculations for these effect sizes. The magnitude of the effect size (i.e., how big it is) is an estimate of the degree to which two conditions (such as intervention versus control) differ in terms of their therapeutic effectiveness. Alternatively, the magnitude is the degree to which involvement in intervention had a more successful or beneficial outcome for research participants than involvement in a control condition. Better average outcomes for the intervention versus control conditions are indicated by a positive effect size, equal average outcomes by a 0 effect size, and worse average outcomes by a negative effect size, regardless of whether the effect size is measured as an *r* or a *d*.

Murphy and Tickle-Degnen (2001) found the average effect size of 16 studies was $r = .26$. The effect size was statistically significant ($p < .0001$), indicating chance was not a reasonable explanation for the effect. The magnitude of effect was essentially the same regardless of whether the measured outcome of the intervention was change in a capacity, such as motor coordination or depression, or an activity performance, such of activities of daily living or functional mobility. This *r* of .26 can be compared to the *r* column in Table 12-10. In that column, there is a *r* of .24, which is very close to .26. Such a magnitude of *r* is considered to be of "moderate" size for intervention effects (Cohen, 1988; Rosenthal & Rosnow, 1991).[3]

The effect size *r* is a point-biserial correlation or partial correlation coefficient that indicates the degree to which the independent variable (intervention versus control) is associated with the outcome scores. Rosenthal and Rubin (1982) have shown that the magnitude of the *r*, when multiplied by 100%, can most easily be understood as an estimate of the change in success rates across two conditions. They created a practical tool, called the Binomial

Table 12-10

EFFECT SIZES AND SUCCESS RATES

Magnitude of Effect[a]		*d Success Rates*				*r Success Rates*		
	d	Control	Intervention	Change	*r*	Control	Intervention	Change
Zero	0.0	50%	50%	0%	0.0	50%	50%	0%
Small	.20	46%	54%	8%	.10	45%	55%	10%
Medium	.50	40%	60%	20%	.24	38%	62%	24%
Large	.80	34%	66%	32%	.37	32%	69%	37%
Very Large	2.00	16%	84%	68%	.71	15%	86%	71%

[a]Based on Cohen (1988) and Rosenthal & Rosnow (1991). See Tickle-Degnen (2001) for ca culation details.

Effect Size Display, for translating the effect size r into intervention success rates. Success is defined here as receiving a score that is higher than the combined average of both conditions, and failure as receiving a lower than average score. Table 12-10 shows that for a moderate size r of .24, 62% of the participants who received intervention had a successful outcome relative to 38% of the participants in the control condition who had a successful outcome. Since 62% minus 38% is equal to 24%, the success rate increases by 24% from the control to the intervention conditions. These success rates, which are essentially equivalent to those for $r = .26$, indicate that rehabilitation intervention was successful for more people with Parkinson's disease than was the control condition, and the failure rate was lower for the intervention than control condition.

The other common effect size in the rehabilitation literature is d, which can be directly converted to or from r (see Tickle-Degnen, 2001 for details) or can be calculated directly from the means and standard deviations of reported outcome findings. The effect size d is the difference between the mean outcomes for two conditions in standard deviation units. A d of .50 means that the average intervention outcome was one-half of a standard deviation higher than the average control outcome. Table 12-10 shows that a d of .50 is equivalent to an r of .24. For the same magnitude of intervention effect, the r-related success rates are slightly different from the r-related rates, but either one gives a useful approximation of the difference in success rates. If Therapist Foster made a practice of noting or calculating effect sizes from research reports, he or she would know that an intervention effect of $d = .50$ or $r = .24$ is of a magnitude often found in effective rehabilitation interventions with older adults (Carlson, Fanchiang, Zemke, & Clark, 1996), including client-centred ones in which clients are involved in developing their own goals (Clark et al., 1997). It is important to note that the effect size found in these studies as well as that found by Murphy and Tickle-Degnen (2001) indicates that there was still a number of older clients, approximately 40%, for whom rehabilitation intervention was not successful, and a number of clients, also approximately 40%, for whom the control condition was successful.

The findings of the meta-analysis offer possible answers to the second question in Table 12-3, the one posed for communication with managers and funders: it is likely that it would be beneficial for Therapist Foster's population of Parkinson's clients to take part in rehabilitation. However, as with many forms of intervention, there is no guarantee that rehabilitation will provide a greater benefit to all clients than no treatment or other forms of treatment.

Interpretation of a Single Study

Therapist Foster may continue to search the literature for evidence specifically related to Mr. Davis' desire to improve functioning in meal preparation. A study by Kondo et al. (1997) examined the use of microwave ovens as an intervention to improve meal preparation functioning among five older adults with disabilities. Although none of the participants had Parkinson's disease, they were disabled and living in the community like Mr. Davis, as shown in Table 12-5. Participants kept a daily log of their frequency of using cooking appliances, number of food items they prepared, and duration of meal preparation during four systematically applied phases of intervention and nonintervention, each of 3 weeks duration. During the first phase, there was no intervention; the participants used their normal cooking appliances. Then they were given a microwave oven and trained in its use. The second phase consisted of having the microwave oven available for use in their homes. In the third phase, the microwave oven was withdrawn, and in the fourth phase it was replaced. The researchers presented the findings with means and standard deviations at each phase, as well as frequency graphs that showed changes in the outcome variables within and across each phase.

This type of study and data presentation can be very useful for evidence-based therapists because the therapist is given access to qualitative and quantitative details about each participant. As a result, the therapist can directly examine similarities and differences in responses across different clients. Therapist Foster would see that, overall, the participants were able to cook more easily and with less time when the microwave oven was available to them than when it was not. In terms of meal preparation time, for example, a visual inspection of the means and graphs shows that cooking time decreased from phases 1 to 2 and 3 to 4, each time with the introduction of the microwave oven. For example, participant 3 took an average of 41 minutes in meal preparation during phase 3 without the microwave oven and 29 minutes with the reintroduction of the appliance. This 12-minute change is a 29% reduction in time. In terms of the effect size d, the average time in the fourth phase was 1.26 standard deviations below the average time in the third phase. Therapist Foster calculated this effect size by dividing the 12-minute difference by the standard deviation of meal preparation time during the nonintervention third phase. This large effect size d is the magnitude of the time decrease relative to participant 3's own normal variation in preparation time.

Among the five participants in general, there was a decrease in preparation time of 17 minutes on the average, ranging from an 8 to 30 minute decrease. The average of the participants' d's was 1, a large effect. On the average, the participants had a preparation time with the microwave that was one standard deviation below their preparation time without a microwave. From these findings, Therapist Foster can derive a possible answer to the first question in Table 12-3, the one addressed specifically to Mr. Davis' goal: a microwave may help Mr. Davis to meet his meal preparation goal.

Communication Examples

The therapist might begin the communication about the intervention evidence in the following manner:

> *Recent research findings have shown that a minority of clients with Parkinson's disease do fine without rehabilitation. However, in these studies, the majority of clients improved or maintained their ability to do daily living activities in response to rehabilitation. I found one study that may be of particular interest to you. In a small study of five older people with movement or fatigue problems similar to your own (although they didn't have Parkinson's disease), microwave ovens had a large positive effect on meal preparation activities. The people had more variety in their meals and took less time to cook their meals when they had a microwave oven than when they did not have one. The studies suggest that you may benefit from a general program of rehabilitation. Also, you may want to consider getting a microwave for preparing your meals. Let's talk more about what we could do to meet your goals in therapy.*

For a communication to managers or funders, the therapist may frame the more formal and statistical communication in the following manner:

> *Recent meta-analyses of rehabilitation intervention with older clients in general and Parkinson's disease clients in particular have found intervention to have a larger positive outcome relative to control interventions [citations]. The effect is of a moderate magnitude, such that 62% of research participants who received intervention had a successful outcome relative to 38% of the participants in the control condition who had a successful outcome. There are many types of individualized interventions that may be effective for clients, dependent upon their own needs and goals. For example, a study with a single-subject design [citation]*

found a large and positive effect of microwave ovens on the meal preparation activities of older individuals with physical disabilities. The meals of these participants had more variety and took less time to prepare when they had a microwave oven available, for which they had received training, compared to when they used their standard cooking appliances. The research evidence supports the provision of rehabilitation services to older individuals with Parkinson's disease.

EVIDENCE-BASED COMMUNICATION IN THE FACE OF UNCERTAINTY

When the search for evidence has turned up a recent and high-quality published literature review or meta-analysis, the integration that is needed has already been completed by the published author. The therapist need only translate the technical language and presentation of these reviews into language understandable to decision makers. However, if no such review has been found, the therapist must make an accurate integration him- or herself. Such integration takes skill, which develops with the study of research methods and the practice of having to communicate clearly about a body of evidence. Among the guidelines to follow when making an integrated interpretation of a body of evidence are the following two (Tickle-Degnen, 2000):

1. Give heavier emphasis to studies that provide more accurate (stronger) evidence than to those studies with weaker evidence. The therapist should refer to standard research methods textbooks (Portney & Watkins, 2000) that address this type of accuracy in their sections on evaluating the internal and external validity of studies.

2. When examining statistics, do not rely solely on significance tests and their p-values for determining what the study found unless the study involved a large sample size, roughly about 60 or more participants. Studies that have large sample sizes have more power to detect a statistically significant effect than studies with small sample sizes (Ottenbacher & Maas, 1999).

It is possible that the findings of two studies may appear to be different. For example, one claims to support the effectiveness of an intervention and the other claims to not support it. The study that claims to fail to support the effectiveness, typically represented as $p > .05$, may have had a small sample size, possibly making it a low power study. The study that claimed to support the effectiveness, with a $p < .05$, may have had a large sample size, enhancing its power to detect a statistically significant effect. Despite the difference in the p-values of the two studies, the actual mean scores of the participants may show that participants in both studies derived benefit more from the intervention than the nonintervention condition. Therefore, the p-value findings may have led to different conclusions about effectiveness, simply because of power issues, not because of underlying differences in true effectiveness. The integrated interpretation of these two studies would be that they appear to support the effectiveness of the intervention.

When the findings are in opposite directions from two large-sample studies of high quality, the therapist will find the task of integration to be more challenging. In this case, the therapist must report to the decision makers that the body of evidence gives conflicting answers to the clinical question. This conflicting evidence will be one factor that therapist and decision makers consider as they discuss the evidence. Conflicts in evidence call upon the therapist to use the highest level of clinical reasoning skills. There is much uncertainty in therapy because every human being is unique and responds to therapy in an individual manner. Nevertheless, there is a great deal of predictable and systematic behaviour in human beings as well. The therapist uses reasoning that brings uniqueness and predictability together to make decisions in the face of uncertainty (Mattingly & Fleming, 1994).

Conflicts in evidence call upon therapists to not only tap into their clinical reasoning skills, but also to start to develop research questions for an on-site research study. This chapter has addressed how the therapist collects and talks about evidence from published research studies undertaken by researchers other than the therapist. The next logical step in evidence-based practice is to design an on-site study for collecting evidence about one's own clinical population and to use that evidence to help resolve the conflicting findings found in the body of published evidence.

EVIDENCE-BASED COMMUNICATION OPPORTUNITIES IN EVERYDAY PRACTICE

Evidence-based practice requires therapists to keep current in the research findings that are relevant to their clinical populations. To keep current, the therapist must incorporate time for literature searching and reading into clinical practice. The communication about evidence with others will not be an additional time burden if the therapist learns to turn everyday communication opportunities into evidence-based ones.

Communication opportunities with clients arise at the first meeting, at assessment and intervention planning sessions, during the provision of treatment, and discharge planning sessions. Whenever the therapist is giving recommendations or involving the client in decision making, there is an opportunity for incorporating evidence into the message. Even if the client is not interested in hearing evidence-based information, the therapist can communicate about it in an indirect manner to support the client's development of knowledge and active involvement in decision making. For example, using evidence from research on the effectiveness of microwave ovens in enhancing participation in meal preparation activities, the therapist might say, "Some people similar to you have found it easier to make meals with a microwave oven. Do you want to try a microwave oven in therapy to see if it works for you?"

With managers and colleagues, group meetings are an ideal forum for disseminating research evidence because the message is discussed among several people at one time in one location. Appropriate types of meetings are team conferences about clients, staff education sessions, and departmental meetings directed at program planning, budget review, and quality assurance. Journal clubs, in which members take turns in reviewing and presenting a summary of a body of research literature, can reduce the individual burden of searching and reading literature. Discussions at journal clubs are relatively unfettered by day-to-day clinical demands. This type of context supports brainstorming and creative thinking that can stimulate the evidence-based modification or development of assessment and intervention procedures.

Any communication with a funder can be an opportunity for the discussion of research evidence, whether it be face-to-face, via telephone, or written documentation. One of the more formal communications might be a funding proposal, which requires tight organization and scholarly citations. The more comfortable therapists become with the published research evidence in their area of clinical expertise, the more skillfully they will be able to communicate about that evidence in a brief and understandable format. There is no need to tell the client, the manager, or the funder everything that is known about the evidence, unless asked to do so. The therapist communicates enough evidence for informed decision-making, yet is prepared to communicate about evidence in na more detailed manner.

Take-Home Messages

Communicating Evidence Effectively
- Message must be relevant, framed to enable decision making and action, and comprehensible.
- Four steps to evidence-based communication:
  - Clinical role of decision maker: client/family member, manager, and funder are all potential decision makers.
  - Decisions involved: determine relevant participation issues, select assessment procedures, and plan and implement intervention. The types of information are descriptive, assessment, and intervention.
  - Gather/interpret evidence: formulate clinical question and research possible answers. Type of evidence being sought; attribute of interest; description of clinical population. Most efficient to search for research synthesis and meta-analysis.
  - Communicate the evidence: for communication with clients use simple language, terms that cross cultures and perspectives, brevity with appropriate amount of detail, repetition and checks for confusion, suggestion for concrete action related to the information.

Interpretation
- Assessment tool should have been tested for the particular form of reliability and validity.
- Studies that provide access to both quantitative and qualitative details help in examining similarities and differences in responses.

Uncertainty
- If no meta-analysis is available, therapist can perform this function, but it takes a great deal of skill.
- Give heavier emphasis to studies that provide more accurate evidence than those with weaker evidence (internal and external validity).
- Do not rely solely on statistical significance tests and their p-values unless there are more than 60 participants in the study; studies with a larger size have more power to detect a statistically significant effect.
- When findings are in contradictory directions, report upon conflict and use reasoning skills; opportunity to develop research questions for on-site study.

Everyday Practice
- Incorporate time for literature searching and reading.
- Take advantage of opportunities for communicating evidence to clients and for utilizing group meetings as a forum for disseminating research evidence.
- Therapists maintain balance of communicating just enough evidence for informed decision making while being prepared to communicate about evidence in a more detailed manner.

ENDNOTES

[1] Susan Berger, MS, OTR/L was very helpful in guiding me to the recent literature on patient education, and Mary Law, PhD, OT(C) to the review of dissemination literature at the National Center for the Dissemination of Disability Research.

[2] It is possible to defend the authors' use of causality language on a couple of grounds, however. First, from a theoretical perspective, the factors studied in the meta-analysis are predicted to have a causal influence on subjective well-being. Second, some of the studies may have had designs that were supportive of a causal explanation, but the meta-analytic authors did not report information about designs in such a manner as to determine the validity of making a causal interpretation. A perusal of the titles on their reference list suggests that most of the designs were correlational in nature.

[3] Cohen (1988) gave two different sets of standards for interpreting the magnitude of r and d. Rosenthal and Rosnow (1991) pointed out that the two sets of standards do not match when r is converted to d and that Cohen applied a stricter criterion to r than d. The d standards are used in this chapter to interpret intervention effect r's since Cohen intended d to be used for comparing the means of treatment and control groups. On the other hand, Cohen's stricter r standards are used in this chapter to interpret descriptive associations since Cohen intended his r standards to be applied primarily to descriptive associations.

LEARNING AND EXPLORATION ACTIVITIES

The purpose of this chapter is to demonstrate the important role that effective communication plays in incorporating evidence into practice. The following exercise builds upon the process developed in the chapter to assist the student interpreting research studies and relating them to the individual.

1. Research and Communication

To complete the following exercises, create a case scenario or think of an actual client in your area of clinical interest. Write down a description of the client. Be sure to specify the diagnosis or presenting reasons for coming to the therapist and other attributes of interest about the client, such as those in Table 12-5.

   a. Create a descriptive, an assessment, and an intervention clinical question for guiding the search for evidence and the development of possible answers to discuss with the client or the client's family members.

   b. Create a table like Table 12-5 and, using the following template, include columns for describing the client and research participants from each of the three types of studies: a descriptive, assessment, and intervention study. Complete a preliminary literature search based upon the three clinical questions, and locate three studies that appear relevant from their titles. Retrieve and read the articles. Fill in the table by summarizing the research participants' attributes.

   c. Interpret the results from the study that you judge to be most relevant for generating possible answers to one of the clinical questions. Based upon the results, what is the possible answer to the clinical question? Is the study of a quality that makes you feel confident that the possible answer is justifiable? Explain.

Client Identity	Disease	Degree of Disability	Age	Gender	Race and Ethnicity	Family and Living Context	Work Status	Socio-economic Status
Study #1 (Descriptive)								
Study #2 (Descriptive)								
Study #3 (Descriptive)								

REFERENCES

Bradshaw, P., Ley, P., Kincey, J. A., & Bradshaw, J. (1975). Recall of medical advice: Comprehensibility and specificity. *British Journal of Social and Clinical Psychology, 14*, 55-62.

Carlson, M., Fanchiang, S., Zemke, R., & Clark, F. (1996). A meta-analysis of the effectiveness of occupational therapy for older persons. *Am J Occup Ther, 50*, 89-98.

Clark, F., Azen, S. P., Zemke, R., Jackson, J., Carlson, M., Mandel, D., et al. (1997). Occupational therapy for independent-living older adults: A randomized controlled trial. *JAMA, 278*, 1321-1326.

Cohen, J. (1988). *Statistical power analysis for the behavioral sciences* (2nd ed.). Hillsdale, NJ: Lawrence Erlbaum.

Davis, T. C., Bocchini, J. A., Fredrickson, D., Arnold, C., Mayeaux, E. J., Murphy, P. W., et al. (1996). Parent comprehension of polio vaccine information pamphlets. *Pediatrics, 97*, 804-810.

Doak, C. C., Doak, L. G., & Root, J. H. (1996). *Teaching patients with low literacy skills* (2nd ed.). Philadelphia, PA: J. B. Lippincott.

Falvo, D. R. (1985). *Effective patient education: A guide to increased compliance*. Rockville, MD: Aspen.

Kondo, T., Mann, W. C., Tomita, M., & Ottenbacher, K. J. (1997). The use of microwave ovens by elderly persons with disabilities. *Am J Occup Ther, 51*, 739-747.

Koplas, P. A., Gans, H. B., Wisely, M. P., Kuchibhatla, M., Cutson, T. M., Gold, D. T., et al. (1999). Quality of life and Parkinson's disease. *Journal of Gerontology: Medical Sciences, 54A*, M197-M202.

Mattingly, C., & Fleming, M. H. (1994). *Clinical reasoning: Forms of inquiry in a therapeutic practice*. Philadelphia, PA: F. A. Davis.

McColl, M. A., & Pollock, N. (2001). Measuring occupational performance using a client-centred perspective. In M. Law, C. Baum, & W. Dunn (Eds.), *Measuring occupational performance: Supporting best practice in occupational therapy*. Thorofare, NJ: SLACK Incorporated.

Murphy, S., & Tickle-Degnen, L. (2001). The effectiveness of occupational therapy-related treatments for persons with Parkinson's disease: A meta-analytic review. *Am J Occup Ther, 55*, 385-392.

National Center for the Dissemination of Disability Research (NCDDR). (1996). *A Review of the Literature on Dissemination and Knowledge Utilization*. Retrieved October 19, 2000, from http//www.ncddr.org/du/products/review/index.html.

Ottenbacher, K. J., & Maas, F. (1999). How to detect effects: Statistical power and evidence-based practice in occupational therapy research. *Am J Occup Ther, 53*, 181-188.

Pinquart, M., & Sörensen, S. (2000). Influences of socioeconomic status, social network, and competence on subjective well-being in later life. *Psychol Aging, 15*, 187-224.

Portney, L. G., & Watkins, M. P. (2000). *Foundations of clinical research: Applications to practice* (2nd ed.). Upper Saddle River, NJ: Prentice Hall Health.

Redman, B. K. (1997). *The practice of patient education* (8th ed.). St. Louis, Mo: Mosby.

Rosenthal, R., & Rosnow, R. (1991). *Essentials of behavioral research: Methods and data analysis* (2nd ed.). New York, NY: McGraw-Hill.

Rosenthal, R., & Rubin, D. B. (1982). A simple general purpose display of magnitude of experimental effect. *Journal of Educational Psychology, 74*, 166-169.

Sackett, D. L., Richardson, W. S., Rosenberg, W., & Haynes, R. B. (1997). *Evidence-based medicine: How to practice and teach EBM*. New York, NY: Churchill Livingstone.

Stolee, P., Stadnyk, K., Myers, A. M., & Rockwood, K. (1999). An individualized approach to outcome measurement in geriatric rehabilitation. *Journal of Gerontology: Medical Sciences, 54A*, M641-M647.

Tickle-Degnen, L. (2000). Evidence-based practice forum—Communicating with clients, family members, and colleagues. *Am J Occup Ther, 54*, 341-343.

Tickle-Degnen, L. (2001). From the general to the specific: Using meta-analytic reports in clinical decision-making. *Evaluation & the Health Professions, 24*, 308-326.

Yip, A. M., Gorman, M. C., Stadnyk, K., Mills, W. G. M., MacPherson, K. M., & Rockwood, K. (1998). A standardized menu for goal attainment scaling in the care of frail elders. *The Gerontologist, 38*, 735-742.

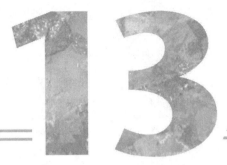

Research Dissemination and Transfer of Knowledge

Mary Law, PhD, OT(C) and Ian Philp, BASc

LEARNING OBJECTIVES

After reading this chapter, the student/practitioner will be able to:

- Distinguish between the various models of research transfer.
- Identify effective research transfer dissemination models.
- Recognize the differences between knowledge-driven models and problem-driven models of evidence-based policy.
- Characterize the roles and challenges of evidence-based policy within evidence-based practice.

INTRODUCTION

Transferring research into practice seems to be the very reason for the existence of evidence-based practice (EBP), and it would be reasonable to assume that it is something at which evidence-based practitioners would be skilled. Despite the need for research transfer, however, the best methods for doing it still remain a mystery for many who embrace EBP. Traditionally, "transfers of health care information" took place through either the undiscriminating distribution of print media (such as a bulletin or a journal article) or through large group seminars. For a long time, this was thought to be enough; however, practitioners have recently realized that these methods are inadequate. The problems were substantial: either the information wasn't reaching those who needed it, it wasn't convenient for the practitioners who wanted to learn, or the format of the material alienated the participants.

In the past decade, there have been major efforts made to create organizations that will ensure effective research transfer. One such institution is HEALNet, a nationwide network of Canadian researchers from various disciplines. These professionals are attempting to improve decision making in the Canadian health care system, thereby enhancing its responsiveness to new innovations. As they state on their web site, HEALNet's research "focuses on enhancing the use and utility of information in health care decision making from analyzing information needs to developing strategies and tools to facilitate effective information use and assess performance" (HEALNet, n.d.) (see the Web Links section on p. 266 for more information).

HEALNet and its partners have created a model of how research transfer works in health care, including many different factors. HEALNet's model, although complex, shows how to perfect the use of research findings and encompasses three major categories: understanding how health care decisions are made, using the evidence/knowledge/information/data available, and linking use of evidence with performance. The model is best conceptualized as a loop in which constant feedback leads to an improvement in the whole process.

Perhaps one of the most important points made by HEALNet is that it gives an idea of the complexity involved in research transfer. There are many more considerations than just the fact that the research has been done correctly (this is also discussed in the chapter on evidence-based policy). We must also examine the characteristics of the different pieces in the research transfer equation. What are the characteristics of the scientific evidence used? Who are the decision makers who will be examining it? In what organizational context do we expect this research information to be used? There are a rich variety of variables that must be considered, and their interplay is discussed in the chapter on evidence-based policy. Effective research transfer can sometimes be more of an art than a science.

In addition to the HEALNet model, another model for research transfer comes from researcher Maureen Dobbins and colleagues (in press), who breaks the research transfer process into five key stages:

1. Knowledge
2. Persuasion
3. Decision
4. Implementation
5. Confirmation

Dobbins et al.'s (in press) model extends to evidence-based policy, as do many larger models of research transfer activities, since the two (research transfer and policy making) interact. Each of Dobbins et al.'s five phases has a specific purpose. The *knowledge* stage begins when research is complete and attempts to identify the best ways for presenting that knowledge to others (discussed later in this chapter on p. 258). The *persuasion* stage is twofold— it includes persuading other practitioners, and policy makers, of the merits of one's research. Third, the *decision* stage leads to evidence-based decision making on whether or not this innovation will be put to use. The fourth and fifth stages, *implementation* and *confirmation*, deal more specifically with evidence-based policy.

The HEALNet and Dobbins et al. models of research transfer are important. On a smaller level, how is research best transferred to individual practitioners? A good systems theory model for research transfer comes from an older article (Goode, Lovett, Hayes, & Butcher, 1987) from the *Journal of Nursing Administration*. It describes the research transfer process as a three-pronged mechanism, consisting of *input*, *throughput*, and *output*, and Goode et al. set out a series of eight steps to research transfer. They are as follows:

1. Identifying problems occurring in the clinical area.
2. Gathering information from research studies that add knowledge regarding the problems.
3. Assuring that the (practitioners) have adequate knowledge to read the research studies critically and understand their implications.
4. Determining if the research is relevant to the type of patients and clinical setting in which it was to be used.
5. Devising ways to transform knowledge so that it can be used in clinical practice.
6. Defining what patient outcomes are expected.
7. Providing education and training that is needed to get the practice change into the system.
8. Evaluating and adjusting or modifying the new practice protocol.

Goode et al.'s (1987) model builds upon the realization that research transfer cannot be a passive endeavor. Once practitioners finish their formal training, health "authorities" dictating what should and what should not be learned underestimate the abilities of individual clinicians. Of course, large agencies will distribute clinical guidelines and evidence-based policy; however, it will be up to individuals to assimilate much of the knowledge on their own. The strategy of teaching practitioners the process and having them perform short, self-directed inquiries into subjects is better than distributing information that will not be used. More important, perhaps, than even the content of the evidence being transferred is the method of transfer. Choosing a research transfer flow that accords practitioners respect for their experience and makes them enthusiastic to use their own critical appraisal skills, while simultaneously encouraging researchers when they see that the fruits of their labour put to good use, is the ultimate goal. Returning to Goode et al.'s model, the input, throughput, and output stages encompass the eight steps quite well.

Input—Steps 1 to 3

At this point of the research transfer process, the emphasis is on preparing the practitioners to gather and assimilate new knowledge. When the research transfer process is started, it begins with a topic that is a current clinical problem in the practitioners' everyday setting. The surest way to alienate new inductees to evidence-based practice is to make them work on esoteric, theoretical cases because they will soon lose interest and respect for the evidence-based process. If practitioners are set to work on improving care in an area that is known to be a clinical problem, however, they will respond much more positively and will see it as a chance to test themselves against real clinical challenges. One must ensure that practitioners feel supported and capable of working with the evidence they have gathered, and if not, they have recourse to experienced help.

Throughput—Steps 4 to 6

The throughput stage is a crucial one and will be discussed again later in this chapter. Especially important is step 5, which concerns transforming knowledge to practice. This can mean interpreting knowledge useful for individuals, but it also includes the practitioner preparing to teach others about what he or she has found. Research and findings into this topic will be discussed later in this summary. Throughput generally encompasses the making of critically appraised topics (CATs) (and possibly systematic reviews) and preparing them for use with clients in a clinical setting.

Output—Steps 7 and 8

In this last step of the model, the findings of the research inquiry are collated, and research has effectively been transferred into practice. At this stage, reflection on the entire process should occur, and thoughts on how research transfer can be improved or further tested should be recorded. The evaluation of the entire process follows a feedback loop and returns to the input step of the process. In this way, Goode et al.'s (1987) research transfer strategy is like a self-cleaning machine: each time this strategy is used by a practitioner, it is further integrated into his or her thinking and becomes open to his or her insights and modifications.

CONCRETE RESEARCH TRANSFER STRATEGIES

As was mentioned before, when a practitioner is undertaking a research transfer project, he or she will need to be able to teach others what he or she has found when finished. It was also stated at the beginning of this summary that conventional speech and print methods were found to be inadequate for effective, long-lasting research transfer. Research transfer dissemination strategies, which are more effective, are those that conform to the personal learning needs of the researcher and utilize two or more different approaches simultaneously.

Evidence from randomized clinical trials (RCTs) and systematic reviews, which examined practitioners' habits, indicates that there is no one optimal way to disseminate research to other practitioners. In their powerful article, "No Magic Bullets: A Systematic Review of 102 Trials of Interventions to Improve Professional Practice," Oxman, Thomson, Davis, and Haynes (1995) conclude that "there are no 'magic bullets' for improving the quality of health care, but there are a wide range of interventions available that, if used appropriately, could lead to important improvements in professional practice and patient outcomes" (p. 142). Table 13-1 is a list of research transfer strategies from Oxman et al.'s article.

Much of Oxman et al.'s (1987) article examines each type of intervention and its particular individual or combined effectiveness. Specific combinations of research transfer dissemination strategies must be made to suit the content being disseminated. Strategies such as "local opinion leaders," "audit and feedback," and "reminders" show that research transfer works well when personalized to individuals practitioners' needs. Reading Oxman et al.'s article in its entirety is recommended, not only for its content, but also to appreciate its systematic review format.

Table 13-1

RESEARCH TRANSFER TEACHING STRATEGIES FOR PRACTITIONERS

Educational Materials

Distribution of published or printed recommendations for clinical care, including clinical practice guidelines, audiovisual materials, and electronic publications.

Conferences

Participation of health care providers in conferences, lectures, workshops, or trainee-ships outside their practice settings.

Outreach Visits

Use of a trained person who meets with providers in their practice setting to provide information, which may include feedback on the provider's performance.

Local Opinion Leaders

Use of providers explicitly nominated by their colleagues to be "educationally influential."

Patient-Mediated Interventions

Any intervention aimed at changing the performance of health care providers for which information was sought from or given directly to patients by others (e.g., direct mailings to patients, patient counselling delivered by others, or clinical information collected directly from patients and given to the provider).

Audit and Feedback

Any summary of clinical performance of health care over a specified period, with or without recommendations for clinical action. The information may have been obtained from medical records, computerized databases, or patients or by observation.

Reminders

Any intervention (manual or computerized) that prompts the health care provider to perform a clinical action. Examples include concurrent or inter-visit reminders to professionals about desired actions such as screening or other preventive services, enhanced laboratory reports or administrative support (e.g., follow-up appointment systems or stickers on charts).

Marketing

Use of personal interviewing, group discussion (focus groups), or a survey of targeted providers to identify barriers to change and the subsequent design of an intervention.

Multifaceted Interventions

Any intervention that includes two or more of the last six interventions described above.

Local Consensus Process

Inclusion of participating providers in discussion to ensure agreement that the chosen clinical problem is important and the approach to managing it appropriate.

Oxman, A. D., Thomson, M. A., Davis, D. A., & Haynes, R. B. No magic bullets: A systematic review of 102 trials of interventions to improve professional practice.—Reprinted from *Canadian Medical Association Journal* 15 November 1995; *153*(10), 1423-1431 by permission of the publisher, © 1995 Canadian Medical Association Journal.

A further application of research transfer dissemination strategies is through organizations known as *journal clubs*. Long popular with physicians, journal clubs are a group of practitioners who split up the literature to be read, with each person focusing on one particular article, journal, or group of journals. When the journal club convenes, practitioners summarize and present what they've garnered from their reading to the other participants, thereby cutting down the amount of slogging through the medical literature that must be done by each practitioner. Jaan Siderov recently wrote an article in which he meta-analyzed the habits of 131 journal clubs for medical residents (1995). His main conclusions were that the crucial elements that make a good journal club include mandatory attendance from participants, meetings with the provision of food, fewer full staff attending (thus giving students the feeling of greater freedom to debate and discuss without being evaluated), and a modest size, to preclude feelings of exclusion.

DIFFERENT MODELS OF RESEARCH TRANSFER

As can be appreciated, the models of research transfer presented here merely scratch the surface of the work that has been done on the subject. There are, however, great similarities between the different models, as Brown and Rodger point out in their 1999 article, "Research Utilization Models: Frameworks for Implementing Evidence-Based Occupational Therapy Practice." Examining nine models of research transfer, Brown and Rodger categorize the similarities between them. Their most important finding was that each model had "a systematic process of analysis to facilitate the incorporation of research findings into clinical practice" (i.e., each had a well-defined process by which it best distributed new knowledge to its client population).

Brown and Rodger (1999) also outline some of the common benefits they found that were gained from research transfer initiatives. The principal seven are:
1. A reaffirmation of current clinical practice.
2. A change in current clinical practice.
3. The establishment of a collaborative network.
4. The enhancement of critical thinking skills.
5. Cost savings.
6. The generation of new research questions.
7. Improvement in client outcomes.

Interestingly, the improvement in client outcomes is only one of the benefits accrued from research transfer, supporting the argument that research transfer enhances the health of not only the client but also the system that treats him or her.

Two other short articles that should be looked at to fully appreciate the challenges of transferring research into practice are those of Grol (1997) and Sheldon, Guyatt, and Haines (1998). Grol's paper, "Beliefs and Evidence in Changing Clinical Practice" is excellently written and laid out and provides more context on research transfer teaching strategies. He outlines four types of strategies: marketing approaches, behavioural approaches, social interaction, and organizational approaches, and discusses when each can be appropriate. Grol also presents his own research transfer model. By contrasting Grol's model with Goode et al.'s (1987), and then examining models such as that of Thomson-O'Brien and Moreland (1998), one can begin to get a feel for the general patterns of research transfer and its intricacies.

The second article to read is, "When to Act on the Evidence" (Sheldon et al., 1988). Again, this article provides yet another perspective on research transfer, its process, and its challenges. The more perspectives you examine, the more you will know where your own understanding of research transfer needs to be fortified, clarified, and improved.

As an evidence-based practitioner, when you are working on understanding research transfer and its methods, you are essentially learning about how others learn best. This knowledge will be of service when communicating with clients, when attempting to understand other health care professionals' presentation of data and hypotheses, and when expressing your clinical thoughts both orally and in writing.

EVIDENCE-BASED POLICY

Evidence-based policy is a relatively new field of study in the realm of EBP. Evidence-based medicine and the work of Archie Cochrane were the inspirations for the movement; however, all of the evidence gathered and analyzed for evidence-based medicine was concentrated on better patient care. The idea that evidence could be used on policy successes and failures could be gathered in the same way did not initially pique the same outpouring of interest and work, but it is becoming increasingly important.

There are reasons why evidence-based policy has been slow to catch on. The material we have covered in EBP up to this point has been primarily logical, rational processes. This makes sense, since EBP is an attempt to introduce a more systematic approach to the use of health care knowledge. When entering into the realm of evidence-based policy, however, logic cannot always be trusted. The creation of policy from research findings is a fundamentally different exercise than the careful synthesis and analysis of academic data. EBP, as a process, is based on individual or small group consideration of knowledge and research information. In contrast, evidence-based policy is based on the consideration of health care research by large groups that must come to a consensus, and by those who may not be experts in the field, namely managers and policy makers. As such, processes that worked in EBP cannot necessarily be completely replicated in the creation of policy.

The differences between how EBP and evidence-based policy are made has been known for some time. One of the major obstacles to policy being made along evidence-based lines is the fact that the two contributors to policy—scientists and managers—perceive and value research differently. A good example of this problem is given by Dr. Francois Champagne, a researcher at Quebec's Université de Montréal. Presenting at a 1999 conference in Toronto, Dr. Champagne discussed the differences by proposing that evidence-based policy making can be perceived through two fundamentally different models (Champagne, 1999).

The first, which Champagne calls the "knowledge-driven model," is one that makes sense in a rationally determined environment. It follows five steps:

1. Research (basic, then applied).
2. Technological development.
3. Use (adoption of technology).
4. Quality of implemented actions.
5. Outcome.

This model is the view most commonly held by scientists, who work primarily in the first steps of the model, doing research that could be directed toward certain ends. This model is built on several inherent assumptions. The knowledge-driven model assumes that once new knowledge exists, it will naturally be pressed toward use. In evidence-based policy making, however, this is not necessarily the case. "Perfect knowledge" would be required for policy making to work in this way.

"Perfect knowledge" implies that all evidence is applied in exactly the most beneficial way. This rests on the idea that policy makers and scientists are able to omnisciently see exactly where basic and applied research could be put to use. Furthermore, it assumes that all relevant knowledge will be adopted in its field without impediments. Unfortunately, however, there are many factors standing in the way of research being used in this manner. Basic and applied research is distributed in health care journals, which grow in number and size each month. Scientists and policy makers are not able to sort through all of the new knowledge, nor see how it could be applied to their work; thus, new findings sometimes go unused. Even when evidence and research findings are identified as important, the process of implementing them into policy is often a long and rocky one. Even the best evidence can be doomed by hasty decision making, poor presentation, or due to political reasons. There are often reasons other than evidence that supports implementation of specific policies. This leads to an important truth of evidence-based policy making: management, or the creation of new policies from research, is inherently based in its context. The environment in which policy is made has a strong hand in shaping its eventual outcome.

A second model of evidence-based policy making, known as the "problem-driven model," takes an alternative approach to the process and avoids some of the idealism of the knowledge-based model (Champagne, 1999). Realizing the contextual nature of health care policy, this model does not begin with research, but rather with a problem or question. This model, a view more commonly held by managers, suggests that evidence-based policy is made according to this logic:

1. Definition of problem.
2. Identification of missing knowledge.
3. Acquisition of knowledge, various possible channels.
4. Interpretation for the problem situation.
5. Use (adoption of technology).

In the problem-driven model, once a problem or information need has been understood, policy makers decide which evidence they will require and use various channels to obtain it. Furthermore, both of the channels by which the model suggests that research knowledge is obtained take note of realities. In the problem-driven model, research findings will generally come from either a pool of knowledge already available to policy makers or through commissioned research into a specific problem. This understanding of the realities of how research findings come to practice acknowledges the fact that evidence distribution is not always perfect and that policy makers do tend to draw upon knowledge already available to them. Once policy makers have the research they require, they will interpret it for the situation at hand and finally use it.

As mentioned, the problem-driven model approximates the "real" processes of policy making better than the knowledge-driven model, but why is that? Why do scientists tend to believe that evidence will be used in a different way than managers do? Investigation into this problem has shown that different groups perceive how research should be used in different ways. In a 1981 article, Weiss and Weiss posed the question, "What is meant by using research for policy making?" (p. 846). While seemingly simple, this question is central to the issue, as it highlights the differences of opinion between groups (researchers and policy makers) and reason why misunderstandings to occur.

What Weiss and Weiss found is that researchers see the use of evidence in policy as a fundamentally rational, linear process. When new evidence is published, they feel it should, and will be, expediently put to use in the most applicable field. Decision makers, on the other hand, see a greater and more varied number of ways to use research and are less willing to act on specific pieces of research alone. Much more is required than just top-notch research for policy makers to implement evidence into policy. They see evidence-based policy making as a holistic, multifaceted, nonlinear process. Champagne (1999) summarizes that "researchers and decision makers belong to separate communities with different values and different ideologies and [thus] these differences impede utilization."

Decision making in complex situations is not necessarily a rational process; decision makers and managers draw in a great deal of evidence and assess it in a holistic manner. Instead of affording evidence weight based purely on its methodology and scientific rigour, policy makers are much more apt to take in and consider a great deal of evidence simultaneously, sometimes placing more emphasis on proximate sources, the opinions of local experts, etc. They also generalize the results of many studies together, working with this accumulated evidence. Finally, managers may not always use research purely for the purposes of making the best policy. As Champagne (1999) says, they may use knowledge "deliberately, politically, tactically, and conceptually" to manipulate or work within the context of their policy environment.

Does this mean that EBP fundamentally breaks down during its final stage? Not necessarily. Although evidence-based policy making is not necessarily a linear exercise, it can still yield valid and useful conclusions. Therefore, is there anything that health care professionals can do to influence policy makers to use our high-quality evidence? Dobbins et al. (in press) suggests that "tailoring" evidence to fit the needs and desires of policy makers is a good way to get evidence heard. They looked specifically at systematic overviews of research and how to get decision-makers to agree to them. Decision makers, it must be remembered, have specific needs for the evidence they use. Among these, as Champagne (1999) says, is the need for data to be available, accessible, valid, and, Dobbins et al. would likely add, engaging. Without these characteristics even the most methodically rigorous study is liable to be given less importance than it may deserve.

In addition to macrolevel work on evidence-based policy, which attempts to understand the entire system, there are also smaller steps that have been taken toward moving research into policy. By examining the literature on evidence-based policy, common trends of the field can be understood. The first article to consider appeared in the journal *Health Policy* and discusses "practice guidelines." The authors (Lohr, Eleazer, & Mauskopf, 1998) contend that practice guidelines are the main format of evidence-based policy today. A practice guideline consists of a series of clinical recommendations or dictates on an issue that has been assembled from the best possible evidence. Practice guidelines are distributed by national clearinghouses to avoid conflict between them and to allow care to be standardized to one high standard. The foremost clearinghouse for evidence-based guidelines is the U.S. Agency for Health Care Policy and Research (AHCPR), which distributes a large volume of information on health care and evidence-based practice on the web (www.ahcpr.gov).

When looking at a specific clinical guideline, for example the clinical guideline on rehabilitation for traumatic brain injury (www.ahcpr.gov/clinic/epcsums/tbisumm.htm), we can see that there are many aspects present. The guideline includes background on the issue, outlines the key questions on the issue, details the most current evidence and its sources, and then describes the critical appraisal that has been done on the issue. The guideline culminates by discussing the findings of the critical appraisal (which may even be a systematic review).

Guidelines, like any health care documents, are subject both to practitioner bias and clinical error. Despite possible flaws, they are and can prove to be a strong initial link between research and policy. Lohr et al. (1998) present suggestions about guidelines themselves. Their suggestions are that guides should be systematic, logical, defensible (i.e., reliable and valid), practical, feasible, clear, and understandable to experts and laypersons alike (within reason). By making guidelines accessible, clients who take an interest in their care can begin to inform themselves as well. Lohr et al. also list benefits or goals of practice guidelines. A good practice guideline should do the following:

1. Improve knowledge by making clinicians aware of the recommendations.
2. Change attitudes about standards of care.
3. Shift practice patterns.
4. Enhance patient outcomes.

In their article "Clinical Practice Guidelines: Between Science and Art," authors Battista and Hodge (1998) also discuss practice guidelines. As they see it, guidelines serve six principle roles:

1. Cost control.
2. Quality assurance.
3. Enhancing access to care.
4. Patient empowerment.
5. Safeguarding professional autonomy and medical liability.
6. Resolving management issues (i.e., rationing, competition, micromanagement).

Once again, we can see that guidelines are expected to fulfill a variety of roles. The pressure put on clinical practice guidelines to fill all of these needs sometimes precludes them being very useful in any one area, and they may end up being only partially useful in many. Chapter 11 of this book discusses guidelines in detail.

In order to be able to form the best possible practice guidelines, Davis and Howden-Chapman's (1996) article, "Translating Research Findings into Health Policy," suggests several insights into the policy making process. Foremost amongst their report is the admission that "the [decision making] process is more one of incremental adjustment to competing pressures than the rational formulation and pursuit of a single goal" (p. xx). Davis and Howden-Chapman suggest that research formed with the express goal of becoming a practice guideline and planned by policy makers as such is much more likely to be used.

As a word of warning, Davis and Howden-Chapman (1996) raise a very important point about the universality of practice guidelines. Although a practice guideline sanctioned by a body such as the AHCPR is a testament to the clinical knowledge that has been accumulated in the field, it runs the risk of segregating smaller local communities from the health care loop. Smaller centres and rural practitioners may feel that the currents of evidence, policy, and research have passed them by, and since they had no hand in crafting this strange guideline, they will not heed it. Guidelines must be rigid enough to make some suggestions on the issue in question while simultaneously allowing flexibility for individual interpretation and adaptation to local surroundings. This is concordant with the goals of evidence-based practice: to take the best available evidence from the health sciences literature and policy and to integrate it into local practices.

A final word on practice guidelines comes from Stephen Birch (1997) at McMaster's Centre for Health Policy Analysis (CHEPA). In a detailed paper entitled, "As a Matter of Fact—Evidence-Based Decision Making Unplugged," Birch lucidly outlines how RCTs, systematic reviews, and evidence-based practice guidelines can all "lie." By failing to consider the socioeconomic class of study participants, for example, the "best evidence" for one population may be totally different from that for another. Practice guidelines can be dangerous, however, if they are used too universally. This speaks to the need for the holistic policy-making process and the contribution and input of local decision makers who attempt to draw many factors into a decision.

Birch's article also raises another interesting point: Are there any characteristics of organizations themselves that can make them more open to considering new policies? Champagne (1999) has worked on the question and suggests that there are. Organizations that have an informal atmosphere, specialize in a particular field of knowledge, and participate in inter-organization networks of knowledge sharing are most likely to adopt new innovations and recommendations with greater ease. In conventional institutions, problems with adopting new ideas may arise, such as the resistance of established health care professionals to new ideas due to their familiarity with the old. In more informal and less hierarchical systems, however, practitioners are more apt to feel as if they have a stake in shaping the use of a policy for their institution; therefore, they may be more willing to follow it.

A comprehensive discussion of evidence-based practice guidelines can be found in Gray and colleagues' (1997) article, "Transferring Evidence from Research Into Practice." Evidence-based policy and clinical guidelines, however, will be most apparent when examined on a case-by-case basis in which the blend of research and politics is evident. A good rule of thumb for all evidence-based policy making is that policies must apply to a wide range of people, be adaptable to the needs of local practitioners, and keep the best evidence at hand while spurring on toward future research.

Take-Home Messages

Research Transfer into Practice
- New innovations to replace usual transfer of research using widespread print media and large conferences.
- HEALNet: National network of Canadian researchers that gives an idea of complexity involved in research transfer.
- Research transfer model as three-pronged mechanism:
  - input—emphasis on preparing practitioners to gather and assimilate new information
  - throughput—interpreting knowledge to be useful for individuals, preparing to teach others the knowledge
  - output—reflection on research process and improvements; feedback loop
- Effective research transfer dissemination strategies conform to personal learning needs of the researcher and utilize at least two different strategies simultaneously.

Evidence-Based Policy
- Not always a logical process, but based on the considerations of health care policy research and the consensus of a group who may not always be experts.
- Knowledge-driven model—requires "perfect knowledge" and assumes knowledge will be adopted without impediment; unrealistic.

- Problem-driven model—alternative approach; begins with a problem rather than research; acknowledges that evidence distribution is not always perfect and that policy makers tend to draw upon previously available information.
- Practice guidelines: consist of series of clinical recommendations that have been assembled from the best possible evidence.
- Researchers see evidence in policy as a fundamentally linear and rational process; decision makers see more variety and are less likely to act on a single piece of evidence.

WEB LINKS

What is a CAT?
http://cebm.jr2.ox.ac.uk/docs/cats/catabout.html
This page at the CEBM is a great overview on CATs, including how they work and how they are put together.

University of Rochester Page on CATs
www.urmc.rochester.edu/medicine/res/CATS/thecat.html
A sample CAT template is posted on this web page, as well as more information about CATs in general.

HEALNet: Health Evidence Application and Linkage Network
http://hiru.mcmaster.ca/nce/default.htm
HEALNet, mentioned in the chapter, is an Ontario-centred organization that attempts to improve health care decision making through the effective networking of health care professionals. Its web site contains a number of resources on research transfer.

US Agency for Health Care Policy and Research
www.ahcpr.gov
This site has a great deal of information on health care policy, as well as a list of practice guidelines, which can be downloaded and examined.

Centre for Health Economics and Policy Analysis
www.chepa.org
CHEPA, home of author Stephen Birch (mentioned previously in the chapter), does a great deal of work on health policy analysis and is on the forefront of new knowledge in the field.

LEARNING AND EXPLORATION ACTIVITIES

The purpose of this chapter is to build upon the previous methods of organizing evidence in order to demonstrate the methods for transferring that evidence into practice and policy. These exercises highlight various sections of the chapter by leading the student through exercises both as an individual and as a group, which allows opportunities to utilize this understanding of the different types of evidence.

1. Research Transfer into Practice
   a. What methods work best when transferring research findings? Oxman et al.'s (1995) chart suggests a number of ways of transferring research. Can you think of any more? Why would some be better than others? At what kind of learners are they primarily aimed? Is there a way to make research transfer strategies that speak equally well to many different learning styles?

   b. Try out your own research transfer. Choose a field, and find a piece of previously (to your knowledge) unapplied research. Through careful examination of the research conclusions, determine which parts of the research can be transferred into practice, and develop ways to do this (again, Oxman et al.'s [1995] methodologies will help here). If working in a group, each participant may attempt this exercise, and all can take turns at teaching others what they have found. Whose research transfer strategy worked "the best" (i.e., was memorable for the most people)? Why?

2. Evidence-Based Policy
   c. This exercise will take some preparation and is best attempted in a group. Choose a topic of clinical interest, and find a current clinical policy related to it. In the reference list of the policy should be a list of articles and academic sources used in its creation. Find two or three of the articles on this list, and assign one to each group member. Have each person read both the policy and their assigned article, then convene together as a group. How was each person's article reflected in the policy? Which articles received more or less weight? Why might this have been? Does this policy make good use of current knowledge?

   d. Attempt the same exercise in reverse: find a number of articles on a subject and convene a "policy conference" around them. You will probably want to assign one article to each person and have them argue for it in the conference, as well as designating some nonaligned administrators and decision makers. Even more complex (and interesting) would be if every member of the group was given a specific interest that they were to support during the meeting, but which they could not directly reveal to others. After you have finished the exercise, evaluate your performance. How did you interact in the conference? What forms of discussion worked best? Were everyone's needs met to their satisfaction? Who "won"?

REFERENCES

Battista, R. N., & Hodge, M. J. (1998). Clinical practice guidelines: Between science and art. *Health Policy, 46*, 1-19.

Birch, S. (1997). As a matter of fact—Evidence-based decision making unplugged. *Health Econ, 6*, 547-559.

Brown, T. G., & Rodger, S. (1999). Research utilization models: Frameworks for implementing evidence-based occupational therapy practice. *Occupational Therapy International, 6*(1), 1-23.

Champagne, F. (1999). *The use of scientific evidence and knowledge by managers. Closing the loop*. Toronto, ON: Third International Conference.

Davis, P., & Howden-Chapman, P. (1996). Translating research findings into health policy. *Soc Sci Med, 43*(5), 865-872.

Dobbins, M., Ciliska, D., Cockerill, R., Barnsley, J., & DiCenso, A. (in press). A framework for the dissemination and utilization of research for health care policy and practice. *Primary Health Care: Research and Development.*

Goode, C. J., Lovett, M. K., Hayes, J. E., & Butcher, L. A. (1987). Use of research based knowledge in clinical practice. *J Nurs Adm, 17*(2), 11-18.

Gray, J. A., Haynes, R. B., Sackett, D. L., Cook, D. J., & Guyatt, G. H. (1997). Transferring evidence from research into practice: 3. Developing evidence-based clinical policy. *Evidence-Based Medicine, 2*(2), 36-8.

Grol, R. (1997). Beliefs and evidence in changing clinical practice. *British Medical Journal, 315*, 418-421.

HEALNet. (n.d.). *About HEALNet.* Retrieved January 15, 2002, from http://healnet.mcmaster.ca/about/mainframe.htm.

Lohr, K. N., Eleazer, K., & Mauskopf, J. (1998). Health policy issues and applications for evidence-based medicine and clinical practice guidelines. *Health Policy, 46*, 1-19.

Oxman, A. D., Thomson, M. A., Davis, D. A., & Haynes, R. B. (1995). No magic bullets: A systematic review of 102 trials of interventions to improve professional practice. *Canadian Medical Association Journal, 153*(10), 1423-1431.

Sheldon, T. A., Guyatt, G. H., & Haines, A. (1998). When to act on the evidence. *British Medical Journal, 317*, 139-142.

Siderov, J. (1995). How are internal medicine residency journal clubs organized and what makes them successful? *Arch Intern Med, 155*, 1193-1197.

Thomson-O'Brien, M. A., & Moreland, J. (1998). Evidence-based practice information circle. *Physiotherapy Canada, 50*(3), 184-189, 205.

Weiss, C. H., & Weiss, J. A. (1981). Social scientists and decision makers look at the usefulness of mental health research. *Am Psychol, 36*(8), 837-847.

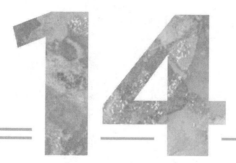

Health Care Delivery of Rehabilitation Services for Postacute Stroke

Home Care Versus Institutional Care—What is the Evidence?

Julie Richardson, MSc

LEARNING OBJECTIVES

After reading this chapter, the student/practitioner will be able to:

- Recognize the limitations in health care delivery research stemming from deficiencies in evidence.
- Understand the challenges within randomized controlled trials, including rapid changes in the delivery of health services.
- Critically evaluate the research studies in postacute stroke rehabilitation and recognize some of the deficiencies.
- Identify the characteristics of stroke that increase the importance of environmental settings in rehabilitation.

BACKGROUND

Introduction

The purpose of this chapter is to provide readers with an example of a review of the evidence in one area of practice. As you are reading this chapter, think about the implications of these findings for consumers, therapists, managers, and policy makers.

There is a dearth of research evidence from health service delivery trials available to direct evidence-based practice. Health service delivery research is an aspect of evidence-based practice that suffers from a paucity of evidence from trials. This is epitomized in relation to the delivery of rehabilitation services in which there is a paucity of evidence to direct how and where rehabilitation practice should be delivered. Health service delivery research has only recently been instituted as a research programme. An example of this is the Cooperative Studies Program at Veterans Affairs (Henderson et al., 1998; James, 1998). Health service delivery research has emanated from clinical trial biomedical research, which focuses on the efficacy and safety of tested interventions with precisely defined endpoints and data collection procedures (James, 1998). Health service delivery research (HSDR) involves more between-centre variation and a less standardized, more applied approach to care than biomedical interventions, although uniformity of the intervention should be a goal. The formulation of interventions in HSDR trials often involves multiple components that enhance the possibility of positive treatment effect; however, this can also create problems with interpretation. The rapid change in delivery of health services, which is part of present health care practice, can occur in the midst of a trial and needs to be anticipated so that the final results are not contaminated by external changes (Henderson et al., 1998). The effect of environment on the practice and relearning of everyday skills and on the resumption and adaptation of roles following stroke is an area in which evidence from health services research can be used to examine the effect of the environmental context on recovery and reintegration.

STROKE: THE PROBLEM

There is a high personal and societal burden associated with stroke. Persons with residual physical, functional, and mobility problems receive rehabilitation in institutional settings and within the home. Most patients would prefer to reside at home following such an event once they are medically stable. Studies to date have failed to clarify which environmental setting produces better outcomes; whether they differ in health care, personal, and financial costs; and whether either outcome or cost differs according to patient characteristics.

Stroke: Definition and Diagnosis

Stroke occurs when blood flow to a part of the brain is interrupted, resulting in symptoms lasting more than 24 hours. Ischaemic stroke can be thrombotic (40% to 55% of all strokes) or embolic (15% to 30%), while haemorrhagic strokes (5% to 20% of all strokes) can be subdivided into intracerebral and subarachnoid in origin (Delaney & Potter, 1993). There is no standardized classification of stroke subtypes. Diagnostic error associated with cerebrovascular disease ranged from 10% to 62% false positives and 5% to 48% false negatives in studies comparing clinical diagnosis to autopsy diagnosis (Bonita, 1992; Ebrahim, 1990; Stehbens, 1991; Terent, 1993). The use of computerized tomography scans only improves diagnostic accuracy by 2% (Leibson, Naessens, Brown, & Whisnant, 1994). Therefore, any stroke treatment study using the clinical or record-based diagnosis of stroke will have a heterogenous sample and include cases whose neurological symptoms have other causes.

Burden of Illness

Hospital stroke rates are often used as a surrogate for stroke incidence rates. Using the ICD codes for haemorrhagic and ischaemic stroke, the Institute for Clinical Evaluative Sciences (ICES) estimates that there were 14,937 strokes in Ontario in 1998 (The Joint Stoke Strategy Working Group [TJSSW Group], 2000). This includes only persons with strokes who were hospitalized. Another 424 strokes occurred while the patient was in the hospital. It has been estimated that there are about 6 stroke survivors per 1,000 people in the population. In 1996, Ontario had a population of almost 8.3 million between 20 to 85+. Therefore, Ontario could have at least 50,000 stroke survivors in any year. The results from the National Population Health Survey (1996 to 1997) report that the point prevalence of the number of persons living in the community in Ontario with stroke is 88,000; as well, there are 22% of institutionalized adults 65 years and older who have had a stroke (TJSSW Group, 2000).

Approximately 30% to 60% of stroke survivors require assistance with basic self-care activities (Gordon, 1993). An estimated average cost of each stroke admission in Toronto was $27,500 (Smurawska, Alexandrov, Bladin, & Norris, 1994). Among long-term survivors, 48% have hemiparesis, 22% cannot walk, 24% to 53% report complete to partial dependence on activity of daily living scales, 12% to 18% are aphasic, and 32% are clinically depressed (World Health Organization, 1989), while 6% show cognitive impairment (Kotila, Waltimo, Niemi, & Laaksonen, 1986).

Although the incidence of stroke appears stable, the magnitude of the problem will grow because it is projected that there will be 6 million Canadians 65+ years by 2021 (Stone, 1986). Therefore, methods of care delivery that will optimize function and minimize burden and cost in this patient group need to be investigated.

Current Care

The average age of persons with stroke admitted to Ontario hospitals was 74 years with 51% being female (Gordon, 1993). The average hospital length of stay was 18 days. Forty-five percent were discharged home and a further 15% went home with home care. The remaining 40% were discharged to another facility: 14% went to rehabilitation hospitals, 12% to chronic care hospitals, 9% to nursing homes, and 5% to acute care hospitals (TJSSW Group, 2000). In Toronto alone, home care access centres see 9,000 individuals per day, of which 8% are referred because of stroke.

Prognostic Factors and Course of Recovery from Stroke

A recent review identified predictors of functional outcome (ADL) poststroke. Kwakkel, Wagenaar, Koelman, Lankhorst, and Koetsler (1997) reviewed 78 studies, of which 13 studies met the specified criteria. The criteria included reliability and validity of measures, inclusion of an inception cohort, uniform endpoint of observation, control for drop-outs during the period of observation, sufficient sample size, and patient characteristics specification. From these studies, only the findings based on pre-established valid and reliable criteria were selected. Between three and five studies identified the following predictors: older age, previous stroke, urinary incontinence, lowered consciousness at onset, disorientation, severity of paralysis, poor sitting balance, low admission ADL score, low level of social support, and low metabolic rate of glucose outside the infarct area. A point estimate for each predictor variable was not given.

Neurological and functional recovery (including spontaneous recovery) occurs most rapidly 1 to 3 months after stroke (Kelly-Hayes et al., 1989; Skilbeck, Wade, Hewer, & Wood, 1983). However, improvement in motor strength and self-care functions continues for up to a year (Ferrucci et al., 1993). The Durham County Study (Duncan, Goldstein, Matchar, Divine, & Feussner, 1992) found dramatic recovery of motor function during the first 30 days, followed by slower but continued improvement, especially in more severely affected and older individuals. The evidence to date would indicate that greater intensity of treatment produces improved function in the first 3 to 4 months poststroke (Keith, 1997; Kwakkel et al., 1997; Ottenbacher & Jannell, 1993).

Home Care Delivery—Health Services Research

Funding of home care programmes as an alternative to institutional care is an important political and economic issue. In January 1996, the Ministry of Health announced reforms to the organizational structure of home care and created 43 Community Care Access Centres (CCACs) (Coyte & Young, 1997). In 1975, total expenditures on home care services were $32.2 million. By 1992, this figure had risen to $915.6 million (Coyte & Young, 1999). Increasing expenditures have been allocated without evidence of service effectiveness. There is no relationship between decreasing inpatient days/1,000 and home care utilization rates (Coyte, Young, & Croxford, 2000). Studies that have examined the associated costs and outcomes of home care have produced inconsistent results (Coyte et al., 2000; Hendrik & Inui, 1986; Jarnio, Ceder, & Thornton, 1984; Thornton, Dunstan, & Kemper, 1988). A recent study found the cost savings associated with early discharge strategies to home care programmes for joint replacement in Ontario was approximately $4,000 (Coyte et al., 2000). However, costs may increase for patients at high levels of functioning and not at risk for institutional care costs (Jarnio et al., 1984; Thornton et al., 1988; Gaumer et al., 1996). Studies concerning the relative benefits and costs of alternative programs would improve the efficiency with which the government spends this large amount of money.

The Effect of Therapy in Stroke Rehabilitation

No study has examined the effects of therapy compared to no treatment. Most trials have compared the intervention to conventional therapy. Duncan (1997) compiled a synthesis of clinical trials that examined various specific targeted interventions, such as neurofacilitation, biofeedback, strength training, forced use, and repetitive training. There was no attempt to combine the effects of the trials. She concluded that therapy interventions benefit moderately to minimally involved stroke patients and the interventions that demonstrated positive results require active participation of the patients, repetitive training, and intensive practice including resistance training (Duncan, 1997). Ottenbacher and Jannell (1993) completed a meta-analysis of stroke rehabilitation research trials. Thirty-six trials met the following criteria: investigated the effects of stroke rehabilitation, included patients whose diagnosis was stroke, measured outcomes related to functional abilities, reported the comparison between two groups, and reported results in a manner that allowed quantitative analysis. A total of 3,717 patients participated in the trials (52% were males and 48% were females). The mean age of the patients was 68.9 +/- 6.78. The mean year of report appearance was 1982 +/- 6.32. The mean *d* index for the 36 trials collapsed across all the functional outcome measures was 0.40 +/- 0.33 (95% CI = 0.35, 0.45). This *d* index was computed from 173 statistical tests included in 36 trials reviewed. The effect size can be translated to a U3 value of 65.5 (Kwakkel, Kollen, & Wagenaar, 1999), which can be interpreted as the average patient in the treatment condition receiving focused rehabilitation performed better than approximately 65% of patients in the comparison conditions (95% CI 63.6% to 67.3%). Finally, a descriptive synthesis by Kwakkel et al. (1999) from randomized and controlled trials also concluded that therapy should be task-oriented and focused. However, there is no conclusive evidence that one therapeutic approach produces superior outcomes in functional status than any other approach (Cohen, 1998). In summary, stroke rehabilitation results in patient return toward normal function.

RANDOMIZED CONTROLLED TRIALS— HOSPITAL CARE VERSUS HOME CARE

In Canada, to date, there has been one prospective study that has compared rehabilitation postacute stroke delivered from home care versus hospital-based services (HBS) (Mayo et al., 2000). This study excluded persons without a caregiver who would normally receive these services (N = 606), as well as persons with significant coexisting conditions and requiring assistance with ambulation from more than one person after 28 days and did not include an economic evaluation. Recruitment was difficult (from the 1,542 persons admitted with stroke over the 2-year period, 114 were recruited). Only a third of the sample were women. Women are less likely to have a caregiver at home and, therefore, may be excluded from trials for this reason.

The effect of the in-home rehabilitation experience on the caregiver was not investigated. The intervention period was only 4 weeks long (N = 10 visits: 6 physiotherapy, 4 occupational therapy), which may be insufficient to deliver the care necessary for older persons discharged home. Treatment trials examining intensity of training following stroke have shown greatest recovery with intensive training over the first 3 to 4 months (Keith, 1997; Kwakkel et al., 1997; Sivenius, Pyorala, Heinonen, Salonen, & Reikkinen, 1985). Although the visits were similar between the intervention and the control group, the proportion of persons receiving visits in the control group was less. For example, 75% of the home care group received physiotherapy compared with only 50% in the HBS group. The length of hospital stay was shorter for the home care group (6 days shorter than the usual care), and there was a statistically and clinically important difference between the two groups' physical health after 3 months, but not on completion of the trial, in favour of the home care group. These methodological problems render the question posed equivocal.

There are seven studies outside Canada; three of these had an accompanying economic analysis. An randomized controlled trial (RCT) involving patients from a stroke registry showed no difference in functional outcomes between home care and HBS (Wade, Langton-Hewer, Skilbeck, Bainton, & Burns-Cox, 1985). Randomization was not successful, contamination and cointervention occurred in the home care group, and there were large drop-out rates at follow-up.

A second trial compared outcomes for patients in either setting over an 8-week period with a 6-month follow-up (Young & Forster, 1991a, 1991b, 1992, 1993). This study found a positive outcome in favour of the home care group on three of the six outcome measures at both assessment times (Barthel Index, motor assessment, and ambulation). Five patients changed treatments after randomization. A cost minimization study showed that the costs associated with home care were significantly less (the median difference in treatment costs was £265, CI, £190 to £340, p<0.01) and there were no differences between the groups for indirect costs (1993).

A more recent study found no difference between groups of patients who were randomly allocated to three treatment settings: stroke unit, home care, or HBS (Gladman, Whynes, & Lincoln, 1994). Contamination occurred when nine home care patients received HBS. Poor prognostic factors were more prevalent in the home care group. There were higher costs overall with home care services, but this was not tested for statistical significance (Gladman, Lincoln, & Barer, 1993).

A Swedish study found no difference between patient groups receiving home care and groups receiving rehabilitation in a hospital, day care, or outpatient care setting over a 3 to 4 month period (Holmqvist et al., 1998; Holmqvist, de Pedro-Cuestas, & Moller, 1996; von Koch, Holmqvist, Kostulas, Almazan, & de Pedro-Cuestas, 2000). This study did not have sufficient statistical power to detect a difference and included persons with transient ischemic attacks (TIA) as well as completed strokes. Baseline differences between groups on patient characteristics such as coping capacity and frequency of associated diseases were recorded. A cost analysis during the pilot study phase found that total direct per capita costs were lower for home care (von Koch et al., 2000). Two further trials have examined the effect of early discharge to home care following stroke (Rodgers et al., 1997; Rudd, Wolfe, Tilling, & Beech, 1997). Neither produced positive results, and both suffered from lack of power, unblinded evaluation, and multiple raters. Finally, an Australian study found no difference between the groups and nonstatistically significant reduction in costs in favour of the home care group (Anderson et al., 2000a, 2000b). The power analysis for this study was based on a 7-point difference in the physical health summary primary outcome of the Short Form 36 (SF-36), which would not necessarily reflect effects of a rehabilitation intervention. Approximately half of patients in either group had an identified caregiver, and home-based caregivers had lower mental health scores on two separate assessments. Descriptive information on these studies follows (see Review of Health Service Delivery: Randomized Controlled Trials by Study).

What Evidence Could be Provided by a Further Canadian Trial Which Would Assist in Answering this Question?

Several studies have found no difference between groups rehabilitated in the home versus the institution. This suggests that a home setting is as good as an institutional setting. There has been only one positive treatment trial, and all studies suffer from the methodological problems discussed that limit the external and internal validity of the results. The Canadian study (Sivenius et al., 1985) excluded persons who may benefit from rehabilitation within the home environment, specifically women who may have been excluded because they did not have a caregiver. Other reports confirm this finding. Data (Canadian Institute for Health Information, 2002) of persons discharged with stroke from acute hospitals in Ontario between 1993 to 1996 showed that women had a longer median length of stay in acute care compared to men (11 days versus 9 days; p<0.001). Men were more likely to be discharged home (40.9% respectively versus 50.6%; p<0.001) (Holroyd-Leduc, Kapral, Austin, & Tu, 2000) and women were more likely to be discharged to chronic care facilities (25.2% versus 16.8%; p<0.0001). The risk of death 1 year after stroke was lower in women (adjusted odds ratio 0.939, 95% CI 0.899, 0.98; P=0.004). These studies have not addressed the potential for women without caregivers to be rehabilitated in the home.

REVIEW OF HEALTH SERVICE DELIVERY: RANDOMIZED CONTROLLED TRIALS BY STUDY

Gladman et al., 1993

Design and Similarity of Groups
- Baseline differences on function

Population (Source, Age, Number per group)
- Hospital sample x = 70 yrs, HCP N = 165, HBP N = 162

Control of Evaluation Bias (Blinding)
- Partial; postal assessments at baseline and 3 months; blinded assessor at 6 months

1 Degree Outcome
- Extended Activities of Daily Living Index (EADLI)

2 Degree Outcome
- Health status, caregiver burden, life satisfaction

Statistical Significance
- No

Clinical Significance
- No

Point Estimates and Confidence Intervals
- EADLI median difference 0.0, 95% CI -1 ,1)

Description of Intervention
- Total numbers of visits similar between groups (not tested); no detailed description of intervention

Time and Numbers at Follow-Up
- 90% HCP 92% HBP 3 and 6 month follow-up

Economic Evaluation
- Yes, cost minimization (cost of HBP 25% higher than HCP)

Holmqvist et al., 1998,

Design and Similarity of Groups
- Baseline characteristics essentially the same

Population (Source, Age, Number per group)

- Stroke registry = 71.7 years, HCP N = 41, HBP N = 40

Control of Evaluation Bias (Blinding)

- Yes, outcome assessors blinded

1 Degree Outcome

- Sickness impact profile

2 Degree Outcome

- Barthel, Katz, walking speed, social activity, health status, patient satisfaction

Statistical Significance

- Not at 3 months but some group differences at 6 months

Clinical Significance

- No

Point Estimates and Confidence Intervals

- 3 months SIP median difference = 2.0; HCP SIP AOR = 0.84 (0.38-1.90); Independence in Barthel ADL AOR = 1.18 (0.56-2.48); walking without an aid AOR = 1.13(0.56-2.26)
- 6 months Barthel mobility median difference = 9 p = 0.0131; Frenchay Activities Index (washing up median difference = 3 p = 0.0371)

Description of Intervention

- Task and context orientated, spouse active participant, goal-directed activities for HBP. HBP = heterogenous based interventions.

Time and Numbers at Follow-Up

- 3 months (100% follow-up); 6 months (97% = HCP; 95% = HBP)

Economic Evaluation

- No (but prior economic evaluation of pilot study cost minimization less costs associated with HCP)

Wade et al., 1985

Design and Comparability of Groups

- Groups essentially similar at baseline except that greater number in HCG had loss of consciousness at onset

Population (Source, Age, Number per group)
- Stroke registry N = 44 trial
- x= 73.25 years, N = 47 control

Control of Evaluation Bias (Blinding)
- Assessors and patients unblinded

Randomization, Contamination, and Cointervention
- Faulty randomization process; contamination and cointervention occurred

1 Degree Outcomes
- Barthel

2 Degree Outcome
- Social functioning; activities index, depression, general health questionnaire, caregiver burden

Statistical Significance
- Explanatory analysis; not intention to treat (no difference between groups)

Clinical Significance
- No

Time and Numbers at Follow-Up
- 6 months 47% HBP, 52% HCP

Description of Intervention
- Description of team given
- No standardized description of intervention

Point Estimates and Confidence Intervals
- Barthel ADL grouping chi-square 0.96; Activities Index mean difference 0.1, Mann Whitney uz = 0.303, depression = 1.5, t = 1.78; p < 0.10.

Economic Evaluation
- No

Young & Foster, 1992

Design and Comparability of Groups
- RCT stratified on function and time; groups essentially similar at baseline

Population (Source, Age, Number per group)
- Hospital sample N = 61 day hospital
- x = 71 years, N = 63 home care

Control of Evaluation Bias (Blinding)

- Outcome assessor blinded

Randomization, Contamination, and Cointervention

- Yes, no contamination or cointervention

1 Degree Outcome

- Barthel

2 Degree Outcome

- Functional ambulation categories, Frenchay Activities index, Nottingham Health Index

Statistical Significance

- Intention to treat analysis; yes (results favour home physiotherapy)

Clinical Significance

- Yes

Time and Numbers at Follow-Up

- 8 weeks and 6 months 85% (controls), 88% (home)

Description of Intervention

- Minimal description—8 week intervention
- Day hospital group median visits = 31
- Home care group median visits = 15

Point Estimates and Confidence Intervals

- Barthel chi-square = 1.9, df = 2, p < 0.25; motor club assessment chi-square = 8.4, df = 2, p < 0.25 in favour of home-based group.

Economic Evaluation

- Yes and cost minimization (home care less associated costs)

Rudd et al., 1997

Design, Sample Size, and Comparability of Groups

- Groups comparable at baseline
- N = 167 HCP, N = 164 HBP, x = 73 years

Population (Source)

- Hospital-based stroke registry
- Eligibility not clearly stated

Control of Evaluation Bias (Blinding)

- Randomization concealed
- Assessments at 2, 4, and 6 months unclear whether assessors were blinded; assessments done at 12 months were blinded
- Blinding not formally assessed

Contamination and Cointervention

- Contamination and cointervention not evaluated

1 Degree Outcome

- Modified Barthel score

2 Degree Outcome

- Frenchay aphasic, depression, MMS, motoricity, 5-metre walk, Nottingham health profile, caregiver strain index

Statistical Significance

- Intention to treat analysis; no difference between groups; power calculations given

Clinical Significance

- No

Description of Intervention

- Team described; intervention or amount of care received not described

Time and Numbers at Follow-Up

- 1 year follow-up
- 87% = HCP, 76% = HBP

Point Estimates and Confidence Intervals

- Barthel mean difference = 0 (CI 0, 1); Frenchay aphasia mean difference = 1 (CI -2.5, 1.6); MMSE mean difference = 0 (CI -1.5, 1.7); 5 metre walk mean difference = 0, (CI -0,1); caregiver strain index mean difference = 1 (CI-0-2)

Economic Evaluation

- No

Rodgers et al., 1997

Design, Sample Size, and Comparability of Groups

- Groups comparable at baseline
- x = 73 years, N = 46, HCP N = 46 HBP

Population (Source)

- Hospital-based sample (UK)

Control of Evaluation Bias (Blinding)

- No, assessors and patients not blinded

Contamination and Cointervention

- Randomization concealed; contamination and cointervention not evaluated

1 Degree Outcome

- Oxford Handicap Scale

2 Degree Outcome

- Nottingham extended ADL scale, health status, GH status, length of stay

Statistical Significance

- Intention to treat analysis; not sufficient power
- HCP = 13 days, HBP = 22 days, p = 0.02

Clinical Significance

- No

Description of Intervention

- Team described; number of visits not recorded and intervention not described

Time and Numbers at Follow-Up

- 7 days, 10 days, and 3 months postdischarge follow-up
- 97% = HCP, 91% = HBP

Point Estimates and Confidence Intervals

- Not reported

Economic Evaluation

- No

Mayo et al., 2000

Design and Comparability of Groups

- No significant differences between groups on any baseline differences

Population (Source, Age, Number Per Group)

- Hospital sample, HC N = 58; HBG N = 56; Canadian (Montreal)

Control of Evaluation Bias (Blinding)

- Randomization concealed
- Yes, outcome assessors blinded

Randomization, Contamination, and Cointervention

- Contamination and cointervention not addressed

1 Degree Outcome

- Short-Form 36

2 Degree Outcome

- Canadian Neurological scale, Stream, Timed Get Up and Go, Barthel Index OARS, Reintegration into Normal Living Index

Statistical Significance

- Intention to treat analysis; not statistically significant at end of trial but was significant at follow-up

Clinical Significance

- Yes

Description of Intervention

- Home care prompt discharge from hospital with PT, OT, speech, dietary consultation and nursing (14.5 visits); usual care PT, OT, and ST in hospital or outpatient setting (20.5 visits); duration 4 weeks
- 75% of HC received physiotherapy but only 50% HBG

Time and Numbers at Follow-Up

- 3 months follow-up from baseline HC = 87%
- HBG = 80% at follow-up

Point Estimates and Confidence Intervals

- 3 months follow-up group differences in favour of home care physical subscale SF-36 = 5 points F = 4.17; p = 0.018; physical role subscale 16 points F = 5.73; p = 0.018; IADL 1.5 points F = 4.18 p = 0.018; RNL 1.7 points F = 5.41, p = 0.006

Economic Evaluation

- No

Anderson et al., 2000a, 2000b

Design and Comparability of Groups

- Groups essentially the same

Population (Source, Age, Number per group)

- Hospital sample, HC N = 42 and HBG N = 44; Australian sample

Control of Evaluation Bias (Blinding)

- Yes, outcome assessors blind; randomization not concealed to patient

Randomization, Contamination, and Cointervention

- Contamination and cointervention not addressed

1 Degree Outcome

- Modified Barthel

2 Degree Outcome

- Mini mental state exam, general health questionnaire, Adelaide Activities Profile, McMaster Family Assessment Device

Statistical Significance

- Intention to treat analysis; no statistically significant differences between the groups

Clinical Significance

- No

Description of Intervention

- Home care: adaptations to home and goal-directed therapy; self-learning and structured practice sessions
- Hospital-based care acute medical unit or stroke unit; stroke pathways used; differences in amount of treatment not described

Time and Numbers at Follow-Up

- 1, 3, and 6 month follow-up.
- 95% follow-up HC group and 100% for HBG

Point Estimates and Confidence Intervals

- Physical functioning SF-36 mean difference -1.2 (-13.8, 11.5) Modified Barthel 0 (-2.0, 2.0); General health profile physical 0.5 (-9.3, 11.8).

Economic Evaluation

- Yes, cost minimization analysis; mean cost per patient and pharmacy costs not measured.
- Home care ($8,040), HBG = ($10,054), no significant difference between groups on cost

In addition, the Canadian study did not examine the effect on the caregiver or the satisfaction experienced by the patient or the caregiver and included only self-report measures. Therefore, future work needs to examine what it would take to provide services for persons who do not have a caregiver, the effect of the care taking process on the health of the caregiver, and the overall cost benefit. It will also be important to isolate what type of patient profile does best within a home care setting and define the subpopulation of patients that will be most impacted by delivery of home care services and how these services can be most efficiently delivered. The establishment of a costing system for these services could also be used for future evaluation.

Take-Home Messages

Background
- Lack of evidence from health service delivery trials available to direct-evidence practice.
- Health service delivery research (HSDR) involves a less standardized approach to care than biomedical research; uniformity of this research should be seen as a goal.
- Multiple components involved in HSDR trials can enhance possibility of positive treatment effect but also create problems of interpretations.
- Rapid change of health care delivery service can occur in the middle of a trial and needs to be anticipated.
- Effect of environmental context on rehabilitation can be studied through HSDR relating to postacute stroke.

Problem
- Studies have failed to clarify which environmental setting (home or hospital) produces better outcomes and where the two settings differ (e.g., outcomes and costs).
- Magnitude of problem with stroke is expected to grow with an aging population.

Health Care Delivery
- Funding of home care programs as an alternative to institutional care is an important political and economic issue; more studies are needed concerning the relative benefits and costs of alternative programs.
- Some of the deficiencies within the studies of stroke include the effect of rehabilitation therapy on the caregiver; outcomes for those without a caregiver; inclusion of women.
- Important to isolate what type of client profile does best within a home care setting to define the population of clients who would most benefit from the efficient delivery of these services.

LEARNING AND EXPLORATION ACTIVITIES

The purpose of this chapter is to provide an example of research into a specific clinical problem and to demonstrate some of the implications drawn from the research on postacute stroke patients.

1. Using the information provided in the chapter and review table, construct a table/paragraph stating the implications of these findings for the following stakeholders: consumers, therapists, managers of services, and policy makers.

REFERENCES

Anderson, C., Rubenach, S., Cliona Ni, M., Clark, M., Spencer, C., & Winsor, A. (2000a). Home or hospital for stroke rehabilitation? Results of a randomized controlled trial I: Costs minimization at six months. *Stroke, 31*, 1024-1031.

Anderson, C., Rubenach, S., Cliona Ni, M., Clark, M., Spencer, C., & Winsor, A. (2000b). Home or hospital for stroke rehabilitation? Results of a randomized controlled trial II: Health outcomes at six months. *Stroke, 31*, 1032-1037.

Bonita, R. (1992). Epidemiology of stroke. *Lancet, 339*(8), 342-347.

Canadian Institute for Health Information. (2002). Retrieved March 22, 2002, from http://www.cihi.ca.

Cohen, J. (1998). *Statistical power analysis for the behavioural sciences* (2nd ed.). Hillsdale, NJ: Lawrence Erlbaum Associates.

Coyte, P. C., & Young, W. (1997). Applied home care research. *Int J Health Care Qual Assur Inc Leadersh Health Serv, 10*(1), 1-5.

Coyte, P. C., & Young, W. (1999). Regional variations in the use of home care services in Ontario, 1993/1995. *Canadian Medical Association Journal, 161*(4), 376-380.

Coyte, P. C., Young, W., & Croxford, R. (2000). Costs and outcomes associated with alternative discharge strategies following joint replacement surgery: Analysis of an observational study using a propensity score. *Journal of Health Economics, 19*, 907-929.

Delaney, G. A., & Potter, P. J. (1993). Disability post-stroke. *Physical Medical Rehabilitation: State of the Art Reviews, 7*(1), 27-42.

Duncan, P. W. (1997). Synthesis of intervention trials to improve motor recovery following stroke. *Top Stroke Rehabilitation, 3*(4), 1-20.

Duncan, P. W., Goldstein, L. B., Matchar, D., Divine, G. W., & Feussner, J. (1992). Measurement of motor recovery after stroke outcome assessment and sample size requirements. *Stroke, 23*, 1084-1089.

Ebrahim, S. (1990). *Clinical epidemiology of stroke*. Oxford: Oxford University Press.

Ferrucci, L., Bandinelli, S., Guralnik, J. M., Lamponi, M., Bertini, C., Falchini, M., et al. (1993). Recovery of functional status after stroke: A post-rehabilitation follow-up study. *Stroke, 24*, 200-205.

Gaumer, G. L., Birbaum, H., Pratter, F., Burke, R., Franklin, S., & Ellingson-Otto, K. (1996). Impact of the New York long-term health care program. *Med Care, 24*(7), 641-654.

Gladman, J. R. F., Lincoln, N. B., & Barer, D. H. (1993). A randomized controlled trial of domiciliary and hospital-based rehabilitation for stroke patients after discharge from hospital. *J Neurol, Neurosurg, Psychiatry, 56*, 960-966.

Gladman, J., Whynes, D., & Lincoln, N. (1994). Cost comparison of domiciliary and hospital-based stroke rehabilitation. *Age Aging, 23*, 241-245.

Gordon, M. (1993). Monograph series on aging-related diseases: III Stroke (cerebrovascular disease). *Chronic Dis Can, 14*(3), 64-89.

Henderson, W. G., Demakis, J., Fihn, S. D., Weiberger, M., Oddone, E., & Deykin, D. (1998). Cooperative studies in health services research in the department of veteran affairs. *Control Clin Trials, 19*, 149-158.

Hendrik, S. C., & Inui, T. S. (1986). The effectiveness and cost of home care: An information synthesis. *Health Serv Res, 20*(6), 851-880.

Holmqvist, L. W., de Pedro-Cuestas, J., & Moller, G. (1996). A pilot study of rehabilitation at home after stroke: A health economic appraisal. *Scand J Rehabil Med, 28*, 9-18.

Holmqvist, L. W., von Koch, L., Kostulas, V., Holm, M., Widsell, G., Tegler, H., et al. (1998). A randomized controlled trial of rehabilitation at home after stroke in southwest Stockholm. *Stroke, 29*, 591-597.

Holroyd-Leduc, J. M., Kapral, M. K., Austin, P. C., & Tu, J. V. (2000). Sex difference and similarities in the management and outcome of stroke patients. *Stroke, 31*, 1833-1837.

James, K. E. (1998). Health services clinical trials: Design, conduct, and cost methodology. *Control Clin Trials, 19*, 131-133.

Jarnio, G. B., Ceder, L., & Thornton, K. G. (1984). Early rehabilitation at home of elderly patients with hip fractures and consumption of resources in primary care. *Scand J Prim Health Care, 2*, 105-112.

Keith, R. (1997). Treatment strength in rehabilitation. *Arch Phys Med Rehabil, 78,* 1298-1304.

Kelly-Hayes, M., Wolf, P. A., Kannel, W. B., Sytkowski, P., D'Agostino, R. B., & Gresham, G. E. (1989). Factors influencing survival and need for institutionalization following stroke: The Framingham study. *Arch Phys Med Rehabil, 69*(6), 415-418.

Kotila, M., Waltimo, O., Niemi, M. L., & Laaksonen, R. (1986). Dementia after stroke. *Eur Neurol, 25,* 134-140.

Kwakkel, G., Kollen, B. J., & Wagenaar, R. C. (1999). Therapy impact on functional recovery in stroke rehabilitation. *Physiotherapy, 85*(7), 377-391.

Kwakkel, G., Wagenaar, R. C., Koelman, T. W., Lankhorst, G. J., & Koetsier, J. C. (1997). Effects of intensity of rehabilitation after stroke—A research synthesis. *Stroke, 28,* 1550-1556.

Leibson, C. L., Naessens, J. M., Brown, R. D., & Whisnant, J. P. (1994). Accuracy of hospital discharge abstracts for identifying stroke. *Stroke, 25,* 2348-2355.

Mayo, N., Wood-Dauphinee, S., Cote, R., Gayton, D., Carlton, J., Buttery, J., et al. (2000). There's no place like home—An evaluation of early supported discharge for stroke. *Stroke, 31,* 1016-1023.

Ottenbacher, K. J., & Jannell, S. (1993). The results of clinical trials in stroke rehabilitation research. *Arch Neurol, 50,* 37-44.

Rodgers, H., Soutter, J., Kaiser, W., Pearson, P., Dobson, R., Skilbeck, C., et al. (1997). Early supported hospital discharge following acute stroke: Pilot study results. *Clin Rehabil, 11,* 280-287.

Rudd, H., Wolfe, D. A., Tilling, K., & Beech, R. (1997). Randomized controlled trial to evaluate early discharge scheme for patients with stroke. *British Medical Journal, 315,* 1039-1044.

Sivenius, J., Pyorala, K., Heinonen, O. P., Salonen, J. T., & Reikkinen, P. (1985). The significance of intensity of rehabilitation of stroke—Controlled trial. *Stroke, 16*(6), 928-931.

Skilbeck, C. E., Wade, D. T., Hewer, R. L., & Wood, V. A. (1983). Recovery after stroke. *J Neurol Neurosurg Psychiatry, 46*(1), 409-417.

Smurawska, L. T., Alexandrov, A. V., Bladin, C. F., & Norris, J. W. (1994). Cost of acute stroke in Toronto, Canada. *Stroke, 25,* 1628-1631.

Stehbens, W. (1991). Validity of cerebrovascular mortality rates. *Angiology, 42,* 261-267.

Stone L. O. (1986). *Seniors boom—Dramatic increases in longevity and prospectives for better health.* Ottawa, Ontario: Statistics Canada & Health and Welfare Canada and The Secretary of the State of Canada.

Terent, A. (1993). Stroke morbidity. In J. P. Whisnant (Ed.), *Stroke: Populations, cohorts, and clinical trials.* Boston, MA: Butterworth Heineman.

Thornton, C., Dunstan, S. M., & Kemper, P. (1988). The evaluation of the national long term care demonstration: Effect of chanelling on health and long-term care costs. *Health Serv Res, 23*(1), 129-142.

The Joint Stroke Strategy Working Group. (2000). *Towards an integrated stroke strategy for Ontario.* Toronto, Ontario: Ministry of Health and Long Term Care.

von Koch, L., Holmqvist, L. W., Kostulas, V., Almazan, J., & de Pedro-Cuestas, J. (2000). A randomized controlled trial of rehabilitation at home after stroke in Southwest Stockholm: Outcome at six months. *Scand J Med, 32,* 80-86.

Wade, D. T., Langton-Hewer, R., Skilbeck, C., Bainton, D., & Burns-Cox, C. (1985). Controlled trial of home care service for acute stroke patients. *Lancet, 1,* 323-326.

World Health Organization. (1989). Task force report on stroke and other cerebrovascular disorders. *Stroke, 20*(10), 1408-1431.

Young, J. B., & Forster, A. (1991a). Methodology of a stroke rehabilitation trial. *Clin Rehabil, 5,* 127-133.

Young, J. B., & Forster, A. (1991b). The Bradford community stroke trial: Eight weeks results. *Clin Rehabil, 5,* 283-292.

Young, J. B., & Forster, A. (1992). The Bradford community stroke trial: Results at six months. *British Medical Journal, 304*, 1085-1089.

Young, J. B., & Forster, A. (1993). Day hospital and home physiotherapy for stroke patients: A comparative cost-effectiveness study. *J R Coll Physicians Lond, 27*, 252-258.

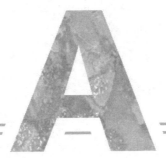

Outcome Measures Rating Form

Developed by CanChild Centre for Childhood Disability Research
School of Rehabilitation Science
McMaster University
Hamilton, Ontario, Canada L8S 1C7
www.fhs.mcmaster.ca/canchild
To be used with: Outcome Measures Rating Form Guidelines (CanChild, 1999)

Name and initials of measure: _____

Author(s): _____

Source and year published: _____

Date of review:_____   Name of reviewer: _____

1. Focus

a. Focus of measurement—Using the modified ICIDH framework

❏ Organic Systems	Any loss or abnormality of psychological, physiological, or anatomical structure or function
❏ Abilities	Ability to perform an activity in an effective manner
❏ Participation/Life Habits	Life situations that individuals participate in and which result from the interaction of an impairment or disability with environmental factors
❏ Environmental Factors	Aspects of the social, cultural, institutional, and physical environments that affect the organization of society and influence what people do.

b. Attribute(s) being measured: Check as many as apply:

This is based on attributes cited in ICIDH, 1980; Quebec and Canadian modification, 1991; and proposed revisions for ICIDH, 1996.

Organic Systems; Impairment

Neurological System

❏ Consciousness	❏ Reflexes	❏ Attention/concentration
❏ Pain	❏ Intelligence	❏ Visual-motor kinesthetics
❏ Sensation	❏ Memory	❏ Perceptual organization and discrimination ability

Voice, Speech, and Hearing

❏ Hearing	❏ Nonverbal communication	
❏ Phonology	❏ Speech articulation	❏ Verbal fluency
❏ Pragmatics	❏ Speech proficiency	❏ Sound production

Vision

❏ Visual acuity	❏ Visual field

Digestive System
- ❏ Chewing and swallowing

Respiratory and Cardiovascular System
- ❏ Heart function
- ❏ Respiratory function
- ❏ Exercise tolerance/ endurance

Musculoskeletal System
- ❏ Body movement
- ❏ Involuntary movement
- ❏ Coordination
- ❏ Muscle strength
- ❏ Range of motion
- ❏ Paralysis
- ❏ Tone
- ❏ Skin integrity
- ❏ Balance
- ❏ Movement patterns/ postures

Urogenital System
- ❏ Sexual functions
- ❏ Continence
- ❏ Urinary/bowel function

Psychosocial
- ❏ Mood/affect
- ❏ Motivation

Abilities/Disabilities; Activities

Personal Care
- ❏ Washing one's self
- ❏ Hygiene
- ❏ Taking medications
- ❏ Toileting
- ❏ Dressing
- ❏ Eating/drinking
- ❏ Managing bowel and bladder

Communication
- ❏ Expressive language
- ❏ Reading
- ❏ Receptive language
- ❏ Writing
- ❏ Telephone communication

Movement
- ❏ Climbing
- ❏ Transfers
- ❏ Manipulation/dexterity of objects
- ❏ Reaching and moving objects
- ❏ Maintaining a body position
- ❏ Functional mobility (indoor)
- ❏ Functional mobility (outdoor)

Management of Home and Environment
- ❏ Driving
- ❏ Shopping
- ❏ Making meals
- ❏ Managing money
- ❏ Using public transport
- ❏ Taking care of others
- ❏ Making appointments
- ❏ Maintaining physical environment
- ❏ Caring for clothing/ household goods

Cognition and Learning
- ❏ Orientation
- ❏ Self-esteem
- ❏ Self-concept
- ❏ Insight
- ❏ Self-efficacy
- ❏ Calculation
- ❏ Problem solving/judgment
- ❏ Knowledge of disability
- ❏ Comprehension/understanding

Social Skills and Social Behaviour
- ❏ Social skills
- ❏ Behaviour problems
- ❏ Social problem solving
- ❏ Coping
- ❏ Social competency

Environmental Factors

Physical

- ❏ Transportation
- ❏ Lighting
- ❏ Safety
- ❏ Size
- ❏ Time

- ❏ Nature/geography
- ❏ Location
- ❏ Equipment/technology/
  appliances/tools

- ❏ Communications
- ❏ Sound
- ❏ Architecture/accessibility/
  design (indoor, outdoor,
  playground, child care,
  school)

Social

- ❏ Attitudes
- ❏ Social rules
- ❏ Social climate
- ❏ Stimulation

- ❏ Community cohesion
- ❏ Social support
- ❏ Communication

- ❏ Family organization
- ❏ Integration
- ❏ Expectations

Cultural

- ❏ Values
- ❏ Roles

- ❏ Ethnicity
- ❏ Cultural norms

- ❏ Degree of diversity

Economical

- ❏ Economic state
- ❏ Income security

- ❏ Work patterns
- ❏ Resources

- ❏ Land use

Institutional

- ❏ Educational services
- ❏ Judicial services
- ❏ Social services
- ❏ Institutional climate
- ❏ Interagency cooperation
- ❏ Other community services (e.g., recreation, religious, cultural)

- ❏ Health services
- ❏ Legislation/regulation
- ❏ Program structure/
  policies

- ❏ Recreational services
- ❏ Government structures
- ❏ Respite services
- ❏ Continuum of services

Familial

- ❏ Financial strain
- ❏ Mastery

- ❏ Family member's stress and coping
- ❏ Family functioning (in the following areas: problem-
  solving, roles, affective responsiveness, affective
  involvement, behaviour control, and general functioning)

Participation (Life Habits)

Self-Management

- ❏ Personal care
- ❏ Mental fitness

- ❏ Nutrition
- ❏ Physical fitness

- ❏ Housing
- ❏ Sleep

Interpersonal Relations

- ❏ Family
- ❏ Marital relations

- ❏ Relatives/friends
- ❏ Sexual relations

- ❏ Social relations with others

Community Life

- ❏ Use of services
- ❏ Voluntary associations

- ❏ Religious practices
- ❏ Citizenship (legal, moral, civic, economic)

- ❏ Community events

Education
- ❐ Preschool/day care   ❐ School   ❐ College/university
- ❐ Vocational training

Work
- ❐ Paid occupation   ❐ Search for employment ❐ Unpaid occupation

Leisure
- ❐ Play   ❐ Arts and culture   ❐ Activity patterns/time use
- ❐ Hobbies   ❐ Sports and games

Mobility
- ❐ In home environment   ❐ Traveling about the ❐ Use of transportation
                               community   (public and private)

c. Does this measure assess a single attribute or multiple attributes?
- ❐ Single
- ❐ Multiple

d. Check purposes that apply and indicate (*) the primary purpose of the measure?
- ❐ To describe or discriminate
- ❐ To predict
- ❐ To evaluative

Comments:

e. Perspective—Indicate possible respondents:
- ❐ Client   ❐ Other professional
- ❐ Caregiver/parent   ❐ Other
- ❐ Service provider

f. Population measure designed for:
   Age: Please specify all applicable ages if stated in the manual
- ❐ Infant (birth to < 1 year)   ❐ Adult (> 18 years to < 65 years)
- ❐ Child (1 year to < 13 years) ❐ Senior (> 65 years)
- ❐ Adolescent (13 to < 18 years)❐ Age not specified

   Diagnosis:
   List the diagnostic group(s) for which this measure is designed to be used:

g. Evaluation context—Indicate suggested/possible environments for this assessment:
- ❏ Home
- ❏ Workplace
- ❏ Other
- ❏ Education setting
- ❏ Community agency
- ❏ Community
- ❏ Rehabilitation centre/
  health care setting

2. Clinical Utility

a. Clarity of Instructions: (check one of the ratings):
- ❏ Excellent: clear, comprehensive, concise, and available
- ❏ Adequate: clear, concise, but lacks some information
- ❏ Poor: not clear and concise or not available

Comments:

b. Format (check applicable items)
- ❏ Interview
- ❏ Task performance
- ❏ Naturalistic observation
- ❏ Other

Questionnaire:
- ○ Self completed
- ○ Interview administered
- ○ Caregiver completed

Physically invasive:	❏ Yes	❏ No
Active participation of client:	❏ Yes	❏ No
Special equipment required:	❏ Yes	❏ No

c. Time to complete assessment: _____ minutes

Administration:	❏ Easy	❏ More complex	*(Consider time,*
Scoring:	❏ Easy	❏ More complex	*amount of training,*
Interpretation:	❏ Easy	❏ More complex	*and ease)*

d. Examiner qQualifications: Is formal training required for administering and/or interpreting?
- ❏ Required
- ❏ Recommended
- ❏ Not required
- ❏ Not addressed

e. Cost (Canadian funds)
   Manual: $_____

   Score sheets: $_____ for _____

   Indicate year of cost information: _____

   Source of cost information: _____

3. Scale Construction

a. Item selection (check one of the ratings):

    ❐ Excellent: included all relevant characteristics of attribute based on compre-
                        hensive literature review and survey of experts

    ❐ Adequate: included most relevant characteristics of attribute

    ❐ Poor: convenient sample of characteristics of attribute

Comments:

b. Weighting

    Are the items weighted in the calculation of total score?   ❐ Yes   ❐ No

    If yes, are the items weighted: ❐ Implicitly ❐ Explicitly

c. Level of measurement: ❐ Nominal   ❐ Ordinal   ❐ Interval   ❐ Ratio

    Scaling method (Likert, Guttman, etc.): _____

    # Items: _____

    Indicate if subscale scores are obtained: ❐ Yes   ❐ No

If yes, can the subscale scores be used alone: Administered: ❐ Yes   ❐ No
                                        Interpreted: ❐ Yes   ❐ No

List subscales: Number of items:

_____ _____

_____ _____

_____ _____

_____ _____

4. Standardization

a. Manual (check one of the ratings):

    ❐ Excellent: published manual that outlines specific procedures for administra-
                        tion, scoring and interpretation, and evidence of reliability and validity

    ❐ Adequate: manual available and generally complete but some information is
                        lacking or unclear regarding administration, scoring and interpreta-
                        tion, and evidence of reliability and validity

    ❐ Poor: no manual available or manual with unclear administration, scoring
                        and interpretaion, and no evidence of reliability and validity

b. Norms available (N/A for instrument whose purpose is only evaluative):

❐ Yes   ❐ No   ❐ N/A

Age: Please specify all applicable ages for which norms are available

❐ Infant (birth to < 1 year)   ❐ Adult (> 18 years to < 65 years)

❐ Child (1 year to < 13 years)   ❐ Senior (> 65 years)

❐ Adolescent (13 to < 18 years)

Populations for which it is normed: _____

_____

Size of sample: n = _____

5. Reliability

a. Rigor of standardization studies for reliability (check one of the ratings)

❐ Excellent: more than two well-designed reliability studies completed with adequate to excellent reliability values

❐ Adequate: one to two well-designed reliability studies completed with adequate to excellent reliability values

❐ Poor: reliability studies poorly completed, or reliability studies showing poor levels of reliability

❐ No evidence available

Comments:

b. Reliability information

Type of reliability	Statistic used	Value	Rating*: excellent, adequate, poor

* guidelines for levels of reliability coefficient (see instructions)

    Excellent: >.80   Adequate: .60 to .79   Poor: <.60

6. *Validity*

a. Rigor of standardization studies for validity (check one of the ratings):
- ❏ Excellent: more than two well-designed validity studies supporting the measure's validity
- ❏ Adequate: one to two well-designed validity studies supporting the measure's validity
- ❏ Poor: validity studies poorly completed or did not support the measure's validity
- ❏ No evidence available

Comments:

_____

_____

b. Content validity (check one of the ratings):
- ❏ Excellent: judgmental or statistical method (e.g., factor analysis) was used and the measure is comprehensive and includes items suited to the measurement purpose
- *Method*: ❏ judgmental ❏ statistical
- ❏ Adequate: has content validity but no specific method was used
- ❏ Poor: instrument is not comprehensive
- ❏ No evidence available

c. Construct validity (check one of the ratings):
- ❏ Excellent: more than two well-designed studies have shown that the instrument conforms to prior theoretical relationships among characteristics or individuals
- ❏ Adequate: one to two studies demonstrate confirmation of theoretical formulations
- ❏ Poor: construct validation poorly completed, or did not support measure's construct validity
- ❏ No evidence available

Strength of association:

_____

_____

_____

_____

d. Criterion validity (check ratings that apply):
- ❏ Concurrent ❏ Predictive
- ❏ Excellent: more than two well-designed studies have shown adequate agreement with a criterion or gold standard
- ❏ Adequate: one to two studies demonstrate adequate agreement with a criterion or gold standard measure

❒ Poor: criterion validation poorly completed or did not support measure's criterion validity

❒ No evidence available

Criterion measure(s) used: _____

_____

Strength of association: _____

_____

_____

e. Responsiveness (check one of the ratings):

❒ Excellent: more than two well-designed studies showing strong hypothe sized relationships between changes on the measure and other measures of change on the same attribute.

❒ Adequate: one to two studies of responsiveness

❒ Poor: studies of responsiveness poorly completed or did not support the measure's responsiveness

❒ N/A

❒ No evidence available

Comments:

_____

_____

Overall Utility (Based on an Overall Assessment of the Quality of This Measure)

❒ Excellent: adequate to excellent clinical utility, easily available, excellent reliability and validity

❒ Adequate: adequate to excellent clinical utility, easily available, adequate to excellent reliability and validity

❒ Poor: poor clinical utility, not easily available, poor reliability and validity

Comments/notes/explanations:

_____

_____

_____

_____

Materials Used for Review/Rating

Please indicate the sources of information used for this review/rating:

❏ Manual

❏ Journal articles (attach or indicate location):

    ○ by author of measure

    ○ by other authors

List sources:

_____

_____

_____

_____

_____

_____

❏ Books—provide reference

❏ Correspondence with author—attach

❏ Other sources:

_____

_____

_____

_____

_____

REFERENCE

CanChild Centre for Childhood Disability Research. (1999). *Outcome measure rating form.* Hamilton, Ontario: McMaster University.

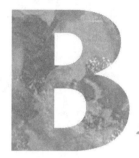

Outcome Measures Rating Form Guidelines

From: CanChild Centre for Childhood Disability Research
School of Rehabilitation Science
McMaster University
Hamilton, Ontario, Canada L8S 1C7
www.fhs.mcmaster.ca/canchild

Prepared by: Mary Law, PhD, OT(C)

General Information: Name of measure, authors, source, and year.

1. Focus

a. FOCUS OF MEASUREMENT. Use the modified ICIDH framework to indicate the focus of the measurement instrument that is being reviewed. The definitions are as follows: ORGANIC SYSTEMS: any loss or abnormality of psychological, physiological, or anatomical structure or function. ABILITIES: ability to perform an activity in an effective manner. PARTICIPATION (LIFE HABITS): life situations that individuals participate in and which result from the interaction of an impairment or disability with environmental factors. ENVIRONMENTAL FACTORS: aspects of the social, cultural, institutional, and physical environments that affect the organization of society and influence what people do.

b. ATTRIBUTE(S) BEING MEASURED. The rating form lists attributes organized using the ICIDH framework. Check as many attributes as apply to indicate what is being measured by this instrument.

c. SINGLE OR MULTIPLE ATTRIBUTE. Check the appropriate box to indicate whether this measure assesses a single attribute only or multiple attributes.

d. List the PRIMARY PURPOSE for which the scale has been designed. Secondary purposes can also be listed, but the instrument should be evaluated according to its primary purpose (i.e., discriminative, predictive, evaluative).

   DISCRIMINATIVE: A discriminative index is used to distinguish between individuals or groups on an underlying dimension when no external criterion or gold standard is available for validating these measures.

   PREDICTIVE: A predictive index is used to classify individuals into a set of predefined measurement categories—either concurrently or prospectively—to determine whether individuals have been classified correctly.

   EVALUATIVE: An evaluative index is used to measure the magnitude of longitudinal change in an individual or group on the dimension of interest (Kirshner & Guyatt, 1985).

e. PERSPECTIVE. Indicate the possible respondents.

f. POPULATION for which it is designed (AGE). If no age is stated, mark as age unspecified. List the diagnostic groups for which the measure is used.

g. EVALUATION CONTEXT refers to the environment in which the assessment is completed. Check all possible environments in which this assessment can be completed.

2. Clinical Utility

a. CLARITY OF INSTRUCTIONS. Check one of the ratings. Excellent: clear, comprehensive, concise, and available. Adequate: clear, concise but lacks some information. Poor: not clear and concise or not available.

b. FORMAT. Check all applicable items to indicate the format of data collection for the instrument. Possible items include naturalistic observation, interview, a questionnaire (self-completed, interview administered, or caregiver-completed), and task performance.

   PHYSICALLY INVASIVE indicates whether administration of the measure requires procedures that may be perceived as invasive by the client. Examples of invasiveness include any procedure that requires insertion of needles or taping of electrodes or that requires clients to take clothing on or off.

   ACTIVE PARTICIPATION OF CLIENT. Indicate whether completion of the measure requires the client to participate verbally or physically.

   SPECIAL EQUIPMENT REQUIRED. Indicate whether the measurement process requires objects that are not part of the test kit and are not everyday objects. Examples of this include stopwatches, a balance board, or other special equipment.

c. TIME TO COMPLETE THE ASSESSMENT. Record in minutes. For ADMINISTRATION, SCORING, and INTERPRETATION, consider the time, the amount of training, and the ease with which a test is administered, scored, and interpreted, and indicate whether these issues are easy or more complex. For ADMINISTRATION, SCORING, and INTERPRETATION to be rated as easy, each part of the task should be completed in under one hour with minimal amount of training and is easy for the average service provider to complete.

d. EXAMINER QUALIFICATIONS. Indicate if formal training is required for administering and interpreting this measure.

e. COST. In Canadian funds, indicate the cost of the measurement manual and score sheets. For SCORE SHEETS, indicate the number of sheets obtainable for that cost. List the SOURCE and the YEAR of the cost information so readers will know if the information is up to date.

3. Scale Construction

a. ITEM SELECTION. Check one of the ratings. Excellent: included all relevant characteristics of the attribute based on comprehensive literature review and survey of experts (a comprehensive review of the literature only is enough for an excellent rating, but a survey of experts alone is not enough). Adequate: included most relevant characteristics of the attribute. Poor: convenient sample of characteristics of the attribute.

b. WEIGHTING. Indicate whether the items in the tool are weighted in the calculation of the total score. If items are weighted, indicate whether the authors have weighted these items implicitly or explicitly. Implicit weighting occurs when there are a number of scales and each has a different number of items and the score is obtained by simply adding the scores for each item. Explicit weighting occurs when each item or score is multiplied by a factor to weight its importance.

c. LEVEL OF MEASUREMENT. State whether the scale used is NOMINAL (descriptive categories), ORDINAL (ordered categories), or INTERVAL or RATIO (numerical) for single and for summary scores. Indicate the SCALING METHOD that was used and the NUMBER OF ITEMS in the measure. Indicate if SUBSCALE SCORES are obtained. Indicate whether the subscales can be administered alone and the scores interpreted alone. In some cases, the scores can be interpreted alone, but the whole measure must be administered first. List the subscales with the number of items and indicate if there is evidence of reliability and validity for the subscales so that the scores can be used on their own.

4. Standardization

Standardization is the process of administering a test under uniform conditions.

a. MANUAL. Check one of the ratings. Excellent: published manual that outlines specific procedures for administration, scoring and interpretation, evidence of reliability and validity. Adequate: manual available and generally complete but some information is lacking or unclear regarding administration, scoring and interpretation, and evidence of reliability and validity. Poor: no manual available or manual with unclear administration, scoring and interpretation, and no evidence of reliability and validity.

b. NORMS. Indicate whether norms are available for the instrument. Please note that instruments that are only meant to be evaluative do not require norms. Indicate all AGES for which norms are available, the POPULATIONS for which the measure has been normed (e.g., children with cerebral palsy, people with spinal cord injuries), and indicate the SIZE OF THE SAMPLE which was used in the normative studies.

5. Reliability

Reliability is the process of determining that the test or measure is measuring something in a reproducible and consistent fashion.

a. RIGOUR OF STANDARDIZATION STUDIES FOR RELIABILITY. Excellent: More than two well-designed reliability studies completed with adequate to excellent reliability values. Adequate: one to two well-designed reliability studies completed with adequate to excellent reliability values. Poor: No reliability studies or poorly completed, or reliability studies showing poor levels of reliability.

b. RELIABILITY INFORMATION.

Internal consistency: the degree of homogeneity of test items to the attribute being measured. Measured at one point in time.

Observer:

i) intra-observer—measures variation that occurs within an observer as a result of multiple exposures to the same stimulus.

ii) inter-observer—measures variation between two or more observers.

Test-Retest: measures variation in the test over a period of time.

Complete the table and reliability information by filling in the TYPE OF RELIABIL-ITY that was tested (internal consistency, observer, test-retest); the STATISTIC that was used (e.g., Cronbach's coefficient alpha, kappa coefficient, Pearson correlation, intra-class correlation); the VALUE of the statistic that was found in the study; and the RATING of the reliability. Guidelines for levels of the reliability coefficient indicate that it will be rated excellent if the coefficient is greater than .80, adequate if it is from .60 to .79, and poor if the coefficient is less than .60.

6. Validity

a. RIGOUR OF STANDARDIZATION STUDIES FOR VALIDITY. Excellent: More than two well-designed validity studies supporting the measure's validity. Adequate: one to two well-designed validity studies supporting the measure's validity. Poor: No validity studies completed, studies were poorly completed or did not support the measure's validity.

b. CONTENT VALIDITY. Check one of the ratings.

Content validity: the instrument is comprehensive and fully represents the domain of the characteristics it claims to measure (Nunnally, 1978).

Excellent: judgmental or statistical method (e.g., factor analysis) was used and the measure is comprehensive and includes items suited to the measurement purpose. *Adequate*: has content validity but no specific method was used. *Poor*: instrument is not comprehensive.

METHOD. Note whether a judgmental (e.g., consensus methods) or statistical method (e.g., factor analysis) of establishing content validity was used.

c. CONSTRUCT VALIDITY.

Construct validity: the measurements of the attribute conform to prior theoretical for-mulations or relationships among characteristics or individuals (Nunnally, 1978).

Excellent: More than two well-designed studies have shown that the instrument con-forms to prior theoretical relationships among characteristics or individuals. *Adequate*: one to two studies demonstrate confirmation of theoretical formulations. *Poor*: No con-struct validation completed.

Indicate the STRENGTH OF ASSOCIATION of the findings for construct validity by listing the value of the correlation coefficients found.

d. CRITERION VALIDITY. Check one of the ratings.

Criterion validity: the measurements obtained by the instrument agree with another more accurate measure of the same characteristic (i.e., a criterion or gold standard measure) (Nunnally, 1978).

Indicate whether the type of criterion validity that was investigated is CONCURRENT, PREDICTIVE, or both.

Excellent: More than two well-designed studies have shown adequate agreement with a criterion or gold standard. *Adequate*: one to two studies demonstrate adequate agreement with a criterion or gold standard measure. *Poor*: no criterion validation completed.

Indicate the STRENGTH OF ASSOCIATION of the evidence for criterion validity by listing the values of the correlation coefficients that were found in the criterion validity studies. Using the information from the assessment that has been completed on this measure, check the appropriate rating to give an overall assessment of the quality of the measure.

e. RESPONSIVENESS. Check one of the ratings (applicable only to evaluative measures).

Responsiveness: the ability of the measure to detect minimal clinically important change over time (Guyatt, Walter, & Norman, 1987).

Excellent: More that two well-designed studies showing strong hypothesized relationships between changes on the measure and other measures of change on the same attribute. *Adequate*: One to two studies of responsiveness. *Poor*: No studies of responsiveness. *N/A*: Check if the measure is not designed to evaluate change over time.

Overall Utility

Excellent: Adequate to excellent clinical utility, easily available, excellent reliability and validity. *Adequate*: Adequate to excellent clinical utility, easily available, adequate to excellent reliability and validity. *Poor*: Poor clinical utility, not easily available, poor reliability and validity.

Materials Used

Please indicate and list the sources of information which were used for this review. By listing sources of information and attaching appropriate journal articles or correspondence with authors, it will be easier to find further information about this measure if it is required.

SUGGESTED READING

Law, M. (1987). Measurement in occupational therapy: Scientific criteria for evaluation. *Can J Occup Ther, 54*, 133-138.

REFERENCES

Guyatt, G., Walter, S. D., & Norman, G. R. (1987). Measuring change over time: Assessing the usefulness of evaluative instruments. *Journal of Chronic Diseases, 40*, 171-178.

Kirshner, B., & Guyatt G. (1985). A methodological framework for assessing health indices. *Journal of Chronic Diseases, 38*, 27-36.

Nunnally, J. C. (1978). *Psychometric theory*. New York, NY: McGraw-Hill.

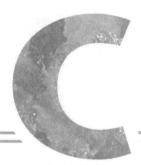

Critical Review Form for Quantitative Studies

These guidelines were developed by the McMaster University Occupational Therapy Evidence-Based Practice Research Group (Law et al., 1998).

Print the full citation of the article:

Comments

STUDY PURPOSE:
Was the purpose stated clearly?
○ Yes
○ No

Outline the purpose of the study. How does the study apply to your research question?

LITERATURE:
Was relevant background literature reviewed?
○ Yes
○ No

Describe the justification of the need for this study.

DESIGN:
○ randomized (RCT)
○ cohort
○ single case design
○ before and after
○ case-control
○ cross-sectional
○ case study

Describe the study design. Was the design appropriate for the study question? (e.g., for knowledge level about this issue, outcomes, ethical issues, etc.)

Specify any biases that may have been operating and the direction of their influence on the results.

SAMPLE:
N =

Was the sample described in detail?
○ Yes
○ No

Sampling (who, characteristics, how many, how was sampling done?) If more than one group, was there similarity between the groups?

Comments

Was sample size
justified?
○ Yes
○ No
○ N/A

Describe ethics procedures. Was informed consent
obtained?

OUTCOMES:

Specify the frequency of outcome measurement (i.e.,
pre, post, follow-up)

Outcome areas   List measures used

Were the outcome
measures reliable?
○ Yes
○ No
○ Not addressed

Were the outcome
measures valid?
○ Yes
○ No
○ Not addressed

INTERVENTION:
Was intervention described
in detail?
○ Yes
○ No
○ Not addressed

Provide a short description of the intervention (focus,
who delivered it, how often, setting). Could the intervention be replicated in practice?

Was contamination avoided?
○ Yes
○ No
○ Not addressed
○ N/A

Was cointervention avoided?
○ Yes
○ No
○ Not addressed
○ N/A

Comments

RESULTS:
Were results reported
in terms of statistical
significance?
○ Yes
○ No
○ N/A
○ Not addressed

What were the results? Were they statistically significant
(i.e., p < 0.05)? If not statistically significant, was the
study big enough to show an important difference if it
should occur? If there were multiple outcomes, was that
taken into account for the statistical analysis?

Were the
analysis method(s)
appropriate?
○ Yes
○ No
○ Not addressed

Was clinical
importance reported?
○ Yes
○ No
○ Not addressed

What was the clinical importance of the results? Were
differences between groups clinically meaningful? (if
applicable)

Were drop-outs reported?
○ Yes
○ No

Did any participants drop out from the study? Why?
(Were reasons given and were drop-outs handled appropriately?)

CONCLUSIONS AND
CLINICAL
IMPLICATIONS:

What did the study conclude? What are the implications of these results for practice? What were the main
limitations or biases in the study?

Were conclusions appropriate
given study methods and
results?
○ Yes
○ No

REFERENCE

Law, M., Stewart, D., Letts, L., Pollock, N., Bosch, J., & Westmorland, M. (1998). *Critical review form for quantitative studies*. Retrieved March 14, 2002, from http://www.fhs.mcmaster.ca/rehab/ebp.

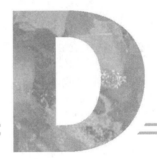

Guidelines for
Critical Review Form

Quantitative Studies

INTRODUCTION

- These guidelines accompany the Critical Review Form for Quantitative Studies developed by the McMaster University Occupational Therapy Evidence-Based Practice Research Group (Law et al., 1998). They are written in basic terms that can be understood by clinicians, students and researchers.

- Where appropriate, examples and justification for the guidelines/suggestions are provided to assist the reader in understanding the process of critical review.

- Guidelines are provided for the questions (left hand column) in the form, and the instructions/questions are provided in the Comments column of each component.

CRITICAL REVIEW COMPONENTS

Citation

- Include full title, all authors (last name, initials), full journal title, year, volume number, and page numbers.

- Providing this information ensures that another person could easily retrieve the same article.

Study Purpose

- Was the purpose stated clearly? The purpose is usually stated briefly in the abstract of the article, and again in more detail in the introduction. It may be phrased as a research question or hypothesis.

- A clear statement helps you determine if the topic is important, relevant, and of interest to you. Consider how the study can be applied to your practice and/or your own situation before you continue. If it is not useful or applicable, go on to the next article.

Literature

- Was relevant background literature reviewed? A review of the literature should be included in an article describing research to provide some background to the study. It should provide a synthesis of relevant information, such as previous work/research, and a discussion of the clinical importance of the topic.

- It identifies gaps in current knowledge and research about the topic of interest, and thus justifies the need for the study being reported.

Design

- There are many different types of research designs. The most common types in rehabilitation research are described next.

- The essential features of the different types of study designs are outlined to assist in determining which was used in the study you are reviewing.

- Some of the advantages and disadvantages of the different types of designs are outlined to assist the reader in determining the appropriateness of the design for the study being reported.
- Different terms are used by authors, which can be confusing, so alternative terms will be identified where possible.
- Numerous issues can be considered in determining the appropriateness of the methods/design chosen. Some of the key issues are listed in the Comments section and will be described below. Diagrams of different designs and examples using the topic of studying the effectiveness of activity programmes for seniors with dementia are provided.
- Most studies have some problems due to biases that may distort the design, execution, or interpretation of the research. The most common biases are described at the end of this section.

Design Types

Randomized

- Randomized controlled trial, or randomized clinical trial (RCT) is also referred to as Experimental or Type 1 study. RCTs also encompass other different methods, such as cross-over designs.
- The essential feature of a RCT is a set of clients/subjects identified and then randomly allocated (assigned) to two or more different treatment "groups." One group receives the treatment of interest (often a new treatment) and the other group is the "control" group, which usually receives no treatment or standard practice. Random allocation to different treatment groups allows comparison of the client groups in terms of the outcomes of interest because randomization strongly increases the likelihood of similarity of clients in each group. Thus, the chance of another factor (known as a confounding variable or issue) influencing the outcomes is greatly reduced.
- The main disadvantage of a RCT is the expense involved, and in some situations it is not ethical to have "control" groups of clients who do not receive treatment. For example, if you were to study the effectiveness of a multidisciplinary inpatient program for postsurgical patients with chronic low back pain, it may be unethical to withhold treatment in order to have a "control" group.
- RCTs are often chosen when testing the effectiveness of a treatment or to compare several different forms of treatment.

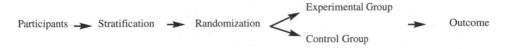

Example: The effects of two different interventions, functional rehabilitation and reactivation, were evaluated using a RCT. Forty-four patients of a long-term care centre were randomly allocated to one of the two types of intervention. Outcomes were measured using a variety of psychometric tests at three different points in time (Bach, Bach, Bohmer, Gruhwalk, & Grik, 1995).

Cohort Design

- A cohort is a group of people (clients) who have been exposed to a similar situation (e.g., programme) or a diagnosis/disease. Whatever the topic/issue of interest, the group is identified and followed/observed over time to see what happens.

- Cohort designs are "prospective," meaning that the direction of time is always forward. Time flows forward from the point at which the clients are identified. They are sometimes referred to as prospective studies.

- Cohort studies often have a comparison ("control") group of clients/people who have not been exposed to the situation of interest (e.g., they have not received any treatment). One of the main differences between a RCT and a cohort study is that the allocation of people (clients) to the treatment and control groups is not under the control of the investigator in a cohort study—the investigator must work with the group of people who have been identified as "exposed" and then find another group of people who are similar in terms of age, gender, and other important factors.

- It is difficult to know if the groups are similar in terms of all the important (confounding) factors; therefore, the authors cannot be certain that the treatment (exposure) itself is responsible for the outcomes.

- Advantages of cohort studies are they are often less expensive and less time-consuming than RCTs.

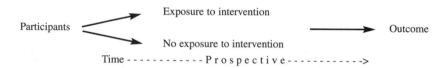

Example: Evaluation of a mental stimulation programme used a cohort design to measure changes in mental status in 30 patients over a 2-month time period. The first 15 patients who were admitted to a day care centre received treatment and composed the "exposed" group. The remaining 15 admissions did not receive treatment immediately and served as a "control" group (Koh et al., 1994).

Single Case Design

- Single subject/case research involves one client, or a number of clients, followed over time or evaluated on outcomes of interest.

- There are different types of methods used in single case designs, with different terms used such *n of 1 studies*, *before-after trial in the same subject*, or single case *series* involving more than one subject/client.

- The basic feature of any single subject design is the evaluation of clients for the outcome(s) of interest both before (baseline) and after the intervention. This design allows an individual to serve as his or her own "control." However, it is difficult to conclude that the treatment alone resulted in any differences, as other factors may change over time (e.g., the disease severity may change).

- It is useful when only a few clients have a particular diagnosis or are involved in a treatment that you want to evaluate. This type of study is easily replicated with more than one client. Its flexible approach makes it particularly appropriate for conducting research in clinical settings.

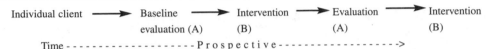

Time - - - - - - - - - - - - - - - - - - P r o s p e c t i v e - - - - - - - - - - - - - - - - - - ->

Example: A study examining the effects of environmental changes during an intervention on a psychiatric ward used a single case design to observe changes in behaviour in 10 individual patients. Observations of each patient's behaviour were made before, during, and after the intervention (Burton, 1980).

Before-After Design

- Before-after design is usually used to evaluate a group of clients involved in a treatment (although as previously mentioned, it is a method also used to study single cases/individuals).

- The evaluator collects information about the initial status of a group of clients in terms of the outcomes of interest and then collects information again about the outcomes after treatment is received.

- This is a useful design when you do not wish to withhold treatment from any clients. However, with no "control" group, it is impossible to judge if the treatment alone was responsible for any changes in the outcomes. Changes could be due to other factors such as disease progression, medication use, lifestyle, or environmental changes.

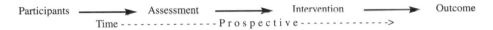

Example: The level of caregiver strain following placement of an elderly family member with dementia in adult day care was evaluated using a before-after design. Outcomes of caregiver strain and burden of care were measured in 15 subjects before and after the day care placement (Graham, 1989).

Case Control Design

- Case control studies explore what makes a group of individuals different. Other terms used are *case-comparison study* or *retrospective study*. *Retrospective* is the term used to describe how the methods look at an issue after it has happened. The essential feature of a case control study is looking backward.

- A set of clients/subjects with a defining characteristic or situation (e.g., a specific diagnosis or involvement in a treatment) is identified. The characteristic or situation of interest is compared with a "control" group of people who are similar in age, gender, and background but who do not have the characteristic or are not involved in the situation of interest. The purpose is to determine differences between these groups.

- It is a relatively inexpensive way to explore an issue, but there are many potential problems (flaws) that make it very difficult to conclude what factor(s) is responsible for the outcomes.

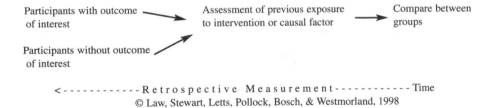

<- - - - - - - - - - - - R e t r o s p e c t i v e   M e a s u r e m e n t - - - - - - - - - - - Time

Example: If a therapist wanted to understand why some clients of a day care programme attended a daily activity programme (which was optional) on a regular basis while other clients did not attend, a case control design could be used to explore differences between the two groups of clients in relation to age, gender, interests, background, and current living situation.

Cross-Sectional Design

- Involves one group of people, and the evaluation of the whole group is carried out at the same time.

- This design is often used to explore what factors may have influenced a particular outcome in a group of people. It is useful when relatively little is known about an issue/outcome.

- Surveys, questionnaires, and interviews are common methods used in cross-sectional studies. They are relatively inexpensive and easy, as evaluation takes place at one point in time.

- It is impossible to know if all factors have been included in the evaluation, so it is difficult to draw cause-effect conclusions from the results beyond the group of people being studied.

Participants   ⟶   Measurement of outcomes and other factors at the same time

Time: All done at one point in time

Example: Clients and their families who have been involved in a new activity programme for seniors with dementia can be surveyed or interviewed upon discharge to evaluate the impact of the programme on their quality of life, activity participation, and level of satisfaction.

Case Study Design

- A case study is carried out in order to provide descriptive information (data) about the relationship between a particular treatment (exposure) and an outcome of interest. It is also called a *descriptive study*, as that is the primary purpose. There is no control group.

- It is often used to explore a new topic or treatment, when there is little knowledge. However, the results can only be considered in terms of describing a particular situation. It may generate information to support further study of the topic of interest.

Participants with condition of interest   ⟶   Information about clinical outcome

Example: Twelve patients on a long-stay geriatric ward were observed over a period of time to determine the effectiveness of providing individual and group activities on the ward. Engagement levels were observed and recorded at 10-minute intervals to determine any differences between no intervention, individual activities, and group activities (McCormack & Whitehead, 1981).

Appropriateness of Study Design

Some of the important issues to consider in determining if the study design is the most appropriate include:

- Knowledge of the topic/issue: If little is known about an issue, a more exploratory method is appropriate (e.g., a case study or a cross-sectional design). As our level of knowledge increases, study designs become more rigorous, where most variables that could influence the outcome are understood and can be controlled by the researcher. The most rigorous design is the RCT.

- Outcomes: If the outcome under study is easily quantified and has well-developed standardized assessment tools available to measure it, a more rigorous design (e.g., a RCT) is appropriate. If outcomes are not fully understood yet, such as quality of life, then a design that explores the different factors that may be involved in the outcomes is appropriate, such as a case control design.

- Ethical issues: It is appropriate to use a research design that uses control groups of people receiving no treatment if there are no ethical issues surrounding the withholding of treatment.

- Study purpose/question: Some designs are well-suited to studying the effectiveness of treatment, including RCT's, before-after designs, and single-case studies. Other designs (e.g., case control and cross sectional) are more appropriate if the purpose of the study is to learn more about an issue or is a pilot study to determine if further treatment and research is warranted.

Biases

- There are many different types of biases described in the research literature. The most common ones that you should check for are described under three main areas:
  1. Sample (subject selection) biases, which may result in the subjects in the sample being unrepresentative of the population in which you are interested.
  2. Measurement (detection) biases, which include issues related to how the outcome of interest was measured.
  3. Intervention (performance) biases, which involve how the treatment itself was carried out.
- The reader is directed to the bibliography if more detailed information is needed about biases.
- A bias affects the results of a study in one direction—it either "favours" the treatment group or the control group. It is important to be aware of which direction a bias may influence the results.

Sample/Selection Biases

a. Volunteer or referral bias

- People who volunteer to participate in a study or who are referred to a study by someone are often different than nonvolunteers/nonreferrals.
- This bias usually, but not always, favours the treatment group, as volunteers tend to be more motivated and concerned about their health.

b. Seasonal bias

- If all subjects are recruited and thus are evaluated and receive treatment at one time, the results may be influenced by the timing of the subject selection and intervention. For example, seniors tend to be healthier in the summer than the winter, so the results may be more positive if the study takes place only in the summer.

- This bias could work in either direction, depending on the time of year.

c. Attention bias

- People who are evaluated as part of a study are usually aware of the purpose of the study and, as a result of the attention, give more favourable responses or perform better than people who are unaware of the study's intent. This bias is why some studies use an "attention control" group, where the people in the control group receive the same amount of attention as those people in the treatment group, although it is not the same treatment.

Measurement/Detection Biases

a. Number of outcome measures used

- If only one outcome measure is used, there can be a bias in the way that the measure itself evaluated the outcome. For example, one ADL measure considers dressing, eating, and toiletting but does not include personal hygiene and grooming or meal preparation.

- This bias can influence the results in either direction (e.g., it can favour the control group if important elements of the outcome that would have responded to the treatment were missed).

- Bias can also be introduced if there are too many outcome measures for the sample size. This is an issue involving statistics, which usually favours the control group because the large number of statistical calculations reduces the ability to find a significant difference between the treatment and control groups.

b. Lack of "masked" or "independent" evaluation

- If the evaluators are aware of which group a subject was allocated to, or which treatment a person received, it is possible for the evaluator to influence the results by giving the person, or group of people, a more or less favourable evaluation. It is usually the treatment group that is favoured. This should be considered when the evaluator is part of the research or treatment team.

c. Recall or memory bias

- This can be a problem if outcomes are measured using self-report tools, surveys, or interviews that require the person to recall past events. Often a person recalls fond or positive memories more than negative ones, and this can favor the results of the study for those people being questioned about an issue or receiving treatment.

Intervention/Performance Biases

a. Contamination

- This occurs when members of the control group inadvertently receive treatment, thus the difference in outcomes between the two groups may be reduced. This favours the control group.

b. Cointervention

- If clients receive another form of treatment at the same time as the study treatment, this can influence the results in either direction. For example, taking medication while receiving or not receiving treatment could favour the results for people in either group. The reader must consider if the other, or additional, treatment could have a positive or negative influence on the results.

c. Timing of intervention
- Different issues related to the timing of intervention can introduce a bias.
- If treatment is provided over an extended period of time to children, maturation alone could be a factor in improvements seen.
- If treatment is very short in duration, there may not have been sufficient time for a noticeable effect in the outcomes of interest. This would favour the control group.

d. Site of treatment
- Where treatment takes place can influence the results. For example, if a treatment programme is carried out in a person's home, this may result in a higher level of satisfaction that favours the treatment group. The site of treatment should be consistent among all groups.

e. Different therapists
- If different therapists are involved in providing the treatment(s) under study to the different groups of clients, the results could be influenced in one direction. For example, one therapist could be more motivating or positive than another, and hence the group that she worked with could demonstrate more favourable outcomes. Therapist involvement should be equal and consistent among all treatment groups.

Sample

- N =   ? The number of subjects/clients involved in the study should be clear.
- Was the sample described in detail? The description of the sample should be detailed enough for you to have a clear picture of who was involved.
- Important characteristics related to the topic of interest should be reported, in order for you to conclude that the study population is similar to your own and that bias was minimized. Important characteristics include:
  a. Who makes up the sample? Are the subjects appropriate for the study question and described in terms of age, gender, duration of a disability/disease, and functional status (if applicable)?
  b. How many subjects were involved, and if there are different groups, were the groups relatively equal in size?
  c. How was the sampling done? Was it voluntary or by referral? Were inclusion and exclusion criteria described?
  d. If there was more than one group, was there a similarity between the groups on important (confounding) factors?
- Was the sample size justified? The authors should state how they arrived at the sample size to justify why the number was chosen. Often, justification is based on the population available for study. Some authors provide statistical justification for the sample size, but this is rare.
- Ethics procedures should be described, although they are often left out. At the very least, authors should report if informed consent was obtained at the beginning of the study.

Outcomes

- Outcomes are the variables or issues of interest to the researcher. They represent the product or results of the treatment or exposure.
- Outcomes need to be clearly described in order for you to determine if they were relevant and useful to your situation. Furthermore, the method (the how) of outcome measurement should be described sufficiently for you to be confident that it was conducted in an objective and unbiased manner.
- Determine the frequency of outcome measurement. It is important to note if outcomes were measured pre- and post-treatment and whether short-term and/or long-term effects were considered.
- Review the outcome measures to determine how they are relevant to practice (i.e., they include areas of occupational performance, performance components, and/or environmental components).
- List the measures used and any important information about them for your future reference. Consider if they are well-known measures or ones developed by the researchers for the specific study being reported. It may be more difficult to replicate the study in the latter situation.
- The authors should report if the outcome measures used had sound (well-established and tested) psychometric properties—most importantly, reliability and validity. This ensures confidence in the measurement of the outcomes of interest.
- Were the outcome measures reliable? Reliability refers to whether a measure is giving the same information over different situations. The two most common forms of reliability are test-retest reliability (the same observer gets the same information on two occasions separated by a short time interval) and inter-rater reliability (different observers get the same information at the same time).
- Were the outcome measures valid? This asks whether the measure is assessing what it is intended to measure. Consider if the measure includes all of the relevant concepts and elements of the outcome (content validity) and if the authors report that the measure has been tested in relationship to other measures to determine any relationship (criterion validity). For example, a "valid" ADL measure will include all relevant elements of self-care and will have been tested with other measures of daily living activities and self-care functioning to determine that the relationship between the measures is as expected.

Intervention

- Intervention described in detail? There should be sufficient information about the intervention for you to be able to replicate it.
- In reviewing the intervention, consider important elements such as:
  a. The focus of the intervention: Is it relevant to practice and your situation?
  b. Who delivered it? Was it one person or different people? Were they trained?
  c. How often was the treatment received? Was it sufficient in your opinion to have an impact? Was the frequency the same if there were different groups involved?
  d. The setting: was treatment received at home or in an institution? Was it the same for different groups of subjects if there was more than one treatment group?

© Law, Stewart, Letts, Pollock, Bosch, & Westmorland, 1998

- These elements need to be addressed if you want to be able to replicate the treatment in your practice.
- Were contamination, cointervention avoided? These two factors were described under Biases (see Design section). Were they addressed? If not, consider what possible issues could influence the results of the study. For example, what could happen if some of the clients in the control group received some treatment inadvertently (contamination) or if some subjects were taking medication during the study (cointervention)? Make note of any potential influences. If there was only one group under study, mark "not applicable (n/a)" on the form.

Results

- Were results reported in terms of statistical significance? Most authors report the results of quantitative research studies in terms of statistical significance to prove that they are worthy of attention. It is difficult to determine if change in outcomes or differences between groups of people are important or significant if only averages, means or percentages are reported.
- Refer to the bibliography if you wish to review specific statistical methods.
- Outline the results briefly in this section, focusing on those that were statistically significant. If the results were not significant statistically, examine the reasons: was the sample size not large enough to show an important, or significant, difference, or were too many outcome measures used for the number of subjects involved?
- Were the analysis method(s) appropriate? Do the authors justify/explain their choice of analysis methods? Do they appear to be appropriate for the study and the outcomes? You need to consider the following:
  a. The purpose of the study: Is it comparing two or more interventions or examining the correlation between different variables of interest? Different statistical tests are used for comparison and correlation.
  b. The outcomes: If there is only one outcome measured to compare two different treatments, a simple statistical test such as a t-test will probably be sufficient. However, with a larger number of outcomes involving different types of variables, more complex statistical methods, such as analysis of variance (ANOVA), are usually required.
- Was clinical importance reported? Numbers are often not enough to determine if the results of a study are important clinically. The authors should discuss the relevance of the results to clinical practice and/or to the lives of the people involved. If significant differences were found between treatment groups, are they meaningful in the clinical world? If differences were not statistically significant, are there any clinically' important or meaningful issues that you can consider for your practice?

Drop-outs

- Were drop-outs reported? The number of subjects/participants who drop out of a study should be reported, as it can influence the results. Reasons for the drop-outs and how the analysis of the findings were handled with the drop-outs taken into account should be reported to increase your confidence in the results. If there were no drop-outs, consider that as "reported" and indicate no drop-outs in the Comments section.

Conclusions and Clinical Implications

- The discussion section of the article should outline clear conclusions from the results. These should be relevant and appropriate given the study methods and results. For example, the investigators of a well-designed RCT study using sound outcome measures could state that the results are conclusive that treatment A is more effective than treatment B for the study population. Other study designs cannot make such strong conclusions, as they likely had methodological limitations or biases, such as a lack of a control group or unreliable measures, that make it difficult to "prove" or conclude that it was' the treatment alone that influenced the outcome(s). In these situations, the authors may only conclude that the results demonstrated a difference in the specific outcomes measured in this study for the clients involved. The results may not be generalizable to other populations, including yours. Further study or research should therefore be recommended.

- The discussion should include how the results may influence clinical practice. Do they offer useful and relevant information about a client population or an outcome of interest? Do they warrant further study? Consider the implications of the results, as a whole or in part, for your particular practice and in general.

BIBLIOGRAPHY

Crombie, I. K. (1996). *The pocket guide to critical appraisal: A handbook for health care professionals*. London: BMJ Publishing Group.

Deptartment of Clinical Epidemiology and Biostatistics, McMaster University Health Sciences Centre. (1981). How to read clinical journals: V: To distinguish useful from useless or even harmful therapy. *Canadian Medical Association Journal, 124*, 1156-1162.

Law, M. (1987). Measurement in occupational therapy: Scientific criteria for evaluation. *Can J Occup Ther, 58*, 171-179.

Law, M., King, G., & Pollock, N. (1994). *Single subject research design. Research report #94-2*. Hamilton, ON: Neurodevelopmental Clinical Research Unit.

Mulrow, C. D., & Oxman, A. D. (Eds.). (1996). *Cochrane collaboration handbook*. Available in The Cochrane Library [database on disk and CD-ROM]. The Cochrane Collaboration: Issue 2. Oxford: Updated Software.

Norman, G. R., & Streiner, D. L. (1986). *PDQ statistics*. Burlington, ON: B. C. Decker Inc.

Sackett, D. L. (1979). Bias in analytic research. *Journal of Chronic Disability, 32*, 51-63.

Sackett, D. L., Haynes, R. B., Guyatt, G. H., & Tugwell, P. (1991). *Clinical epidemiology. A basic science for clinical medicine* (2nd ed.). Toronto, ON: Little, Brown and Co.

Streiner, D. L., Norman, G. R., & Blum, H. M. (1989). *PDQ epidemiology*. Toronto, ON: B.C. Decker Inc.

Articles of Activity Programmes for Seniors With Dementia (Referred to in Examples of Study Designs)

Bach, D., Bach, M., Bohmer, G., Gruhwalk, T., & Grik, B. (1995). Reactivating occupational therapy: A method to improve cognitive performance in geriatric patients. *Age Aging, 24*, 222-226.

Burton, M. (1980). Evaluation and change in a psychogeriatric ward through direct observation and feedback. *Br J Psychiatry, 137*, 566-571.

Graham, R. W. (1989). Adult day care: How families of the dementia patient respond. *Journal of Gerontological Nursing, 15*(3), 27-31, 40-41.

Koh, K., Ray, R., Lee, J., Nair, T., Ho, T., & Ang, P. C. (1994). Dementia in elderly patients: Can the 3R mental stimulation programme improve mental status? *Age Aging, 23*, 195-199.

Law, M., Stewart, D., Letts, L., Pollock, N., Bosch, J., & Westmorland, M. (1998). *Critical review form for quantitative studies.* Retrieved March 14, 2002, from http://fhs.mcmaster.ca/rehab/ebp.

McCormack, D., & Whitehead, A. (1981). The effect of providing recreational activities on the engagement level of long-stay geriatric patients. *Age Aging, 10*, 287-291.

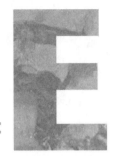

Critical Review Form for Qualitative Studies

Print the full citation of the article:

Comments

STUDY PURPOSE:
Was the purpose stated
clearly?
O Yes
O No

Outline the purpose of the study.

LITERATURE:
Was relevant background
literature reviewed?
O Yes
O No

Describe the justification of the need for this study.

What area(s) of occupational
therapy was studied?

How does the study apply to your research question?

STUDY DESIGN:
What was the design?
O Ethnography
O Grounded theory
O Participatory action research
O Phenomenology
O Other

What was the study design? Was the design appropriate
for the study question? (e.g., for knowledge level about
about the issue, ethical issues)

_____

Comments

Was a theoretical
perspective identified?
○ Yes
○ No

Describe the theoretical perspective for this study.

Method(s) used:
○ Participant observation
○ Interviews
○ Historical
○ Focus groups
○ Other

_____

Describe the method(s) used to answer the research
question.

SAMPLING:
Was the process of purpose-
ful selection described?
○ Yes
○ No

Describe sampling methods used. Was flexibility in the
sampling process demonstrated?

Sampling was done until
redundancy in data was reached
○ Yes
○ No
○ Not addressed

Was informed consent
obtained?
○ Yes
○ No
○ Not addressed

Describe ethics procedure.

DATA COLLECTION:
Descriptive Clarity
Clear & complete
description of:
  Site: ○ yes   ○ no
  Participants: ○ yes   ○ no
  Researcher's credentials:
            ○ yes   ○ no

Describe the context of the study. Was it sufficient for
understanding the "whole" picture?

Comments

Role of researcher and
relationship with
Participants   ○ yes   ○ no
Identification (bracketing)
of assumptions of researcher
   ○ yes   ○ no

Describe how elements of the study were documented.
What was missing?

Procedural Rigor
Procedural rigor was used in
data collection strategies
○ Yes
○ No
○ Not addressed

Describe data collection methods. How were the data
representative of the "whole" picture? Describe any
flexibility in the design and data collection methods.

DATA ANALYSIS:
Analytical Preciseness
Data analysis was inductive
○ Yes   ○ No
○ Not addressed

Describe method(s) of data analysis. Were the methods
appropriate? What alternative explanations were
explored?

Findings were consistent with
and reflective of data
○ Yes   ○ No

Auditability
Decision trail developed
and rules reported
○ Yes   ○ No
○ Not addressed

Describe the decisions of the researcher regarding
transformation of data to themes/codes. Outline the
rationale given for development of themes.

Process of transforming data
into themes/codes was
described adequately
○ Yes   ○ No
○ Not addressed

Comments

Theoretical Connections
Did a meaningful picture of
the phenomenon under study
emerge?
○ Yes
○ No

How were concepts under study clarified and refined
and relationships made clear? Describe any conceptual
frameworks that emerged.

TRUSTWORTHINESS
Triangulation was reported for
Sources/data   ○ Yes ○ No
Methods   ○ Yes ○ No
Researchers   ○ Yes ○ No
Theories   ○ Yes ○ No

Member checking was used to
verify findings
○ Yes   ○ No
○ Not addressed

Describe the strategies used to ensure trustworthiness
of the findings.

CONCLUSIONS and
IMPLICATIONS

Conclusions were
appropriate given the
study findings
○ Yes   ○ No

The findings contributed
to theory development
and future practice/research
○ Yes   ○ No

What did the study conclude? What were the implications of the findings for rehabilitation (practice and research)? What were the main limitations in the study?

Guidelines for Critical Review Form

Qualitative Studies

INTRODUCTION

- These guidelines accompany the Critical Review Form for Qualitative Studies developed by the McMaster University Occupational Therapy Evidence-Based Practice Research Group (Law et al., 1998). They are written in basic terms that can be understood by researchers as well as clinicians and students interested in conducting critical reviews of the literature.
- Guidelines are provided for the questions in the left hand column of the form and the instructions/questions in the Comments column of each component.

CRITICAL REVIEW COMPONENTS

Citation

- Include full title, all authors (last name, initials), full journal title, year, volume number, and page numbers.
- Providing this information ensures that another person could easily retrieve the same article.

Study Purpose

- Was the purpose stated clearly? The purpose is usually stated briefly in the abstract of the article and again in more detail in the introduction. It may be phrased as a research question.
- A clear statement helps you determine if the topic is important, relevant, and of interest to you.

Literature

- Was relevant background literature reviewed? A review of the literature should be included in an article describing research to provide some background to the study. It should provide a synthesis of relevant information such as previous work/research and discussion of the clinical importance of the topic.
- It identifies gaps in current knowledge and research about the topic of interest, and thus justifies the need for the study being reported.
- What areas of rehabilitation were studied? Indicate the area(s) of practice that are of interest to the researcher or how this study applies to practice.
- Consider how the study can be applied to practice and/or your own situation before you continue. If it is not useful or applicable, go on to the next article.

Study Design

- There are many different types of research designs. These guidelines focus on the most common types of qualitative designs in rehabilitation research.
- The essential features of the different types of study designs are outlined to assist in determining what was used in the study you are reviewing.

- Numerous issues can be considered in determining the appropriateness of the design chosen. Some of the key issues are listed in the Comments section and are discussed on the next page.

Design Types

Ethnography

- Ethnography is a well-known form of qualitative research in anthropology and focuses on the question, "What is the culture of a group of people?" The goal of ethnographic research is to tell the whole story of a group's daily life by identifying the cultural meanings, beliefs, and patterns of the group. Culture is not limited to ethnic groups, and ethnographers study the culture of organizations, programmes, and groups of people with common social problems such as smoking and drug addiction. In the area of health care, Krefting (1989) described a disability ethnography, which is a strategic research approach focusing on a particular human problem and those aspects of group life that impact on the problem.

Example: A qualitative ethnographic study was conducted to explore the process and outcomes of a program for seniors with dementia. Data from observations, interviews with patients and staff, and field notes were analyzed to discover the opportunities and barriers to conducting an occupational program in a day hospital unit (Borell, Gustavsson, Sandman, & Kielhofner, 1994).

Phenomenology

- Phenomenology answers the question, "What is it like to have a certain experience?" It seeks to understand the phenomenon of a lived experience. This may be related to an emotion, such as loneliness or depression, to a relationship, or to being part of an organization or group. The assumption behind phenomenology is that there is an essence to shared experience. It comes from the social sciences and requires a researcher to enter into an individual's life and use the self to interpret the individual's (or group's) experience.

Example: A phenomenological approach was chosen to explore the lived experiences of student occupational therapists during their first year of fieldwork placements. The focus of the study was on the acquisition of cultural competencies. Data were collected through individual interviews at baseline and after placement, supplemented by the students' journal entries. Two main themes emerged related to definitional issues about the concept of culture and the students' own identification within a culturally complex society (Dyck & Forwell, 1997).

Grounded Theory

- Grounded theory focuses on the task of theory construction and verification. The inductive nature of qualitative research is considered essential for generating a theory. It searches to identify the core social processes within a given social situation. Glaser and Strauss (1967) developed a research process that takes the researcher into and close to the real world to ensure that the results are "grounded" in the social world of the people being studied. This type of qualitative design is popular in the field of nursing research.

Example: The grounded theory approach to data analysis (Glaser & Strauss, 1967) was used to explore enjoyment experiences of persons with schizophrenia. Interviews with nine participants focused on their descriptions of enjoyment. The themes that emerged from the data analysis helped therapists gain a better understanding of enjoyment experiences of persons with schizophrenia, and the factors that characterized their enjoyment experiences (Emerson, Cook, Polatajko, & Segal, 1998).

Participatory Action Research

- Participatory action research (PAR) is an approach to research and social change that is usually considered to be a form of qualitative research. PAR involves individuals and groups researching their own personal beings, sociocultural settings, and experiences. They reflect on their values, shared realities, collective meanings, needs, and goals. Knowledge is generated and power is regained through deliberate actions that nurture, empower, and liberate persons and groups. The researcher works in partnership with participants throughout the research process.

Example: A PAR study involved researchers working with parents of children with physical disabilities to discover environmental situations that presented substantial challenges to their children. Through focus groups and individual interviews with 22 families, participants identified environmental factors that supported or hindered the daily activities of their children. The participants came together after the interviews were completed to form a parent support and advocacy group, which has continued to advocate for change to environmental constraints in their community (Law, 1992).

Other Designs

- These are many other qualitative research designs described in the literature. They come from different theoretical traditions and disciplines, and some are extensions of the more popular ethnographic and phenomenological designs. Some of the most frequently described designs in qualitative literature include heuristics, ethnomethodology, hermeneutics, ecological psychology, and social interactionism. Readers interested in further inquiry of qualitative research designs are directed to the bibliography at the end of this document.

Appropriateness of Study Design

The choice of qualitative research designs should be congruent with the following:
- The beliefs and world views of the researcher (i.e., the qualitative researcher usually expresses an interest in understanding the social world from the point of view of the participants in it, and emphasizes the context in which events occur and have meaning).
- The nature of the end results desired (i.e., the qualitative research is seeking meaning and understanding, which is best described in narrative form).
- The depth of understanding and description required from participants (i.e., qualitative research usually involves the exploration of a topic or issue in depth with emphasis on seeking information from the people who are experiencing or are involved in the issue).
- The type of reasoning involved: qualitative research is oriented toward theory construction, and the reasoning behind data analysis is inductive (i.e., the findings emerge from the data).

- Crabtree and Miller (1992) suggest that the best way to determine if the choice of a particular qualitative research design is appropriate is to ask how the particular topic of interest is usually shared in the group or culture of interest. For example, if information about how clients responded to treatment is usually shared through discussion and story-telling among individual therapists, then a phenomenological approach may be the most appropriate way to study this experience.

- Was a theoretical perspective identified? The thinking and theoretical perspective of the researcher(s) can influence the study. The researcher knows something conceptually of the phenomenon of interest and should state the theoretical perspective up front.

Qualitative Methods

- A variety of different methods are used by qualitative researchers to answer the research question. The most common ones are described here, with advantages and disadvantages of each.

Participant Observation

- A participant observer uses observation to research a culture or situation from within. The observer usually spends an extended period of time within the setting to be studied and records "fieldnotes" of his/her observations. This type of research may be called *fieldwork*, which comes from its roots in social and cultural anthropology.

- Participant observation is useful when the focus of interest is how activities and interactions within a setting give meaning to beliefs or behaviours. It fits with the assumption that everyone in a group or organization is influenced by assumptions and beliefs that they take for granted. It is therefore considered the qualitative method of choice when the situation or issue of interest is obscured or hidden from public knowledge and there are differences between what people say and what they do.

- Participant observation can be time-consuming and costly, as it can take a long time to uncover the hidden meanings of the situation/context.

2. Interviews

- An interview implies some form of verbal discourse. The participant provides the researcher with information through verbal interchange or conversation. Nonverbal behaviours and the interview context are noted by the researcher and become part of the data.

- Another term used frequently in qualitative research is *key informant interviews,* which refers to the special nature of the participant being interviewed. He or she is chosen by the researcher because of an important or different viewpoint, status in a culture or organization, and/or knowledge of the issue being studied.

- Qualitative interviews place an emphasis on listening and following the direction of the participant/informant. A variety of open-ended questions are chosen to elicit the most information possible in the time available.

- Interviews can be done relatively quickly, with little expense, and are useful when a particular issue needs to be explored in depth. However, the drawback to interviewing is related to the constraints imposed by language. The types of questions asked will frame the informants' responses, and this should be taken into account by the researcher.

Focus Groups

- Focus groups are a formal method of interviewing a group of people/participants on a topic of interest.
- The same principles used for individual interviews apply with focus group interviews (e.g., the use of open-ended questions, the focus on listening and learning from the participants).
- Focus groups are useful when multiple viewpoints or responses are needed on a specific topic/issue. Multiple responses can be obtained through focus groups in a shorter period of time than individual interviews. A researcher can also observe the interactions that occur between group members.
- The disadvantages of focus groups relate to the potential constraints that a group setting can place on individual's responses. Furthermore, the facilitator of the focus group must be skilled in group process and interviewing techniques to ensure the success of the group.

Historical

- Historical research involves the study and analysis of data about past events. The specific methods used are flexible and open because the purpose is to learn how past intentions and events were related due to their meaning and value. The historian learns about particular persons at particular times and places that present unique opportunities to learn about the topic of interest.
- Historical research can provide important information about the impact of the past on present and future events.
- It is a difficult research approach that requires the researcher to enter into an indepth learning process, to become intimately involved in data collection and to be a critical editor of texts. The researcher as historian must make explicit all observations and interpretations.

Other

- Other forms of qualitative research methods include mapping cultural settings and events; recording, using either audio or visual techniques; life histories (biographies); and genograms. Some researchers consider surveys and questionnaires that are open-ended in nature to be qualitative methods if the primary intent is to "listen" to or learn from the participants/clients themselves about the topic of interest.

Sampling

- Was the process of purposeful selection described? Sampling in qualitative research is purposeful, and the process used to select participants should be clearly described. Purposeful sampling selects participants for a specific reason (e.g., age, culture, experience), not randomly.

- There are numerous sampling methods in qualitative research. The sampling strategies used by the researcher should be explained and relate to the purpose of the study. For example, if the purpose of the study is to learn about the impact of a new treatment programme from the perspective of all clients involved in the programme and their families, the purposeful sampling method should be broad to include maximum variation in perspectives and views. On the other hand, if the purpose is to explore an issue indepth, such as the numerous factors and interactions that are involved in a family deciding when and where to place an elderly member in a nursing home, an individual, "key informant" approach may be appropriate.
- Was sampling done until redundancy in data was reached? The main indicator of sample size in qualitative research is often the point at which redundancy, or theoretical saturation of the data, is achieved. The researcher should indicate how and when the decision that there was sufficient depth of information and redundancy of data to meet the purposes of the study was reached.
- The sampling process should be flexible, evolving as the study progresses, until the point of redundancy in emerging themes is reached.
- Was informed consent obtained? The authors should describe ethics procedure, including how informed consent was obtained, and confidentiality issues.

Data Collection

Descriptive Clarity

- Clear and complete descriptions? In qualitative research, the reader should have a sense of personally experiencing the event/phenomenon being studied. This requires a clear and vivid description of the important elements of the study that are connected with the data, namely the participants, the site or setting, and the researcher.
- The researcher includes relevant information about the participants, often in the form of background demographic data. The unique characteristics of key informants help to explain why they were selected. The credibility of the informants should be explored. Particular to qualitative research, the types and levels of participation of the participants should also be described.
- Qualitative research involves the "researcher as instrument," wherein the researcher's use of self is a primary tool for data collection. Documentation of the researcher's credentials and previous experience in observation, interviewing, and communicating should be provided to increase the confidence of the reader in the process. The researcher's role(s), level of participation, and relationship with participants also needs to be described, as they can influence the findings.
- The researcher should declare his or her assumptions about the topic under study ("bracket assumptions") to make his or her views about the phenomenon explicit.
- A vivid description of the participants, site, and researcher should provide the reader with an understanding of the "whole picture" of the topic or phenomenon of interest. Any missing elements should be noted.

Procedural Rigor

- Was procedural rigor used in data collection strategies? The researcher should clearly describe the procedures used to ensure that data were recorded accurately and that data obtained is representative of the "whole" picture. All source(s) of information used by the researcher should be described.
- The reader should be able to describe the data-gathering process, including issues of gaining access to the site, data collection methods, training data gatherers, the length of time spent gathering data, and the amount of data collected.

Data Analyses

Analytical Preciseness

- Were data analyses inductive? The researcher(s) should describe how the findings emerged from the data.
- The authors should report on the flexibility of the data collection process, as it responded to changes or trends in the data.
- Different methods are used to analyze qualitative data. The reader should be able to identify and describe the methods used in the study of interest and make a judgment as to whether the methods are appropriate given the purpose of the study.
- Were findings consistent with and reflective of data? The themes that were developed by the researcher(s) should be logically consistent and reflective of the data. There should be an indication that the themes are inclusive of all data that exists, and data should be appropriately assigned to themes/codes.

Auditability

- Decision trail developed and rules reported? The reasoning process of the researcher during the analysis phase should be clearly described. The process used to identify categories or common elements, patterns, themes, and relationships from the data is important to understand as it is complex. This process is best articulated through the use of a decision or "audit" trail, which tracks decisions made during the process, including the development of rules for transforming the data into categories or codes.
- Was the process of transforming data into themes/codes described adequately? The decision trail should also report on how data was transformed into codes that represented the emerging themes and interrelationships that provide a picture of the phenomenon under study. Often a qualitative researcher will use a specific analysis method, such as an editing style or a template approach (Crabtree & Miller, 1992). The methods used should be fully reported.
- The rationale for the development of the themes should be described.
- These steps in auditing the analysis process provide evidence that the findings are representative of the data as a whole.

Theoretical Connections

- Did a meaningful picture of the phenomenon under study emerge? The findings should clearly describe theoretical concepts, relationships between concepts, and integration of relationships among meanings that emerged from the data in order to yield a meaningful picture of the phenomenon under study. The reader should be able to understand concepts and relationships, including any conceptual frameworks, that the researchers propose. The findings should make sense with current knowledge about the phenomenon under study and the knowledge base of rehabilitation in general.

Trustworthiness

- Establishing trustworthiness ensures the quality of the findings. It increases the reader's confidence that the findings are worthy of attention. Many different strategies are employed in qualitative research to establish trustworthiness (Krefting, 1991), and the researchers should report on the methods they employed.
- Was triangulation reported? A critical group of strategies used to enhance trustworthiness is triangulation. It involves using multiple sources and perspectives to reduce the chance of systematic bias. There are four main types of triangulation:
  - By source—data is collected from different sources (e.g., different people, resources)
  - By methods—different data collection strategies are used such as individual interviews, focus groups, and participant observation
  - By involves the use of more than one researcher to analyze the data and develop and test the coding scheme
  - By theories—multiple theories and perspectives are considered during data analysis and interpretation.
- Was member checking used to verify findings? Participants should validate the findings of the researcher. This can be done in several ways, including mailing a written copy of the findings to each participant or holding a follow-up meeting or focus group. The method(s) used to verify the findings should be reported.

Conclusions

- Were conclusions appropriate given the study findings? Conclusions should be consistent and congruent with the findings as reported by the researchers. All of the data and findings should be discussed and synthesized.
- The findings contributed to theory development and future practice? The conclusions of the study should be meaningful to the reader and should help the reader understand the theories developed. It should provide insight into important professional issues facing occupational therapists. The authors should relate the findings back to the existing literature and theoretical knowledge in rehabilitation. Implications and recommendations should be explicitly linked to practice situations and research directions.

Bibliography

Burns, N. (1989). Standards for qualitative research. *Nursing Science Quarterly, 2*(1), 44-52.

Denzin, N. K., & Lincoln, Y. S. (Eds.). (1994). *Handbook of qualitative research.* Thousand Oaks, CA: Sage Publications, Inc.

Forchuk, C., & Roberts, J. (1992). *How to critique qualitative health research articles.* Working Paper Series 92-2. Hamilton, ON: McMaster University System-linked Research Unit.

Patton, M. Q. (1990). *Qualitative evaluation and research method* (2nd ed.). Newbury Park, CA: Sage Publications, Inc.

Smith, S. E., & Williams, D. G. (Eds.). (1997). *Nurtured by knowledge: Learning to do participatory action-research.* Ottawa, ON: International Development Research Centre.

Articles from Occupational Therapy Literature (Referred to in Examples of Study Design)

Borell, L., Gustavsson, A., Sandman, P., & Kielhofner, G. (1994). Occupational programming in a day hospital for patients with dementia. *Occupational Therapy Journal of Research, 14*(4), 219-243.

Crabtree, B. F., & Miller, W. L. (1992). *Doing qualitative research. Research methods for primary care* (Vol 3). Newbury Park, CA: Sage Publishing.

Dyck, I., & Forwell, S. (1997). Occupational therapy students' first year fieldwork experiences: Discovering the complexity of culture. *Can J Occup Ther, 64*, 185-196.

Emerson, H. A., Cook, J. A., Polatajko, H., & Segal, R. (1998). Enjoyment experiences as described by persons with schizophrenia. *Can J Occup Ther, 65*, 183-192.

Glaser, B., & Strauss, A. L. (1967). *The discovery of grounded theory.* New York, NY: Aldine.

Krefting, L. (1989). Disability ethnography. A methodological approach for occupational therapy research. *Can J Occup Ther, 56*, 61-66.

Krefting, L. (1991). Rigor in qualitative research: The assessment of trustworthiness. *Am J Occup Ther, 45*, 214-222.

Law, M. (1992). *Planning for children with physical disabilities: Identifying and changing disabling environments through participatory research.* Unpublished dissertation, University of Waterloo, Ontario.

Law, M., Stewart, D., Letts, L., Pollock, N., Bosch, J., & Westmorland, M. (1998). *Critical review form for qualitative studies.* Retrieved March 14, 2002, from http://www.fhs.mcmaster.ca/rehab/ebp.

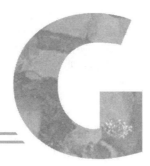

Instructions for the Use of the Functional Independence Measure Decision Trees

Many clinicians have found the decision trees useful tools to determine Functional Independence Measure (FIM) scores as they observe subject behaviors. A separate decision tree for each item may be found on the facing page for that item.

To use the FIM decision tree, begin in the upper left hand corner. Answer the questions and follow the brances to the correct score. You will notice that behaviors and scores above the dotted line indicate that NO HELPER is needed and that behaviors and scores below the dotted lines indicate that a HELPER is needed.

GENERAL DESCRIPTION OF FIM INSTRUMENT LEVELS OF FUNCTION AND THEIR SCORES

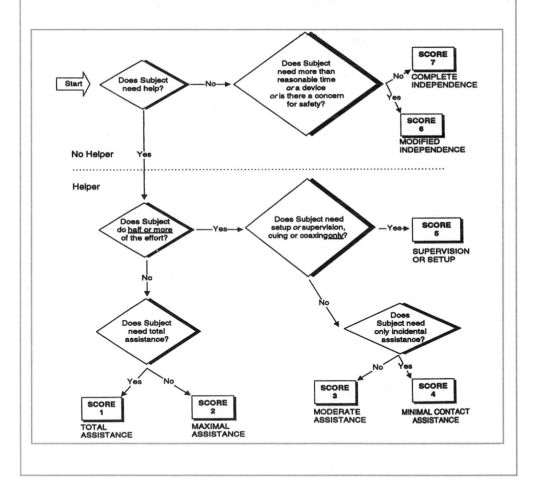

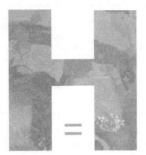

Clinical Pathway Example

KEY

THR: Total hip replacement
TKR: Total knee replacement
HIP: Hip
Nsg: Nursing
CM: Case manager
DVT: Deep venous thrombosis
LTC: Long-term care
SW: Social work
Nutr: Nutrition
HSW: Home support worker
PWB: Partial weight bearing
OPD: Out-patient department
LT: Long term

ADP: Assistive devices program
ADL: Activities of daily living
PT: Physiotherapy
OT: Occupational therapy
L: Left
R: Right
Hx: History
D/C: Discharge
H.C.: Home care
ROM: Range of motion
FWB: Full weight-bearing
SLP: Speech language pathology

<u>**Anticipated visit frequency:**</u>
THR, TKR
PT: 1x/week for 5 wks
Nsg (if req'd): 1x/week for 2 to 3wks
OT (if req'd): 1x/wk for 1 to 3 wks
 # HIP
PT: 1x/wk for 8 to 10 wks
Nsg and OT as required

Ottawa-Carleton Community Care Access Centre Care Pathway

> ### ORTHOPEDIC/LOWER EXTREMITY
>
> **Diagnosis:** _____ **(L) (R)** *(circle)*
> **Date of surgery:**_____
> **Hospital D/C date:**_____

Case Management	Components	INITIAL VISIT	WEEK 2
CM: admission screening assessment: - medical condition, support systems, functional status, behavior/cognition, sociocultural status - suitability of client for care plan - risks (history of falls, poly-pharmacy, use of alcohol, dizziness, environmental hazards) - assess need for other services (SW, Nutr, Nsg, OT, HSW) CM teaching re: - care plan and program expectations - roles (service provider and CM) - develop service goals CM on D/C, review: - equip't (ongoing need, funding) - LTC needs (respite, HSW, alternate care)	OBSERVATIONS/ ASSESSMENTS TESTS/ MEASUREMENTS	☐ PT review: - medications - wound healing - circulatory status (DVT) ☐ Nsg (if client frail & elderly) assess: bathing/transfer, medication management, pain control, remove staples ☐ PT measure: - walking tolerance - stairs (if a requirement) - swelling - pain - strength and ROM	☐ PT review: exercise program ☐ Nsg (if required) assess: progress with self/assist bathing, medication management, return to independence ☐ OT (if required): assess toilet/bath equipment/ transfers, ADL/IADL ☐ PT measure: - ↑walking tolerance - stairs - ↓ swelling, - ↓ pain
		☐ gait (walker) PWB	☐ → walker → cane(s)
Note to service provider: On final visit, transfer client outcomes from teaching brochure to care pathway (below) and return pathway to CCAC **Outcomes**	INTERVENTION/ FUNCTIONAL RESTORATION	☐ PT assess: - toilet/bath equipment - bathing practices - toilet/bed/chair transfers - need for other services or supports eg. HSW: (if required) for bathing, household activities ☐ Nsg (if required): assist with bath transfer	☐ PT (or ☐ OT if required): - screen ADL/IADL (simple meal preparation, bath transfers) - introduce/recommend assistive devices - screen need for energy conservation, work simplification techniques - review need for HSW (if in place)
1.Before the program I managed my walking and activities: ☐ not well ☐ with difficulty ☐ quite well ☐ very well 2.This program helped me improve how I manage walking and activities: ☐ not at all ☐ a little ☐ quite a bit ☐ a great deal	SAFETY/ ENVIRONMENT	☐ PT assess: - safety/environment - regular support systems (ie. caregiver, neighbour) - home access	☐ PT (or ☐ OT if required) assess: - safety in transfers - lifting, carrying
3.I now use community resources: ☐ never(0 used) ☐sometimes (1or2 used) ☐ often (3 used) ☐ always (4 or more) 4.My safety at home has improved: ☐ not at all ☐ a little ☐ quite a bit ☐ a great deal	TEACHING/ CONSULTATIONS	☐ PT ☐ Nsg: discuss client goals ☐ PT: review hospital teaching pkg. or give H.C. pkg. - identify present exercise program - teach re: positioning, restrictions - review pain management	☐ PT: - review client outcomes - provide written exercise program - discuss restrictions in sexual activity (see resource file) ☐ Nsg ☐ OT teach: - client/caregiver/HSW safe bathing
	D/C PLANNING	prepare for self-management	instruct in self-management

Reproduced with permission of the Ottawa-Carleton Community Care Access Center.

	Progress corresponds to care pathway **Report VARIANCES to CM and on Variance Tracking Record**	Physiotherapy Visit # _____ ☐ Yes ☐ No Sig._____ Date: _____	Physiotherapy Visit # ____ ☐ Yes ☐ No Sig._____ Date: _____
CM sig.:_____ CM Code:_____		_____ Visit # ☐ Yes ☐ No Sig._____ Date: _____	_____ Visit # ____ ☐ Yes ☐ No Sig._____ Date: _____
Date: _____		_____ Visit # ☐ Yes ☐ No Sig._____ Date: _____	_____ Visit # ____ ☐ Yes ☐ No Sig._____ Date: ___

Service Provider printed name:(PT)_____

(Nsg)_____

(OT)_____

WEEK 3	WEEK 4	FINAL VISIT
☐ PT: - progress exercise program - assess suitability for OPD ☐ Nsg (if required) ☐ OT (if required): assess self-bathing, need for continued support (HSW); D/C	☐ PT: - progress exercise program - check shoes/leg length discrepancy	☐ PT: - complete exercise program progression
☐ PT measure: - ↑ walking tolerance - stairs - outdoor ambulation - ↑ROM	☐ PT measure: - ↑ walking tolerance - ↑ ROM- flexion, extension - ↑ strength hip, knee	☐ PT measure: - functional walking tolerance - safe on stairs with/without aid - hip: 90 degree fl., neutral extension - hip: gr.3 vs. gravity abduction - knee: 90 degree fl., -10 degree to 0 degree ext.
☐ walker→ cane(s)	☐ progress to 1 cane	☐ →FWB, heel-toe pattern
☐ PT(or ☐ OT if required): - consider ParaTranspo application/ Disabled Parking Permit - screen client's ability to do self-care, household activities without HSW (if in place) ☐ Nsg (if required): assist/delegate bathing	☐ PT (☐ OT if required) review/ resolve: - bath, toilet, bed, chair/car transfers - equipment needs - driving, transportation, community access/activities - meal preparation	☐ PT (or ☐ OT if required): - transfers functional and safe - independent or assisted ADL - functional IADL
☐ OT (if required) review: - in-home safety - bath safety		☐ PT (or ☐ OT if required) review: - all safety concerns in/around home - ensure all necessary supports in place including equipment
☐ prepare for MD recheck ☐ PT: - discuss with CM: length of stay, LTC needs, LT goals, preliminary D/C plan - teach restrictions in driving, sitting in car - discuss LT equipment needs/funding (ADP eligibility)	☐ MD recheck visit date:_____ (complete communication form, progress note) ☐ PT review: client outcomes	☐ PT review: - knowledge of exercise/activity program - limitations, restrictions - bending/lifting/carrying techniques - client outcomes
reinforce self-management	begin to finalize d/c planning	☐ notify MD and CM re: D/C

Reproduced with permission of the Ottawa-Carleton Community Care Access Center.

Physiotherapy Visit # _____	Physiotherapy Visit #	Physiotherapy Visit # ____
☐ Yes ☐ No Sig._____ Date: _____	_____ ☐ Yes ☐ No Sig._____ Date: _____	☐ Yes ☐ No Sig._____ Date: _____
_____ Visit # _____ ☐ Yes ☐ No Sig._____ Date: _____	_____ Visit # _____ ☐ Yes ☐ No Sig._____ Date: _____	_____Visit # ____ ☐ Yes ☐ No Sig._____ Date: _____
_____ Visit # ____ ☐ Yes ☐ No Sig._____ Date: _____	_____ Visit # ____ ☐ Yes ☐ No Sig._____ Date: _____	_____ Visit # ____ ☐ Yes ☐ No Sig._____ Date: _____

Reproduced with permission of the Ottawa-Carleton Community Care Access Center.

Variance Record Example

KEY

Nsg: Nursing
SW: Social work

Nutr: Nutrition
SLP: Speech language pathology

Multidisciplinary Variance Tracking Record

Name _____

ID # _____

Caf # _____

CM code _____

Variance codes (VC):   **Provider codes:**

+98 (-099) Client Condition/Decision   (Nsg) (PT) (OT)

+499 (-500) Family/Caregiver Concern/Issue   (SLP) (Nutr) (SW)

+599 (-600) Health Care Provider/Other Agency Decision/Availability

+749 (-750) Supplies/Equipment/Information/Data Issue/Availability

 800—Off Map

(+) Event occurred **in advance** of plan (–) Event **delayed** compared to plan

Visit Number	Date	VC +/–	Description of Variance	Actions Taken	Signature and Provider Code

General comments/observations (nonvariance-related information):

Date   Signature

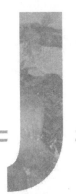

Client Outcomes Example

Ottawa-Carleton CCAC

Client Outcomes

ORTHOPEDIC: ☐ UPPER EXTREMITY
☐ LOWER EXTREMITY

Client name _____
ID# _____
Caf # _____
CM code _____

(label)

Service Provider: _____
Phone# _____
Client
Signature _____

WEEK 1 Date: _____	WEEK 2 → WEEK 4 Date: _____	FINAL VISIT date: _____
I understand: ☐ how to manage pain ☐ my home exercise program ☐ the precautions I need to follow ☐ how to walk safely including stairs using my walker/cane (if required) ☐ how to get on and off my chair, bed, and toilet ☐ how to position myself in bed ☐ how much weight I can put on my leg now that I am home ☐ the safety measures and precautions I should use in my home	I know: ☐ my goals for the program ☐ which items I need to buy to help me walk, dress, bathe, and do meal preparation and how to use them ☐ the funding resources available for purchasing my equipment ☐ my written exercise program I can: ☐ get on and off my chair, bed, and toilet ☐ attend to my personal hygiene ☐ dress/undress with or without assistance ☐ walk safely within / around my home and on stairs _____ meters ☐ walk outdoors _____ meters ☐ stand to prepare light meals ☐ I practise home safety measures/precautions	☐ I understand the importance of my exercise program ☐ I practise the safety measures and precautions in my home and within my community I can: ☐ manage my household activities and self-care (i.e., bathe, dress) ☐ go out in my community safely ☐ pursue my leisure activities ☐ walk safely and independently using a walker, cane, or no aids _____ meters ☐ stand for: _____ minutes

Goals

I would like to be able to:

_____
_____
_____
_____
_____
_____

My concerns:

_____
_____
_____
_____
_____
_____

I know:
☐ my case manager's name _____
☐ my case manager's phone number _____
☐ how and when to contact my case manager

I understand:
☐ the role of my case manager and service providers
☐ how I will participate in the program and the care plan to be followed

I have met my Home Care program goals:
☐ Yes ☐ No
Comments: _____

Mark Pathway as follows: (✓)= completed   N/A= not applicable   N/C= not completed

(0114*)

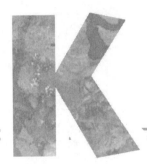

Key Indicator
Record Example

Durham Access to Care
Mastectomy Case Path and
Key Indicators
Target Length of Stay (LOS) = 10 days
Target Number of Nursing Visits = 10

Client Name:

HCN:

KEY INDICATORS	MET at TARGET DATE (Initial)	DATE MET: (if not met at target) (Date and Initial)	COMMENTS (If met before or after target date)
Post-op Day 0 Hospital 9			
1. Pain controlled			
2. Nausea controlled			
3. Stage 1 exercises initiated			
Post-op Day 1 Hospital 9			
4. Pain controlled			
5. Stage 2 exercises initiated			
6. Teaching-drain/exercises initiated			
Post-op Day 2 and 3 Hospital 9			
7. Able to discuss fears and anxieties			
8. Information given regarding support groups			
Post-op Day 4 to 6			
9. Independent with care of drain			
10. Independent with arm exercises			
Post-op Day 7 to 9			
11. Drain out			
12. Progress to stage 3 exercises			
13. Verbalizes understanding of strategies to prevent trauma and infection			
Post-op Day 10 (Discharge)			
14. Independent with wound care			
15. Client has viewed incision			
16. Shoulder range of motion functional			
17. independent with exercises or referred to Out Patient Physiotherapy			

COPY TO BE RETURNED TO CASE PATH COORDINATOR, DATC AT END OF *SURGICAL* EPISODE

AUTHORIZED BY:
Initials: Full Signature: Print Full Name and Discipline:

Reprinted with permission of Durham Access to Care.

Template for the Development of Clinical Pathways

Key Indicators

Clinical Pathway _____ ICD-9 Code(s) _____

(name of pathway-condition/group pathway will address)

Client Name _____ ID# _____ HCN _____

Expected Length of Stay _____ Expected # of Visits: _____

Date Admitted to Pathway _____ Date Discharged from Pathway _____

Date Noted	Visit #	Goals/Expected Outcomes	Date Met	Not Met	Variance Code	Date Variance Noted and Reported	Comments

Variance Codes:	Team Member Signatures:	Case Manager Signature:
1. Patient/client related 2. Situation related 3. Systems related	RN _____ PT _____ OT _____ SLP _____ Nutritionist _____ SW _____	_____ Patient/Client (involved in care planning) Signature _____

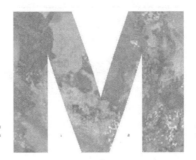

Template for the Development of Clinical Pathways

Timeline

Case type (description) _____

Length of stay: _____

Frequency of visits: _____

Focus	Visit 1	Visit 2	Visit 3
Observations/Assessments			
Tests/Measurements			
Functional Level Safety			
Treatments			
Teaching/Education			
Discharge Planning			
Consultation/Referral			

Admission Criteria:
1.

2.

3.

4.

Discharge Criteria:
1.

2.

3.

4.

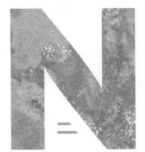

Developing Outcomes

Complete the outcome statements listed below for the following client conditions:

A. Cardiovascular accident (CVA)
B. Congestive heart failure
C. Major joint replacement
D. Bipolar disorder
E. Parkinson's disease
F. Early onset dementia

The client understands and demonstrates knowledge of _____
_____
_____ by visit number _____.

The client's status is stabilized as evidenced by _____
_____
_____ by visit number _____.

The client's family/caregiver understands and demonstrates knowledge of _____
_____
_____ by visit number _____.

The client and caregiver can identify the following safety precautions or prevention factors:
_____
_____
_____

The client and caregiver can identify the following risks related to the health concern:
_____
_____
_____

Index

abilities, 288, 300

ABPI (ankle brachial index pressure index), 214

activities
learning and exploration, 26
reflection, 41–43

ADL (activities of daily living), 174, 239

Agency for Health Care Research & Quality, 197

AHCPR (Agency for Health Care Policy and Research). *See also* Agency for Health Care Research & Quality
clinical practice guidelines, 196–198
evidence-based guidelines, 263–264
online resources, 266

Alberta Clinical Practice Guidelines Program, 217

Alberta WellNet, 211, 216

algorithms
clinical practice guidelines, 201–203, 212
definition, 214

All About Outcomes CD-ROMs, 86

American Occupational Therapy Association, 86

American Occupational Therapy Foundation, 86

analytical preciseness, 336

ankle brachial index pressure index (ABPI), 214

appraisal instrument for clinical pathways, 209

assessment evidence, 225–226

assessment information, 224

assessment questions, 233

assessment tools, for clients with Parkinson's Disease, 236–243

assumptions, 34–35

auditability, 336

Australian National Health and Medical Research Council Clinical Practice Guidelines, 216

barrier-free design, 19

Barthel Index, 239

before-after design, 313

Best Evidence database, 87

biases, 315–317

bimodal samples, 63

biostatistics, 103

Canadian Centres for Health Evidence, 87

Canadian Cochrane Centre, 124

Canadian Medical Association InfoBase, 215

Cancer Care Ontario Practice Guidelines Initiative, 215

care pathway systems, 217

CareMap model, 204, 205

case control studies, 100–101, 313–314

case mixed groups, 204–205, 214

case reports, 101

case study design, 314

CATs (critically appraised topics), 186–193, 258, 266. *See also* randomized controlled trials; systematic reviews

causation, 65–66, 67

CCACs (Community Care Access Centres), 272

CCTR (Cochrane Controlled Trials Register), 86, 122

CDSR (Cochrane database of systematic reviews), 85

CEBM (Center for Evidence-Based Medicine), 105, 188, 192

Center for Case Management, 216
Center for Evidence-Based Emergency
    Medicine, 190
central tendency measures, 60, 62–63
Centre for Health Economics and Policy
    Analysis, 264–265, 266
cerebral palsy, conductive education tech-
    niques, 15–16
charting by exception, 214
CHEPA (Centre for Health Economics
    and Policy Analysis), 264–265, 266
CHID (Combined Health Information
    Database), 87
chronic pain. *See* cognitive-behavioral
    interventions for chronic pain
CINAHL database, 85
citation reviews, 130
client/population intervention, 73
clinical governance, 213
clinical implications, critical review form
    guidelines, 320
clinical judgment, 9, 37–38, 176, 249
clinical outcomes. *See* cognitive-behav-
    ioral interventions for chronic pain
    cognitive-behavioral interventions for
        chronic pain, 129, 165–166
    example, 348
    hospital care versus home care,
        273–282
    key indicators, 205, 210
    measuring, 50–51, 56–65, 67
    medical models, 51–56
    outcome measures rating form,
        288–297
    outcome measures rating form guide-
        lines, 300–320
    reporting and interpreting with statis-
        tics, 59–64
    scenarios, 74–75
    selecting proper outcome measures, 118
clinical pathways. *See also* CPGs
    definition, 214
    development template, 352, 354
    evaluation, 209
    example, 341–344
    historical perspectives, 203–205
    legal implications, 211–213
clinical practice guidelines. *See* CPGs

clinical utility, 301
CMA (Canadian Medical Association)
    clinical practice guidelines, 196–198
    CMA ePractice Tools, 215
Cochrane Collaboration, 86, 112, 118,
    121–123, 124, 215
Cochrane Database of Systematic
    Reviews and Best Evidence, 87
Cochrane Fields/Networks, 122
Cochrane Library, 68, 86, 124
cognitive-behavioral interventions for
    chronic pain
    approaches, 128, 162–165, 166
    materials and methods, 129–162, 166
    objectives, 128–129
    results, 165–166
cohort studies, 100, 188–189, 312
communication techniques
    with clients and family members, 223
    clinical role, 223–224
    considerations, 222–223, 250
    decision makers and, 227–229
    examples
        interpretation of a single study,
            234–236
        interpretation of a synthesis of
            studies, 230–234
        intervention information, 247
    gathering and interpreting evidence,
        224–227, 228, 250
    opportunities in everyday practice,
        249–250
    quality of life considerations, 229–230
    scenario, 222
    uncertainty and, 248–249, 250
computer-based decision support sys-
    tems, 209–210
concurrent variance analysis, 214
conductive education techniques, for
    cerebral palsy, 15–16
confidence interval, 118, 162–163
confirmation stage, research transfer
    process, 257
CONSORT statement, 105, 114–115, 124
content evidence, 240
contextual factors of health conditions, 53
cost-benefit analysis, 174, 176, 180

cost-consequence analysis, 173, 174, 175, 180
cost-effectiveness analysis, 174, 175, 176, 180
cost-minimization analysis, 173–174, 175, 180
cost-utility analysis, 174, 176
covariation, 66
CPGs (clinical practice guidelines)
    algorithms, 201–203, 212, 214
    case types, 205–206
    clinical pathways, 203–205, 209, 211–213
    computer-based decision support systems, 209–210
    decision trees, 201, 204
    definition, 196–198, 214
    development strategies, 206, 208
    development teams, 207
    documentation system, 208–209
    evaluation, 199–201
    implementation, 199
    legal implications, 211–212
    online resources, 215–217
    outcomes, 209
    postimplementation review, 209
CQIN (Clinical Quality Improvement Network), 211
CRGs (Collaborative Review Groups), 122
criteria list, 58–59
criterion-related evidence, 240–241
CRMD (Cochrane Review Methodology Database), 122–123
cross-sectional studies, 101, 314
customized ongoing measurements, 57

DARE (Database of Abstracts of Reviews of Effectiveness), 86, 122
data analysis, 336–337
data collection, 104, 335–336
decision stage, research transfer process, 257
decision trees, 201, 204, 340
deinstitutionalization, 14
descriptive clarity, 335
descriptive evidence, 239
descriptive information, 224, 225
descriptive questions, 233

descriptive review, 165
descriptive statistics, 59–60, 67
developmental coordination disorder, 51
deviation scores, 64
diagnosis/screening, with CATs, 186–188
diagnostic related groups, 205, 214
disabilities
    community awareness, 14–15
    definition, 55–56
discriminative index, 300
disease guidance systems, 211
documentation system, for clinical pathways, 208–209
DRGs (diagnostic related groups, 205, 214
drop-outs, critical review form guidelines, 319
duration measurements, 59

E-model
    definition, 33
    environment, 35, 38
    ethics, 36–37, 39
    evidence, 37–38, 39
    expectations, 34–35, 38
    experience, 35–36, 38–39
economic evaluation, 172–179
eGuidelines, 217
electronic bibliographic databases, 77–81, 91, 130
eligibility criteria, 114
environment factor, E-model, 38
environmental factors, 35, 288, 300
ethics factor, E-model, 36–37, 39
ethnography, 104, 331
evaluation context, 300–301
evaluative evidence, 239
evaluative index, 300
evidence-based clinical practice (EBCP), 8–9
evidence-based communication. *See* communication techniques
evidence-based knowledge, 14, 20–25
evidence-based medicine
    historical perspectives, 37
    learning resources, 11
    online resources, 124
Evidence-Based Medicine Resource Center, 217

Evidence-Based Medicine Reviews, 87
evidence-based policy, 261–266
evidence-based practice. *See also* clinical outcomes; systematic reviews
  CATs (critically appraised topics), 186–193
  challenges, 237
  clinical scenarios, 74
  concepts, 8–10
  definitions, 4–6, 10
  economic evaluation, 172–179
  evaluating evidence
    biostatistics, 103
    classification systems, 101–102
    considerations, 98, 103
    qualitative methods, 103–105
    quantitative methods, 98–101
  goals, 256–257
  myths, 6–8
Evidence-Based Practice Internet Resources, 87
evidence classification systems, 101–102
evidence factor, E-model, 37–38, 39
evidence search
  clinical scenarios, 73–75
  formulating questions, 72–75
  identifying sources, 75–77, 91, 130
  process, 87–90
existing published research, 72
existing theory, 72
expectations factor, E-model, 34–35, 38
experience factor, E-model, 35–36, 38–39
experienced professional period, knowledge development, 16–18
expert professional period, knowledge development, 16–18
exposure, 73
external validity, economic evaluations, 178

factor analytic studies, 21
false-negatives, 102
false-positives, 102
focus groups, 334
forest plot, 118–119
frequency distribution, 60–61
frequency measurements, 59

functional independence measure decision trees, 340
functional limitations, 55

GAP (Guideline Appraisal Project), 217
GAS (Goal Attainment Scaling). *See also* statistics
  study with geriatric rehabilitation population, 237
  tracking achievements, 243–244
  validity, 242–243
GERGIS-German Guideline Information Service, 215
Goal Attainment Scaling. *See* GAS
"gold standard" of evidence, 190. *See* randomized controlled trials
graphic rating scales, 58
grounded theory, 104, 331–332
Guideline Appraisal Project (GAP), 217

hand searching, 130
HBS (hospital-based services), 273
health care. *See also* clinical practice guidelines; HSDR
  continuum pathways, 207
  emerging trends, 196
HEALTHnet, 256–257, 266
HEED (Health Economic Evaluations Database), 179
heterogeneity, 119–121
HIRU (Health Informatics Research Unit)
  definition of evidence-based practice, 8–9
  online resources, 11
historical research, 334
hospital care versus home care, 273–282, 281
HRQL (health-related quality of life), 174
HSDR (health care delivery research)
  hospital care versus home care, 273–282, 281
  for postacute stroke
    definition and diagnosis, 270–271
    home care delivery, 272
    incidence statistics, 271
    prognostic and recovery, 271–272
    therapy, 272–273

hypotheses
  statistics and, 65
  testing, 21, 22

ICES (Institute for Clinical Evaluative
    Sciences), 271
ICIDH-2 model, contextual factors of
    health conditions, 53
ICIDH (International Classification of
    Impairment, Disability, and
    Handicap) framework, 87
if-then statements, 34–35
impairment, 55
implementation stage, research transfer
    process, 257
INAHTA (International Network of
    Agencies for Health Technology
    Assessment), 86
indirect measurements, 56
inferential statistics, 60, 65–66, 67
input, research transfer process, 257–258
interdisciplinary collaboration, 19, 37, 128
internal validity, economic evaluations, 178
International Classification of Functioning
    (ICF) Model, 51–53, 67, 68
International Federation of Pharmaceutical
    Manufacturers Association, 179
intervention information, 224, 226,
    318–319
intervention/performance biases, 316–317
intervention questions, 233
intervention studies, 189
interviews, 333

Journal of Integrated Care Pathways, 216

key indicators, 205, 210, 214, 350
knowledge-driven model, evidence-based
    policy, 262
knowledge stage, research transfer
    process, 257

latency measures, 59
learning and exploration activities
  CATs (critically appraised topics), 191
  clinical practice guidelines, 213
  cognitive-behavioral interventions for
    chronic pain, 167

communication techniques, 251–252
economic evaluation, 180–181
evaluating evidence, 106
evidence-based knowledge, 26
evidence-based practice, 68
evidence search, 91–93
HSDR (health care delivery research),
    281
research transfer process, 266–267
systematic reviews, 125
levels of evidence, 101–102, 114
life satisfaction, 229

MACTAR (McMaster-Toronto Arthritis
    Patient Preference Disability
    Questionnaire, 34
magnitude of evidence, 233, 245
The Markers of Quality in Paths, 209
mean values, 62–63
measurement
  assessment tools, 103
  focus, 300
  levels, 302
  statistical methods, 65–66
measurement/detection biases, 316
median values, 62–63
Medic8, 216
MEDLINE database, 83–84
meta-analyses
  approaches, 123
  definition, 99, 102, 117–118
  gathering and interpreting evidence,
    227, 230
  heterogeneity, 119–121
  online resources, 124
  reporting and interpreting, 118–119
  statistics and, 244
Methods Groups, 122
mode values, 62–63
multimodal samples, 63

narrative reviews, 110, 111
National Guidelines Clearinghouse, 197,
    215
National Information Centre on Health
    Services Research and Health Care
    Technology, 178–179
National Library of Medicine, 178

National Pathway Association (U.K.), 216
NCDDR (National Center for the Dissemination of Disability Research, 222
NCMRR (National Center for Medical Rehabilitation Research Model), 54, 67
negative variance, 214
"next generation" pathways, 205
NGC (The National Guideline Clearinghouse), 197, 215
NHS (National Health System)
    Centre for Reviews and Dissemination (CRD), 86
    clinical governance guidelines, 213
    Independent Appraisal Service, 200
    levels of evidence, 102
    NHSEED (NHS Economic Evaluations Database), 86, 179
    NNT (Number Needed to Treat), 189
    SROTOS (Systematic Reviews of Trials and Other Studies), 111–112, 119–120
NNT (Number Needed to Treat), 189
norm-referenced interpretation, 64
normal distribution, 64–65
novice professional period, 33
novice professional period, knowledge development, 16–18
null hypothesis, 65

OARS (Older Americans Resources and Services) Index, 239, 242
observational measures, 59
Office of Health Economics, 179
Older Americans Resources and Services (OARS) Index, 239, 242
organic systems, 288, 300
OT Bibsys, 86
OTDBASE database, 86
Ottawa Ankle Rule, 197
outcomes, 73, 214, 318, 356. See also clinical outcomes
Ovid database, 85
Ovid Technologies, 87

p-value, 248
paraphysiology, 55

Parkinson's Disease
    assessment tools, 236–243
    interventions, 243–248
participant observation, 333
participation (life habits), 288, 300
participatory action research, 332
PEDro (The Physiotherapy Evidence Database), 87
percentiles, 64
"perfect knowledge", 262
persuasion stage, research transfer process, 257
phenomenology, 104, 331
positive variance, 214
Practice Guideline Evaluation and Adaptation Cycle, 200
predictive evidence, 239
predictive index, 300
preference indicators, 214
preservice experience phase, knowledge development, 16–18
problem-driven model, evidence-based policy, 262
procedural rigor, 336
professional knowledge development, phases, 16–18
professional practice, questions, 72
professional trends, questions, 72
protocol, 214
PT Manager, 11
published research, 72, 75–77, 116

qualitative methods, 103–105, 324–327, 330–337
quality of life, 229
quantitative methods
    assessment tools, 103
    considerations, 98
    critical review form, 306–308
    critical review form guidelines, 310–320
    evaluating evidence, 98–102
questions
    elements, 224
    search terms for, 228
    sources of, 72
    structure of, 189–190
    types of, 233

well-built, 72–73, 90
QUORUM (Quality of Reporting of
    Meta-analyses), 121

randomized controlled trials. *See also*
    research transfer process
    critical review form guidelines, 311
    with definitive results, 99–100
    levels of evidence, 101–102, 114
    with nondefinitive results, 100
    online resources, 105, 124
    systematic reviews, 102
range, in variability measures, 63
rating scales, 57–58
RCT. *See* randomized controlled trials
reflective process, 32–33
rehabilitation models
    International Classification of Fun-
        ctioning (ICF) Model, 51–53, 67,
        68
    NCMRR (National Center for Medical
        Rehabilitation Research Model),
        54, 67
rehabilitation professionals. *See also* clin
    ical judgments; HSDR
    across disciplines, 19–25
    assessing the value of services, 172–179
    within a discipline, 18–19
    process of reflection, 32–33
reliability, 238, 243, 302–303. *See also*
    clinical outcomes
renaissance period, 23–25
representative samples, 99
research transfer process
    models, 256–258, 260–261, 265
    online resources, 266
    teaching strategies, 258–260
results, critical review form guidelines, 319
retrospective variance analysis, 214
risk, in cohort studies, 188–189
Royal College of Nursing Professional
    Clinical Guidelines, 216

sample/selection biases, 315–316
sampling, 104, 317, 334–335
scale construction, 301–302
scholarly publications, 75–77
scientific strategies, 110

Scottish Intercollegiate Guidelines
    Network (SIGN), 215
SD (standard deviation), 63–64
sensitivity analyses, 177, 187–188
sensory integrative performance
    historical perspectives, 23
    identifying problems, 21
SIGN (Scottish Intercollegiate Guidelines
    Network), 215
single case design, 312–313
skewed distributions, 65
societal limitations, 56
Southwestern Ontario Regional
    Academic Health Science Network
    CATs, 192
specificity, 187–188
SROTOS (Systematic Reviews of Trials
    and Other Studies), 111–112,
    119–120
standard deviation, 63–64
standard scores, 63
standardization, 302
standardized assessments, 57
standardized test scores, 64
standards of care, 211–212, 214
statistics. *See also* GAS; meta-analyses
    descriptive, 59–60, 67
    errors in, 102
    inferential, 60, 65–66, 67
    measurement, 65–66
    online resources, 106
    reporting and interpreting, 59–64
Steering Committee on Clinical Practice
    Guidelines for the Care and
    Treatment of Breast Cancer,
    101–102
StrokeNet, 211
study designs, 103–104
subjective well-being, 230
SUMSearch database, 87
syntheses, 227
systematic reviews. *See also* meta-analysis
    analyzing and quantifying data, 115
    approaches, 110–113, 123
    of cognitive-behavioral studies, 165
    definition, 110
    of effects of computer-based decision
        support systems, 210–211

flowchart, 113
information resources, 115–116
meta-analyses and, 99, 102
online resources, 124
preparation, 113–115
published research, 116
reporting findings, 115
selection criteria, 129

tacit knowledge, 32
temporal ordering, 66
test scores, interpreting, 64
theoretical connections, 337
theories
    for causal interpretation, 66
    existing, 72
    if-then statements, 34–35
TJSSW Group (The Joint Stroke Strategy
    Working Group), 271
trustworthiness, 337
Type I error in statistics, 102
Type II error in statistics, 102

universal design, 19
University of Leicester, 111
University of Michigan CATs, 192
University of North Carolina CATs, 192
University of Rochester Medical Center,
    192
University of York, National Health
    Service Centre for Reviews and
    Dissemination, 110–111

validity, 239, 240, 243, 303–304. *See also*
    clinical outcomes
variability measures, 60, 61–62
variance, 214, 346
variance analysis, 214
visual analog scales, 58
VNA First-Home Care Steps, 216

"web of belief", 23
weighting, 301
WHO (World Health Organization),
    International Classification of
    Functioning (ICF) Model, 51–53
WMD (weighted mean difference),
    162–165
World Wide Web
    research resources, 77, 91, 178
    search strategies, 81–83
    Web sites
        evaluating, 79–81
        types of, 78

Z-scores, 63–64, 65

Build Your Library

Along with this title, we publish numerous products on a variety of topics. We are sure that you will find the below titles to be an essential addition to your library. Order your copies today or contact us for a copy of our latest catalog for additional product information.

OCCUPATION-BASED PRACTICE: FOSTERING PERFORMANCE AND PARTICIPATION

Mary Law, PhD, OT(C); Carolyn M. Baum, PhD, OTR/L, FAOTA; and Sue Baptiste, MHSc, OT(C)

160 pp., Soft Cover, 2002, ISBN 1-55642-564-3, Order #35643, **$34.00**

Occupation-Based Practice: Fostering Performance and Participation is an exceptional text designed to offer the student, instructor, and practitioner opportunities to integrate occupation into the client-centered treatment plan. With real-life scenarios and active learning principles, students are able to experience and learn up-to-date and emerging practice in occupational therapy. The workbook format will support occupational therapists as they seek to implement a person, environment, and occupation framework in planning client-centered care.

MEASURING OCCUPATIONAL PERFORMANCE: SUPPORTING BEST PRACTICE IN OCCUPATIONAL THERAPY

Mary Law, PhD, OT(C); Carolyn M Baum, PhD, OTR/L, FAOTA; and Winnie Dunn, PhD, OTR, FAOTA

320 pp., Soft Cover, 2000, ISBN 1-55642-298-9, Order #32989, **$36.00**

This extraordinary text begins with a background of measurement concepts and issues and explores the central theoretical concept of occupational therapy, occupation, and occupational performance outcomes facilitated by person-environment-occupation. Measurement in the context of client-centered approach is a central theme. Strategies for using the assessment information for different purposes, such as individual client outcomes, program evaluation, and quality improvement are covered.

EVIDENCE-BASED REHABILITATION: A GUIDE TO PRACTICE

Mary Law, PhD, OT(C)

400 pp., Soft Cover, 2002, ISBN 1-55642-453-1, Order # 44531, **$37.00**

Specifically written for rehabilitation practitioners, this exceptional text is not designed to teach students how to do research, but rather how to become critical consumers of research, therefore developing skills to ensure that their rehabilitation practice is based on the best evidence that is available. Much of the text focuses on how knowledge is developed, making it an essential tool for both students and practitioners.

Contact us at

SLACK Incorporated, Professional Book Division
6900 Grove Road, Thorofare, NJ 08086
1-800-257-8290/1-856-848-1000, Fax: 1-856-853-5991
Email: orders@slackinc.com or www.slackbooks.com

ORDER FORM

QUANTITY	TITLE	ORDER #	PRICE
	Occupation-Based Practice	35643	$34.00
	Measuring Occupational Performance	32989	$36.00
	Evidence-Based Rehabilitation: A Guide to Practice	44531	$37.00
		Subtotal	$
		Applicable state and local tax will be added to your purchase	$
		Handling	$4.50
		Total	$

Name _____

Address: _____

City: _____ State:_____ Zip: _____

Phone:_____ Fax: _____

Email: _____

- Check enclosed (Payable to SLACK Incorporated)_____
- Charge my: ____ [AMEX] ____ [VISA] ____ [MasterCard]

Account #: _____

Exp. date: _____ Signature _____

NOTE: *Prices are subject to change without notice.*
Shipping charges will apply.
Shipping and handling charges are Non-Returnable.

CODE: 328